Ethan Russo, MD

Handbook of Psychotropic Herbs
A Scientific Analysis
of Herbal Remedies
for Psychiatric Conditions

Pre-publication
REVIEWS,
COMMENTARIES,
EVALUATIONS . . .

"Ethan Russo has written a comprehensive and scientifically sound handbook of psychotropic herbs. It is encyclopedic in its scope, and quite readable: It is a must read for those interested in herbs with psychotropic properties."

Lester Grinspoon, MD
Associate Professor of Psychiatry,
Harvard Medical School

"Here is a remarkable reference source for factual information on over a score of medicinal herbs. This presentation covers botany, history of use, preparation of extracts, animal toxicology, human responses, and established medical values —all with excellent references to the published literature. A fine balance is maintained in answering the questions asked by the researcher (what is in there and what is its action), and by the herbalist (how can it be used to heal and maintain a patient)."

Alexander T. Shulgin, PhD
Experimental Neurochemist

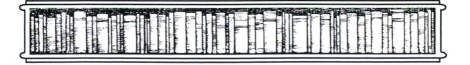

More pre-publication
REVIEWS, COMMENTARIES, EVALUATIONS . . .

"**T**he main part of the book, including monographs of relevant phytomedicines to be used in psychopharmacological practice (e.g., against depression, insomnia) is preceded by chapters with definitions and very useful remarks on quality, regulations, and study design. The monographs focus on critical reviews and compare published studies. The natural traditional alternatives to the established, modern synthetic psychopharmaceuticals are discussed profoundly, and are scientifically correct according to today's knowledge. The systematic structure chosen by the author results in a neat and understandable presentation of the discussed topics, and the psychiatric diseases are clearly diagnostically differentiated. Despite the scientific style of the book's language, it can be understood by the interested nonspecialist too. The case studies in the last part of the book impressively illustrate the potential and the limits of phytopharmaceutical interventions in the field of psychic disturbances. Finally, the extensive bibliography facilitates access to the fascinating use of psychotropic plants."

Rudolf Brenneisen, PhD
Professor,
Department of Clinical Research,
University of Bern, Switzerland

"**P**sychological problems have plagued humanity since the beginning of time. The successful treatment of psychiatric conditions has often eluded Western allopathic medicine. It is no wonder that the consideration of herbal remedies for the treatment of such conditions is now at hand. The *Handbook of Psychotropic Herbs* gives a thorough overview of herbal remedies and their current regulatory status, specific psychological conditions for their use, current research as to their effectiveness, and case studies of their clinical applications. Dr. Russo has done an excellent job of providing health care practitioners with exactly what is needed—a comprehensive, practical handbook that helps them and their patients achieve a better health care outcome through the use of herbal remedies for psychiatric conditions."

Constance Grauds, RPh
President, Association
of Natural Medicine Pharmacists,
San Rafael, California

The Haworth Herbal Press®
An Imprint of The Haworth Press, Inc.

Handbook
of Psychotropic Herbs
A Scientific Analysis
of Herbal Remedies
for Psychiatric Conditions

Handbook
of Psychotropic Herbs
A Scientific Analysis
of Herbal Remedies
for Psychiatric Conditions

Ethan Russo, MD

The Haworth Herbal Press®
An Imprint of The Haworth Press, Inc.
New York • London • Oxford

Published by

The Haworth Herbal Press, an imprint of The Haworth Press, Inc., 10 Alice Street, Binghamton, NY 13904-1580

DISCLAIMER
Medicine is an ever-changing science. As new research and clinical experience broaden our knowledge, changes in treatment and drug therapy are required. While many suggestions for drug usages are made herein, the book is intended for educational purposes only, and the author, editor, and publisher do not accept liability in the event of negative consequences incurred as a result of information presented in this book. We do not claim that this information is necessarily accurate by the rigid, scientific standard applied for medical proof, and therefore make no warranty, expressed or implied, with respect to the material herein contained. Therefore the patient is urged to check the product information sheet included in the package of each drug he or she plans to administer to be certain the protocol followed is not in conflict with the manufacturer's inserts. When a discrepancy arises between these inserts and information in this book, the physician is encouraged to use his or her best professional judgement.

Cover design by Marylouise E. Doyle.

Library of Congress Cataloging-in-Publication Data

Handbook of psychotropic herbs : a scientific analysis of herbal remedies for psychiatric conditions / Ethan Russo.
    p. cm.
   Includes bibliographical references and index.
   ISBN 0-7890-0718-5 (alk. paper) — ISBN 0-7890-1088-7 (alk. paper)
    1. Mental illness—Nutritional aspects—Case studies—Handbooks, manuals, etc. 2. Herbs—Therapeutic use—Case studies—Handbooks, manuals, etc. 3. Psychopharmacology—Case studies—Handbooks, manuals, etc. I. Russo, Ethan.

RC455.4.N8 H36 2000
615′.788—dc21
                                          00-038294

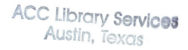

CONTENTS

ABOUT THE AUTHOR

Ethan Russo, MD, is a child and adult neurologist at Montana Neurobehavioral Specialists. He is Board Certified in Neurology with Special Qualification in Child Neurology. He has had a lifetime interest in medicinal plants.

Dr. Russo holds a faculty position in the Department of Pharmaceutical Sciences as an Adjunct Associate Professor at the University of Montana, where he regularly lectures to undergraduate and graduate students in pharmacy, psychology, sports medicine, interpersonal communications, and physical therapy. He is actively engaged in bench research on the serotonin receptor activity of natural products, especially with application to migraine treatment. Dr. Russo is also Clinical Associate Professor in the Department of Medicine at the University of Washington.

Dr. Russo has published numerous peer-reviewed articles on ethnobotany, herbal medicine, and cannabis, and has lectured nationally on those subjects. He has been a seminar leader in the American Botanical Council's "Pharmacy from the Rainforest" program in Peru.

He is the founding editor of *Journal of Cannabis Therapeutics: Studies in Endogenous, Herbal, and Synthetic Cannabinoids,* and is the American Editor for Franjo Grotenhermen's book *Cannabis and Cannabinoids* (both forthcoming from Haworth).

CONTRIBUTORS

Chanchal Cabrera, MNIMH, AHG, is a member of the National Institute of Medical Herbalists (United Kingdom), the Canadian Herb Association, and the American Herbalists Guild. She runs a clinical practice and herbal products manufacturing facility in Vancouver, British Columbia, and divides her time between there and an organic herb farm in Virginia.

Loren D. Israelsen, JD, is president of the LDI Group in Salt Lake City, Utah, a consulting firm specializing in the regulatory and commercial development of herbs, dietary supplements, and other natural products. Mr. Israelsen has previously served as president of Nature's Way Products, Inc., and as an advisor to the National Institutes of Health (NIH), Food and Drug Administration (FDA), and foreign governments on dietary supplement policy.

Robert Velin, PhD, is a neuropsychologist and clinical psychologist with Montana Neurobehavioral Specialists in Missoula, Montana, and a faculty affiliate with the University of Montana, Department of Psychology.

Rebecca A. Wittenberg, a clinical herbalist who has been involved in herbal businesses since 1991, studied ethnobotany and mathematics in college and has formal training including the Southwest School of Botanical Studies with Michael Moore and an apprenticeship with Tiaraona Low-Dog. In 1996, she started Root Laughter Herbals, an herbal manufacturing company dedicated to bringing traditional medicinal herbs into food forms.

Foreword

The explosive growth of the herb industry in the United States in the past decade has been accompanied by a virtual epidemic of herbal publications. Although a few titles stand out, many herb books are basically regurgitations of old data from earlier publications, covering a wide range of herbal materia medica, folklore, personal experience, and, more recently, scientific literature. Many of these books are sometimes indistinguishable from one another.

This book, however, is a first and is truly unique. While some books have focused on herbs for specific ranges of use (e.g., men's health, women's health, herbs for children, tonic herbs, etc.), this book is the first compilation of scientific and clinical data solely on herbs with central nervous system (CNS) effects.

There is a joke that runs in medical circles that many of my physician friends find hits very close to home: "How do you keep a secret from a neurologist or a neurosurgeon? Answer: You publish it!" Apparently, some professionals in this field are characterized as somewhat smug and as having little interest in learning new information. Not this author. Unlike a growing number of writers on the herbal scene who are physicians (or other conventional health care practitioners) with little experience with herbs, Dr. Russo, a neurologist, is no stranger to herbal medicine, having used phytomedicines in his clinical practice and having studied much of the contemporary scientific data available on these natural products. What's more, Dr. Russo has spent a period of time with the indigenous Machiguenga tribe in the Peruvian Amazon, a testament to his insatiable willingness to learn new information from a variety of sources. Thus, the author brings his strong clinical experience in conventional medicine and pharmacotherapy in neurological disorders to the subject of herbs and CNS activities.

The author employs the term *psychotropic* for these agents, that is, literally, agents that "turn" the mind. They are not to be confused with *psychedelic* or *hallucinatory* agents—referring to plants and derived substances previously associated with ritual use and/or abuse—the so-called "recreational" drugs. In the sense that Dr. Russo uses the term, psychotropic herbs can be employed as stimulants, sedatives, anxiolytics, etc., both in clinical medicine as well as in self-medication. Most of these herbs are relatively mild and, when used responsibly, relatively safe, especially when compared to their pharmaceutical counterparts.

With his vast clinical experience, Dr. Russo is well aware of the potential and actual effects of conventional pharmaceutical drugs as well as the relative safety of appropriately used, gentle herbal remedies. He offers numerous case studies that provide examples of rational clinical applications of botanical preparations with positive outcomes—resulting in the overall benefit of the patient.

Dr. Russo's treatment of St. John's wort *(Hypericum perforatum)* is one of the most complete reviews of the clinical literature currently available in the English language. The same can be said of his sections on passion flower *(Passiflora incarnata)*, German chamomile *(Matricaria recutita)*, ginkgo *(Ginkgo biloba)*, kava-kava *(Piper methysticum)*, lavender oil *(Lavandula officinalis)*, and even the controversial, yet clinically useful, marijuana *(Cannabis sativa)*.

The issue of substances that influence the central nervous system and mental functions has either fascinated or repelled people throughout history. Human experience is inextricably linked to the use of psychotropics, whether for religious and ceremonial use or, later, for medically approved therapeutic applications, as well as for their more controversial recreational uses.

Andrew Weil, MD, and Ronald Siegel, PhD, have written about the universal human drive for altering the normal waking state of consciousness. This need has manifested in the use of plants for a wide variety of effects: stimulants such as coffee *(Coffea arabica)* and khat *(Catha edulis)*, narcotics such as opium (from opium poppy, *Papaver somniferum)*, and radically mind-altering psychedelic or "entheogenic" substances such as mescaline (from peyote cactus, *Lophophora williamsii)* and psilocybin (from "magic mushrooms, *Psilocybe* spp.).

Unfortunately, for serious researchers and clinicians, in the realm of public opinion, psychotropic plants are sometimes shrouded in the mysteries of the stereotyped anorexic opium addict curled upon the floor of some Far Eastern opium den, or the half-crazed, hopped-up, hashish-eating "assassins" of *Tales of the Arabian Nights.* As anyone familiar with the ubiquitous "war on drugs" in America knows, it has been virtually impossible to hold a rational public discourse about the potential benefits of psychotropic agents. Anyone suggesting such is often shouted down as being someone who has a far more nefarious agenda: the legalization of illicit drugs.

However, there is another, possibly more gentle aspect of the discussion about psychotropic agents that, until recently, has been virtually ignored in the medical literature in the United States—the safe and responsible use of commonly sold herbal preparations that affect central nervous system activity. Products made from the plants in this book are found on the shelves of health food stores, supermarkets, drugstores, mass market retailers, mail-order catalogs, e-commerce Web sites, and from a growing number of health practitioners, both conventional and alternative.

To the bibliophile interested in the history of psychoactive plants and their derivative drugs, this book can be viewed as joining with some of the classics of the genre: Ernst Von Bibra's *Plant Intoxicants* (1855), Mordicai Cooke's *The Seven Sisters of Sleep* (1997), Louis Lewin's *Phantastica* (1924), Marek Kohn's *Narcomania* (1986), and Jonathan Ott's opus magnum *Pharmacotheon* (1993). It also joins a more recent volume on the subject, written by the contemporary physician Andrew Weil, *From Chocolate to Morphine* (1998).

Similar to his predecessors, Dr. Russo has compiled a comprehensive review of each botanical agent. However, unlike its predecessors, this book deals with plants that are not considered, by today's norms, as being controversial, illicit, addictive, or the domain of the morally depraved. In these pages is sound advice on the rational use of safe and effective herbs to help alleviate a wide range of neurological disorders, from migraine headache to anxiety and mild or moderate depression. Health professionals and laypeople can use this book as an authoritative guide in an area where solid, reliable information is often difficult to obtain.

Mark Blumenthal
Founder and Executive Director,
American Botanical Council
Editor, HerbalGram

Acknowledgments

I would like to thank numerous individuals, foremost among them, my family, for their support and understanding of the time and commitment necessary to this effort.

Next, I would like to thank Varro Tyler for his confidence in me to pursue this task, as well as his counsel, wisdom, and support. Bill Cohen and the enthusiastic and energetic staff of The Haworth Press have been wonderful.

Paulette Cote of the Western Montana Clinic and the staff of the interlibrary loan office of the Mansfield Library provided countless hours of service in pursuit of obscure references. The PubMed database of the National Library of Medicine, the HerbClip service of the American Botanical Council, and the NAPRALERT (Natural Products Alert) database were also key resources.

I would also like to thank my many capable mentors and teachers over the past decade: Richard Schultes, Mark Plotkin, Dennis McKenna, Jim Duke, Mark Blumenthal, Hardy Eshbaugh, Rosita Arvigo, James Castner, don Antonio Montero of the Amazon Center for Environmental Education and Research (ACEER), and the entire Machiguenga tribe of *Parque Nacional del Manú* (Manú National Park).

In addition, I would like to voice my appreciation for the many friends and colleagues I have made in creating this work, especially Keith Parker, Rustem Medora, Chuck Thompson, and Cathy Bartels of the University of Montana, Penny King, Marie-Josée Thibault, Deborah Somerville, and Connie Grauds. Their understanding and support made this effort a true labor of love.

Ultimately, to all the indigenous healers and others who aspire to medicine in accord with nature, my best wishes and hopes go with you.

PART I:
INTRODUCTORY MATERIAL

Chapter 1

Introduction: Why Herbs?

AN ARCHETYPAL SCENE

An herb hunter rises early in the morning and sets out in search of medicinal plants. The quarry may be known, or, rather, the hunter-gatherer may peruse the landscape to survey the bounty of possible harvest, without preconception. New and different plants may appear at any time. She stops frequently, to run her fingertips over the bark of one tree, smell the dew-fringed blossom of a flower, or nibble on the leaf of a spreading ground cover. She uses all of her senses to scrutinize for the best medicine.

Some plants are left in place, while she puts seasonal items in her collecting bag in quantity, leaving enough in the ground to ensure that each will thrive and remain in time of need, weeks, months, or years hence.

She travels far over the course of a few hours but returns home before the sun is too hot, to prepare each plant for its use. Some are set to dry, while others are placed in clay pots to steep. Her task has been successful; she smiles and rests.

This scene is as old as history but could occur anywhere or anytime in the world today, portrayed by a woman or a man. The hunt may have been for food or, just as likely, for medicine.

Many readers may recall the story of the "Ice Man," a Neolithic hunter who, in 1991, was found frozen, high in the Alps, after some 5,000 years. Among his meager belongings were several items that have proven to represent medicinal plants. These included samples of birch fungus, *Piptoporus betulinus,* which possesses laxative and vermicidal effects, precisely what one would need to purge the intestinal parasites he harbored (Capasso, 1998).

Our opening scene represents a "natural order" that many in our modern societies would view as quaint and outmoded. The fact remains, however, that a majority of the world's people pursue similar practices of primitive agriculture and herbal medicine. According to Farnsworth (Farnsworth et al., 1985), 88 percent of the world population continues to rely primarily on traditional medicine.

A compelling force in medicine has always involved the human drive to feel better. An important part of feeling better concerns psychopharmacology, the treatment of disorders of mind and mood. This might pertain to efforts to uplift the spirits of the downtrodden or to banish unwarranted fears. For most cultures, medicine has included the search for enlightenment or higher meaning through the use of sacramental plants. Herbs that fulfill these purposes are called psychotropic, literally, "turning the mind." Herbal medicines that turn the mind for therapeutic purposes are the subject of this book.

FACTS AND FIGURES

Estimates of plant species on our planet range upward of 250,000. About 5 percent, or 13,000 plants, have been employed medicinally and qualify as traditional plant medicines (Tyler, 1993). Indigenous pharmacopoeias range in size from a very few items to the over 1,000 herbal items in the armamentarium of Mayan tribes (Arvigo and Balick, 1993). Similarly, the Ayurvedic system of medicine in India has referred to over 1,000 herbs from ancient times, while traditional Chinese medicine (TCM) has employed 5,000 native plants (Robbers, Speedie, and Tyler, 1996).

About 1,000 plants have been employed more universally in modern times. Over half of those, or 550, are commercially available in the United States. The Food and Drug Administration (FDA) approves 279 as foods or food ingredients (Cott, 1995). The *United States Pharmacopeia* (USP) contained 191 plant drugs in 1905, and those items are frequently referred to as the classic drug plants (Tyler, 1993).

Botanical medicine has been in a steady state of decline in the United States for the bulk of this century, as synthetic biochemistry came into its own. The advent of computer modeling, in which an identified receptor may be mimicked through construction of a novel molecule, became a preferred approach to new drug development. The search for pharmaceuticals in plants was relegated, in turn, to a scientific backwater by the 1970s, and orthodox medicine often tends to look askance at its offerings.

In Germany, Japan, and Italy, in particular, botanical research never fell out of the mainstream. This has led to some ironic eventualities. Thus, the scientific investigation and development of phytopharmaceuticals from Native American remedies such as echinacea *(Echinacea purpurea)* for immune protection, saw palmetto *(Serenoa repens)* for benign prostatic hyperplasia, and others occurred in Europe. These agents are extremely popular in Germany, whereas their rediscovery in their country of origin has been only a very recent event.

That tide has turned, however. Early this decade, Eisenberg and his colleagues published a groundbreaking article that established the great extent to which American citizens have turned to alternative medicine (Eisenberg et al., 1993). Among their findings were the following: 34 percent of persons who responded to a survey had used at least one "unconventional therapy" in the previous year, and one-third of those had seen specific providers for such administration; 3 percent had used herbal medicine in the prior year, and 10 percent had seen an herbal practitioner; about 45 percent of respondents were seeking alternative treatment of anxiety, and 35 percent, depression. These figures provide compelling evidence that conventional medicine did not provide adequate relief to such patients.

In a more recent review, Astin explored reasons that patients pursued alternative treatment (Astin, 1998). He concluded that such users were more educated and reported poorer health status. Most did not express dissatisfaction with conventional medicine but, rather, practiced therapies more in tune with their personal philosophies of life and health. Once again, anxiety and depression figured in the top ten complaints for which patients sought care, and they frequently chose herbal medicines for corresponding treatment.

The growth of herbal medicine in the United States has been explosive in the past decade. Whether cause or effect, it has paralleled an increase in solid scientific investigation of many such agents. In effect, a rational basis has now been provided for many herbal claims. This has promoted the acceptance of those therapies by the public and, to a lesser degree, their physicians.

Recently, Blumenthal stated (Blumenthal et al., 1998, p. 9), "An estimated 30 percent of American adults—60 million—are reported to be using herbs and phytomedicinal products, spending an estimated $3.24 billion in 1996." This trend has been noticed by the business community and has led to a correspondingly rapid growth in the number of start-up companies offering herbal products. Even popular multivitamin brands are marketing products that could be termed "botanically enhanced."

Economic figures on herbal use are impressive. Estimates of the domestic herbal market in the United States were $1.6 billion in 1994 (Brevoort, 1996) but had risen to $3.24 billion in 1996 (Johnston, 1997). By that year, one-third of adult Americans were using herbal medicines, with an average annual outlay of $54. In terms of public expenditure, four of the top thirteen best-selling agents sold in food, drug, and retail outlets in 1997 were psychotropics: ginkgo (number 1), St. John's wort (number 5), valerian (number 10), and kava-kava (number 13) (Blumenthal et al., 1998, p. 11).

Polling data on public acceptance of herbal medicine by the journal *HerbalGram* in 1996 (Anonymous, 1996c) provide additional insight into the motivation behind these trends. When people were asked why they chose herbal treatment, 41 percent replied, "Because it can't hurt and might help." Another 34 percent said, "Because nothing else has helped my condition." Only 4 percent of Americans said that they would not ever consider herbal treatment.

Herbal psychopharmacology has been recently reviewed in an article citing 303 references (Wong, Smith, and Boon, 1998). These authors examined many of the same agents included in this book but concluded that only St. John's wort, for depression, and ginkgo, for dementia, were effective. This book will delve into the topic in greater detail, and with different conclusions.

DRUG DESIGN

At the beginning of the last century, medicine turned from plants to synthetic chemistry to supply its tools of treatment. Shortly before this, Bavarian scientists had chemically manipulated natural salicylates to produce aspirin, acetylsalicylic acid. Many similar examples followed, each an "improvement" over the natural pharmacy. The trend continued, such that many pharmaceutical companies have come to feel that plants, nature's own chemists, are inferior to their human counterparts, and nothing is left to learn from them. More recently, the prototype of drug development has become even more sophisticated. The key to many maladies, particularly disorders of brain chemistry, lies in the identification of a cellular receptor. If the receptor structure has been elucidated, it then becomes possible to fashion a drug molecule on a computer screen to precisely fit that receptor, analogous to a "lock and key" model. The human element of hunting and gathering has been altered substantially by this scheme, while the plant connection has been removed entirely. It then remains to be established whether the synthetic drug candidate is effective at its assigned task in altering human pathophysiology, and, equally important, whether it produces toxicity of its own. Such difficulties attendant to drug use are known as side effects.

The process of drug design is long and tortuous. Current estimates in the United States yield a time of ten years and a cost of $350 million to $500 million to bring a chemical from inception, through its various animal and human trials, to the market shelf and consumer (Blumenthal et al., 1998).

Certain exceptions to the prevailing trend have appeared in recent times, and, to an interesting degree, this "return to nature" has paralleled a social movement that began in the 1960s. Notwithstanding the current methods of pharmaceutical synthesis, fully 25 percent of our current prescription drugs derive directly or indirectly from plants (Farnsworth et al., 1985; Soejarto and Farnsworth, 1989). Every few months, some new, important, and promising therapeutic agent is identified from the plant kingdom, often from a forgotten, "worthless" species. As the author is fond to remark, "One man's weed is another man's medicine."

The Pacific yew *(Taxus brevifolia)* is a good example. This Northwest U.S. denizen, largely ignored by foresters, has yielded taxol, a valuable chemotherapeutic agent in the treatment of breast and ovarian malignancies. The taxol molecule is extremely complex and, to date, has resisted de novo synthesis. Initial fears of the impending doom of the species to harvest its taxol-yielding bark have been allayed somewhat by the newly acquired ability to synthesize the drug from a precursor chemical in the needles of a related, but nonthreatened, species. The fact remains, however, that the taxol molecule is so unusual and novel in its architecture that no chemist or computer design scheme would likely have stumbled upon it without nature's pointing the way, nor is this humbling example an isolated one.

Morphine is a natural plant medicine derived from the Oriental poppy, *Papaver somniferum.* It has a documented history of human use in Asia for thousands of years. Morphine was isolated from the poppy in 1806 and was the first recognized alkaloid, an important group of bitter chemicals derived from plants that impact normal animal chemistry and its pathophysiology. The reasons for morphine's ability to allay pain, halt cough, slow gut motility, or lead to the insatiable drive we call addiction remained a mystery until a generation ago, when the keys to its effects were discovered. As it turns out, our nervous systems, both in brain and gut, contain natural chemicals called enkephalins and endorphins (endogenous morphine) that affect cellular receptor function. After a long delay, while technology attempted to catch up, the poppy has led us to a deeper understanding of our own human functions.

It is the author's belief that many other promising "plant teachers" remain to be discovered. Some will be novel finds in distant deserts or exotic rainforests, while others will come from forgotten neighborhood weeds. The folklore of the past often contains seeds of truth that continue to offer benefits for the modern world. As Hänsel (1968, p. 312) observed, "natural products have always been models and examples for new medicinal agents in biochemical research."

Examination of our plant-derived pharmaceuticals reveals that 75 percent are employed for indications that support their traditional or folkloric usage (Farnsworth et al., 1985). As Cott has stated so eloquently (Cott, 1995, p. 10):

> A significant scientific constraint is placed on drug development when we must limit our search to synthetic chemicals that interact with known biological systems in predicted ways.

Truly unique medications are unlikely to emerge. This is especially true for research in areas where there are no effective drug treatments, such as for cognitive disorders.

Our herbal history must be mined for its unrecognized wisdom. It would seem as important to review what we have forgotten as it is to step out onto new uncharted ground. In so doing, we need not turn off our computers to advance but merely incorporate them in the search, while returning to our basic senses of sight and smell and to our hunter-gatherer instincts to research the psychotropic herbs.

ABOUT THIS BOOK

This volume is designed to introduce the concepts of herbal treatment of mental or nervous conditions, and to serve as a reference of current research on such agents. The book's audience will hopefully include psychologists, social workers, pharmacists, and other counselors in a position to advise patients about psychotropic herbal remedies. Presumably, it may also attract a few enlightened psychiatrists, other physicians, medical students, naturopaths, herbalists, and laypersons seeking additional herbal information.

The book will attempt to inform concerning technical topics but, hopefully, present the material in a manner that allows understanding of its peculiar language. The first time a new concept is presented, it will be defined and, perhaps, abbreviated. Subsequently, it will appear in a glossary. An extensive current bibliography is appended so that the reader may consult original sources or investigate key concepts in greater depth.

The observant reader will note frequent referral to certain texts. Preeminent among these are *Rational Phytotherapy: A Physicians' Guide to Herbal Medicine* (Schulz, Hänsel, and Tyler, 1998), *The Complete German Commission E Monographs: Therapeutic Guide to Herbal Medicines* (Blumenthal et al., 1998), and Varro Tyler's newly revised works, *Tyler's Honest Herbal* (Foster and Tyler, 1999) and *Tyler's Herbs of Choice* (Robbers and Tyler, 1999). That they have been widely quoted and cited will serve as testament to their utility as reference works.

No longer can contemporary physicians honestly say to their patients, "I cannot prescribe ginkgo because its safety is not proven," or "There are no controlled studies on St. John's wort." Such statements are misinformation that can be rectified through the dissemination of current scientific articles and reference books.

Clinical case studies by herbalists and physicians are provided to offer insight into the actual practice of treating patients with psychotropic herbs. These should not necessarily be taken as templates of the best herbal applications, however.

What It Is Not

This volume is not designed to be a "self-help manual," despite its possible placement under that bookstore heading. It cannot replace consultation with a properly trained herbalist, naturopath, or open-minded physician.

The authors and publisher cannot be responsible for misuse or abuse of herbal remedies discussed in the text. Every country has regulations (or lack of regulations) in regard to herbal medicines (see Chapter 2). Although the book includes information on this topic in the U.S. market and abroad, some readers may wish to investigate appropriate federal statutes, which are continually in a state of flux.

The narrative will pertain generally to commercially available herbs employed in the treatment of psychiatric conditions. Thus, agents whose usage is primarily recreational or visionary, or those termed hallucinogenic, psychedelic, or entheogenic (becoming divine within), will not be covered, with the exception of cannabis. The interested reader is referred to several excellent reviews (Ott, 1996; Schultes, 1988; Schultes and Hofmann, 1980, 1992; Schultes and Raffauf, 1990; Schultes et al., 1992; Schultes and Smith, 1976).

HERBS, ACTIVE INGREDIENTS, BOTANICALS, AND PHYTOMEDICINES

The reader may be confused by a profusion of loosely defined terms in the herbal literature. Classically, herbs are nonwoody plants, often with culinary or medicinal usage. Herbal medicine is usually defined more broadly, however, and would include the use of any plant, or plant part or product, in a healing context. This usage may be for symptomatic relief of symptoms or as a daily preventative, prophylactic, or tonic, such as *Panax ginseng.* Herbal agents may be adjuncts, or medicines added on to a regimen to complement the conventional pharmacopoeia.

Some plants have specific active ingredients that have been adopted into the standard pharmacopoeia. Digoxin, a heart tonic from the foxglove plant, *Digitalis purpurea,* is one example. Because of the inherent toxicity and narrow window of therapeutic safety of this agent, its parent plant is rarely employed as a botanical in modern practice. The absence of standardization renders use of the raw herb a clear and present danger to the patient. Digoxin is instead used as a refined pharmaceutical and is not considered an herbal remedy.

In contrast, botanicals, or phytomedicines, are agents employed medicinally as whole plants, parts, or refined extracts thereof. Many have only mild acute effects and may require a period of usage before benefits are manifested. In contrast to digoxin, such preparations do not necessarily contain a single active ingredient. Rather, they produce a synergy from two or more actions of the chemical components. This synergy, or combined action, postulates an interaction of different herbal components that produces a phenomenon in which the end effect is greater than the sum of its parts. This concept is a popular one but has remained controversial and under-recognized, particularly in a regulatory environment such as the U.S. FDA, which emphasizes single-chemical pharmaceutical prescriptions. A couple of examples, subsequently discussed more fully in the text, will suffice.

Ginkgo biloba contains several components with proven therapeutic actions. Use of these chemicals in isolation produces effects more meager than those of the combination. This, then, is a synergistic effect.

Despite intensive investigation, the active ingredient in *Hypericum perforatum,* St. John's wort, remains unidentified. Many believe that there is none. Its clinical efficacy is proven, so how, then, does it work? It may only be through some synergism of various components with little individual effect that a useful clinical response is obtained. As an analogy, the military genius of Alexander the Great could not be manifest without phalanx after phalanx of willing troops.

About Extracts

An extract is a refined preparation that "pulls from" an herb or plant component its essential activity. A variety of forms are possible. Fluidextracts are most often a 1:1 mixture of herb and water, herb and ethanol, or herb with ethanol and water. Trained herbalists frequently employ this form of medicine because it greatly eases the task of formulating an individualized compound prescription according to the patient's need. Quality varies, however, and, particularly in the United States, tinctures (alcoholic mixtures less concentrated than fluidextracts) may not be standardized.

Liquid preparations may also be extracted in glycerol. The latter, termed glycerites, are most often marketed for pediatric usage or for individuals eschewing alcohol. They are generally weaker and more perishable than alcoholic tinctures and are best refrigerated.

Increasingly popular, however, are dry extracts, powdered preparations in capsules or tablets prepared by drying liquid extracts. Through this process, which is often every bit as sophisticated as that employed in conventional pharmaceuticals, it is possible to concentrate desired components and remove undesirable ones, as necessary.

Another type of extraction is the production of essential (or volatile or ethereal) oils, the *huiles essentielles* of the French literature. This "up and coming" branch of herbal medicine will be briefly examined in the discussion on aromatherapy (see Chapter 9).

The process of extraction makes possible a standardization of the end product, a key concept in modern herbal application. With standardization, the research scientist and herbal consumer alike can ensure that the product they employ today will be qualitatively and quantitatively similar to that available next week or next year. It is only in this manner that proper safety and efficacy claims, and fair comparisons of one agent to another, can be made.

Anyone who tills the soil knows results will vary when nature is running the show. One year the garden produces rich red tomatoes, bursting with flavor. Another year, most remain green, lack flavor, or are watery. This demonstrates the concept of quality control. In modern herbalism, humankind attempts to produce a consistent, quality product. Initial production efforts, in this regard, frequently include cultivation of herbs, particularly of selected genetic strains. Variation from wild-type plants is thus reduced.

The next step is the extraction, which may emphasize the isolation of water-soluble (nonpolar) or ethanol-soluble (polar) components, according to the desired chemical composition. Certain substances in the herb may serve as markers of activity. For example, it has frequently been represented that hypericin is the active ingredient of St. John's wort *(Hypericum perforatum)* in the treatment of depression. Recent experiments (Chatterjee, Noldner, et al., 1998; Laakmann et al., 1998) undermine the contention that hypericin is active, but it remains a useful marker of an extract that may be clinically effective. Presumably, the true active ingredient in the extract travels along with hypericin, and its presence in the result ensures clinical activity in some measure.

High-tech assays, such as high-performance liquid chromatography (HPLC), gas chromatography (GC), and mass spectrometry (MS), are employed to analyze herb sources and to provide a chemical fingerprint of the resulting extracts. These efforts result in the ability to maintain high levels of quality control. Some companies even print graphs of their products' results on the packaging as a promotional gimmick.

As will be evident in the text, most controlled studies of herbal psychotropic agents have employed standardized extracts of correctly identified botanical species. Consumers who purchase herbal preparations of known standardized composition have a distinct advantage, clinically, in their expectation of safety, efficacy, and relative freedom from side effects.

To quote Schulz and colleagues (Schulz, Hänsel, and Tyler, 1998, p. 14), "Rational phytomedicines are herbal medicines whose safety and efficacy conform to current testing standards as fully as conventional drugs." For the do-it-yourself consumer, who eschews clinical guidance in herbal treatment, use of standardized preparations would certainly be the safest course of action.

In many countries, regulation ensures standardization, but not in the United States. Caveat emptor! The buyer may be lured by the touted benefits of a small amount of a standardized extract, supplemented by addition of "whole herb." Such supplementation may be counterproductive, by diluting the content of important components in the end result, or, in the case of *Ginkgo biloba,* by including ginkgolic acids, potential allergens that are absent from the best commercial products (Blumenthal et al., 1998).

Legal repercussions prevent the inclusion in this book of endorsements of specific brands. However, the reader will be informed as to what "buzzwords" or standardized extract names are appropriate to seek while comparing brands for suitable herbal psychotropic remedies.

HELPFUL HINTS

Herbal medicines are perishable. It may be most appropriate for the purchaser to purchase quantities that may be consumed within a year or two, although some preparations retain potency longer than that. Good quality products should be expiration dated.

All herbal products are best kept in a cool, dry, and dark location to reduce oxidation of their contents. Refrigeration will vastly prolong the working life of essential oils.

Herbal medicines should be taken with a generous amount of liquid to avoid gastrointestinal irritation by concentrated components. Most should be consumed with food, although package markings, when present, are a good guide to proper use. In the United States, however, these may be quite generic. Therapeutic claims on labels are prohibited, unless accompanied by a disclaimer indicating that the FDA has not approved the statement. As with any medication, dosage guidelines should not be exceeded except under the advice of a qualified practitioner.

Some herbal formulations may be encapsulated or enteric-coated, so as to allow passage through the stomach and subsequent release farther down the digestive tract. Timing of dosage is particularly important for such preparations, often advised before a meal.

Most herbal dosages are two or more times a day when regularly used, due to a short half-life. The half-life refers to the time it takes for 50 percent of the drug to be metabolized, or used up by the body. In general, dosing should occur at a frequency equal to or less than the half-life to maintain steady levels of the drug in the body. This avoids "peaks and valleys" of drug effect. Thus, although hypericin in St. John's wort has a half-life of twenty-four hours, the half-life of the true active component(s) is unknown. It is most often recommended that hypericum be administered three times a day with meals.

Pediatric research on herbs has lagged far behind that in adults, in a manner analogous to that of conventional drugs. Suitable caution is warranted in giving any herbal preparation to children without professional direction. In general, people in their midteens and older may take adult dosages. Children eight to thirteen years of age may receive two-thirds of an adult daily dosage, and children ages five through eight may receive one-third. *The author does not recommend consideration of any agent discussed in this book to children under five years of age without appropriate consultation.*

Many herbal agents for psychotropic use are best taken regularly for a few weeks before significant results can be expected. Chronic conditions require long-term administration. Episodic complaints, such as acute anxiety, may be treated symptomatically at the time of onset.

Herbal Combinations: More Is Better, Right?

In scientific medicine as approved by the FDA, there is a premium on single-compound medicines. This is a continuation of a trend started by Paracelsus in sixteenth-century Switzerland. Exceptions do exist, however. For example, L-dopa, one of the mainstays of treatment of Parkinson's disease, is quickly eliminated from the body and poorly effective unless accompanied by carbidopa, an added component that serves to disrupt enzymatic breakdown of the former.

The role of synergism was mentioned previously. Many *herbal remedies are de facto combinations* due to this synergism of ingredients.

The aspiring herbal consumer is apt to be confronted by a dizzying array of combination preparations, particularly in the United States. Thus, we may see ginkgo and hypericum offered together in one easy-to-take capsule. This trend, often pejoratively labeled as polypharmacy, is inadvisable. Economy of medication is often the wisest policy. When more than one agent is required, it is almost always preferable for patients to take single agents concurrently, following professional guidance.

Rational combinations certainly occur in herbal as in conventional medicine. Galen (129-c. 199) emphasized such mixtures, called theriaca. Historically, these were combinations of many ingredients offered as antidotes to poisoning. The philosophy of theriaca is perpetuated in aromatherapy, in which it is traditional to combine two or many essential oils of similar therapeutic benefit in one treatment of purported greater benefit to the patient.

SAFETY

Public health requires that available medicines be safe. That situation is not necessarily the case in the United States under current (lack of) regulations. The commonly held conception is that "natural" or "organic" labels render a product innocuous. This may or may not be true. After all, hemlock is organic, and still it killed Socrates. Any agent may become toxic in sufficient dosage.

Our bodies truly contain an awe-inspiring innate wisdom, but when confronted by a given molecule, our cells do not distinguish organic from synthetic. They will attempt to incorporate, break down, metabolize, any drug presented into their internal biochemical machinery. It is definitely true that well-standardized phytomedicines have an enormous therapeutic range, or safety margin. The chances of a toxic result with most of the agents discussed in this book are quite low, unlike those of the tricyclic antidepressants, where even a moderate overdose can lead to coma, convulsions, or cardiac arrhythmias.

The safety of botanicals has often been established through a track record of historical usage but also, and more important, by formal toxicity studies and controlled clinical trials. Although anecdotal information is frequently offered as proof of safety or efficacy, such information in isolation is not considered sufficient for scientific standards. When combined with sound clinical and laboratory data, anecdotal usage may be helpful in illustrating appropriate and inappropriate herbal practices in real-life patients. Although herbal medicine may have some catching up to do in this area, this book aims to dispel the notion that a scientific basis is lacking for such agents.

Strong prejudices remain in some quarters against herbal medicine, but these biases are frequently no more justified than the counter-notion, or natural backlash, that all synthetic medicines are inherently evil.

HOW ABOUT HOMEOPATHY?

Homeopathy is a branch of medicine popularized by Samuel Hahnemann in Germany in 1840. It employs techniques of dilution of plant, animal, or mineral agents, sometimes to the point of disappearance of any molecular trace. Controlled studies of homeopathy are notably sparse. An extensive review was undertaken by Kleijnen and colleagues in the Netherlands in 1991 (Kleijnen, Knipschild, and ter Riet, 1991), in an effort to identify well-designed studies from a scientific point of view. Out of a total of 107 controlled trials in 96 published reports, his team found one study for each of the following conditions that demonstrated positive results via homeopathic treatment: behavior in children, depression, nervous tension, and agitation. However, none of these studies approached the authors' threshold for better-designed methodology. As such, it is difficult to draw supportive conclusions.

In 1997, Linde and his colleagues in Germany revisited the topic (Linde et al., 1997). They reviewed 186 clinical trials of homeopathy and identified 119 that met inclusion criteria for their meta-analysis. Although some studies demonstrated positive results that could not be explained merely through a placebo effect, they stated, "However, we found insufficient evidence from these studies that homoeopathy is clearly efficacious for any single clinical condition. Further research on homoeopathy is warranted provided it is rigorous and systematic" (Linde et al., 1997, p. 838). Of note, none of the studies meeting their criteria dealt with psychiatric conditions, the issue at hand.

Most recently, the archconservative *Medical Letter* has weighed in on the topic (1999b, p. 21). Their ultimate pronouncement was that "[t]hese [homeopathic] products have not been proven to be effective for any clinical condition. There is no good reason to use them."

The subject of this book is, rather, the use of biochemically relevant biochemical agents and their therapeutic use in psychopharmacological practice. Homeopathy has its passionate advocates but will not be considered here in detail. Some may consider this a political evasion, abdication of responsibility, or cowardly confinement of the subject matter. So be it. Dissent is the essence of democracy. Let all seek their own soapbox.

A WORD ABOUT WILDCRAFTING

One of the author's fondest memories of his teen years was the quest for jewelweed, *Impatiens capensis*, a folk treatment for poison ivy. Even the mental consideration of that affliction still fills him with dread. Much as in the opening scene of this book, he traveled the woods with a trusted herbal savant, like some latter-day Euell Gibbons (Gibbons, 1966), to find the succulent herb, whose juices were purported to prevent and heal that cutaneous scourge. Science has largely derogated its therapeutic claims (Long, Ballentine, and Marks, 1997), but it worked beautifully. So, what is wrong with this scenario? Nothing, perhaps.

The personal search and harvest of botanicals, known as wildcrafting, will remain one of the hallmarks of human medicine, but it is currently being abused, and badly so. In the author's adopted state of Montana, the purple coneflower, *Echinacea purpurea*, is on the verge of extinction due to the legions of pickers who, for a reward of $8 a pound, have all but torn the last roots from the landscape. Legislation is required to ensure that the newfound popularity of this Native American immune booster does not contribute to its disappearance from the wild.

Cultivation of medicinal herbs, in contrast, offers a buffer against overharvesting in the field. In addition, it allows the selective breeding of "chemovars," varieties of known chemical composition, as well as the provision of higher levels of quality control.

Wildcrafting, except perhaps in the hands of the most experienced herbalist or indigenous tribesman, is a gamble. How do you know what you are getting? Is it really the right species? Is the chemical content adequate and proper? Is it safe? Is it effective? Answers may be assumed, but they are not assured.

Because of these dual concerns of conservation and quality control, this book will emphasize the use of cultivated standardized herbal preparations.

DISCLAIMER

Medicine is art and science. No information herein should be construed as encouraging self-treatment of any medical condition. The author, contributors, and publisher cannot be held accountable for deleterious effects that result from use of any agent discussed in this book. Rather, the interested consumer should discuss treatment options with a qualified herbal practitioner, naturopath, or open-minded, educated physician.

Chapter 2

Regulation of Botanicals in the United States

Loren D. Israelsen

INTRODUCTION

Surprisingly, no U.S. law or regulation defined the term *herb* or *botanical* until the Dietary Supplement Health and Education Act did so in 1994 (U.S. Congress, 1994). Prior to this, herbs were a regulatory pinball bounced from one legal category to another. This is not unexpected, given the astonishing diversity of pharmacological activity and cultural use of herbs in this country. One hundred years ago, herbs were well established as medicines, widely listed in the *United States Pharmacopeia* (USP), and prescribed by physicians. Herbal tinctures, extracts, salves, concoctions, and so forth, were the materia medica of the day. The Food and Drug Administration (FDA), as we know it, would not exist for another forty years, and the first federal law to seriously regulate foods or medicines would not come into existence until 1938.

Federal authority to regulate herbs was embedded in the Food, Drug and Cosmetic Act of 1938, which gave the FDA responsibility to prosecute the adulteration or misbranding of foods, drugs, and cosmetics. Yet the standards of safety, effectiveness, and purity did not exist for many foods or drugs. This absence of meaningful safety and efficacy standards became the central issue as the science of synthetic organic chemistry came into its own. World War II created a demand for more powerful drugs of all kinds, particularly antibiotics and trauma treatment agents. The federal government urged drug companies, then largely botanical crude-drug houses, such as Merck, Lilly, and Parke-Davis, to invest in new synthetic chemistry-based research. The incentives to pursue this new science included patent protection, the government as a prime customer, and the enticingly fast results that such synthetic drugs offered. Those botanicals which could effectively compete in this new world of synthetic chemistry were often the powerful alkaloid derivative botanicals, such as the opiates and other highly active psychotropic plants.

Other botanicals were increasingly seen as the beginnings of drug research and served as useful models for synthetic analogues or derivatives, but not as end products themselves. Thus, the transformation of botanicals in America began. Popular and widely used remedies and crude-drug extracts fell into disuse or were relegated to the world of folklore medicine, ultimately finding refuge in health food stores.

In 1962, the FDA issued strict guidelines on safety and efficacy testing requirements for new drugs. A new drug now required the FDA's prior approval before marketing under a new drug application (NDA). Old drugs were permitted to remain on the market as long as their ingredients and labeling remained unchanged. A handful of such products still exist. Many of them are of botanical origin; however, virtually none are of commercial importance. Two familiar and interesting products, Lydia Pinkham's Pure Vegetable Compound and Absorbine Jr., remain available either as dietary supplements or as grandfathered medicines.

The rapid decline of herbs in commerce ultimately led to the removal, or delisting, of botanicals in the USP. At the turn of the century, hundreds of plants could be found in the USP or the *National Formulary,* but by 1990, only a handful remained. The steady withdrawal of botanicals from the USP sealed the fate of botanical medicines, as the FDA could not, and would not, approve a new drug without an official compendial standard. The last frontier for herbs became the over-the-counter (OTC) drug marketplace. Thousands of OTC medicines included herbal ingredients such as cascara sagrada, senna, psyllium, echinacea, black cohosh, goldenseal, and so on. In 1972, the FDA began a comprehensive review of all OTC products to assess their safety and efficacy. A system of expert advisory panels was established to review therapeutic categories of products, such as analgesics, sleep aids, laxatives, and so forth. All drug ingredients in each category were cataloged, and the relevant industries were invited to submit data in support of individual ingredients' safety or efficacy. With few commercial sponsors left, virtually all botanicals were relegated to Category II status, meaning they were not recognized as safe or effective. Many were also placed in Category III, which was a holding tank for all ingredients whose safety and efficacy were yet undetermined. Although the OTC drug review is not yet complete, it is clear that few botanicals will remain as over-the-counter active ingredients.

The modern herb industry (defined herein as companies or products that came into existence after 1965) held the FDA in great suspicion and avoided involvement in any rule-making or policy discussions with the agency. As a result, many herbs found in older OTC medicines, such as valerian, hops, ginger, saw palmetto, and ginseng, for example, were scientifically orphaned, being without industry or government sponsorship or support. The result has been a steady and inevitable removal of herbal ingredients from OTC drug products in the United States.

HERBS AS FOODS

With herbs now out of the new drug and OTC drug business, the botanical industry has no option but to offer their products as foods. A fair number of herbs were included on the 1968 GRAS (Generally Recognized As Safe) list, but largely as flavorings to alcoholic beverages, which did little to protect these products from an increasingly hostile FDA. At this time, the FDA also recognized that herbs had been herded into the food category and began a series of actions intended to further limit the availability of botanicals and to strictly limit any claims as to the uses or benefits of such products.

In 1980, the FDA issued the now infamous memorandum "Safe and Unsafe Herbs for Use in Herbal Teas." This memorandum took the form of a compliance policy guideline (CPG) that was intended to provide guidance to FDA's field staff in conducting inspections and in carrying out other regulatory duties. In effect, this document became a blacklist of herbs that the FDA used to bring regulatory action against companies offering these specific herbs for sale. This memorandum was broadly criticized by experts and the industry as lacking scientific or botanical integrity or credibility. Notwithstanding, the FDA continued to use this list until 1986, when a federal court challenged the validity of the FDA's policy and practices toward botanicals.

At this time, the agency began using the food additive provisions of the 1958 federal food additive amendment to the Food, Drug and Cosmetic Act to regulate botanicals. The concept of food additives grew out of the scientific and commercial renaissance following World War II. Advances in food technology led to the development of thousands of chemicals that found their way into foods as preservatives, surfactants, foaming agents, and stabilizers and were very useful in adding shelf life, texture, and color to processed and packaged foods. However, questions arose as to the long-term safety of such additives when used in the human food supply. Congress held extensive hearings on this subject and ultimately passed the well-known food additive amendments; these require that any substance added to foods be tested for safety and approved by the FDA prior to its being used in foods. No one questions the wisdom of this policy as it relates to ensuring a safe food supply. However, in the late 1970s, the FDA developed a novel interpretation of the food additive provision, whereby any substance that was used as a food or a food component could be challenged as a food additive at the discretion of the FDA. This became a convenient means of forcing botanicals off the market, by asserting that commonly used herbs were, in fact, food additives and therefore required FDA approval prior to marketing. In a series of bitterly fought court cases, the FDA challenged important botanicals, essential fatty acids, and other dietary ingredients as food additives. The FDA ultimately lost many of these cases but, in the process, left a legacy of deep animosity.

While these skirmishes continued, Congress passed the Nutrition Labeling Education Act of 1990 (NLEA) to reform food labeling and to allow, for the first time, a new class of health claims based on disease-nutrient relationships. The large conventional food industry had championed much of this legislation, but the herb industry saw little relevance to its products or future and so did not participate in these negotiations. However, the FDA's proposed regulations implementing NLEA clearly threatened any future health claims for herbs. Essentially, the FDA proposed that unless a food product or ingredient had received an authorized health claim, no other type of benefit claim or statement could be made for any food product including herbs. A series of public comments and meetings with FDA officials failed to change the agency's proposed regulation.

THE BIRTH OF DSHEA

By late 1991, the herb industry was in a state of siege. Relations with the FDA were at an all-time low. Menacing regulations were imminent, and lawsuits by and against the FDA seemed commonplace. Against this bleak scenario, a group of leading herb companies met to consider their future. Seeing no alternative but corrective legislation, these companies approached Senator Orrin G. Hatch (R-Utah) to address their deep-seated concerns. A lifelong believer in natural health and healing, Senator Hatch agreed to sponsor a Senate bill to resolve these issues once and for all, Congressman Bill Richardson (D-New Mexico) sponsored the House version, and, together, they introduced the Health Freedom Act of 1992. What followed is now regarded as one of the most significant changes to the Food, Drug and Cosmetic Act in this century.

What began as the Health Freedom Act in 1992 ended as the Dietary Supplement Health and Education Act of 1994 (DSHEA) (U.S. Congress, 1994), passed by unanimous consent of the Congress and signed into law by President Clinton on October 24, 1994. What no one had anticipated—including the FDA, Congress, and the herb industry—was an unprecedented outpouring of public support and concern by average citizens demanding unfettered access to dietary supplements and the right to have information as to their use and benefits. Millions of consumers called, wrote, and visited members of Congress, urging their support of DSHEA. It is now widely believed that Congress received more correspondence on this issue than any other topic except the Vietnam War.

DSHEA EXPLAINED

As with most federal laws, the legislative language of DSHEA is arcane, if not mystifying. The core provisions of the act, however, are straightforward and create an expansive framework for all dietary supplements. Botanicals presented a particularly difficult challenge to the drafters of the bill because of the convoluted and largely inconsistent regulatory history of herbs, addressed in earlier sections of this chapter. Should herbs be treated similar to vitamins with respect to, for example, safety standards, claims, and food additive status? In the end, all dietary ingredients were accorded the same status, and the law was written in such a way as to reflect this homogeneity. Unfortunately, this uniformity blurs the clear understanding of how herbs are now regulated. The following summary of DSHEA is an "herbs only" adaptation that provides a useful tool for those wishing to see how DSHEA creates a new architecture for the manufacture, sale, and promotion of herbs.

Botanical Summary of DSHEA

1. (Section 3) *Definition.* The term *dietary supplement* means an herb or other botanical or a concentrate, constituent, extract, or combination of any botanical that is intended for ingestion as a tablet, capsule, or liquid; is not represented for use as a conventional food or as a sole item of a meal or the diet; and is labeled as a dietary supplement. This includes new drugs that were marketed as botanicals prior to such approval; it does not include a botanical approved as a new drug or authorized for investigation as a new drug for which substantial clinical investigations have begun, and have been made public, and which was not previously marketed as a dietary supplement.

2. Botanicals are not Food Additives.

3. (Section 4) A botanical is considered unsafe for one of two reasons: (a) it presents a significant or unreasonable risk of illness or injury under conditions of use recommended or suggested in labeling, or (b) it is a new botanical for which inadequate information exists to provide reasonable assurance that it does not present a significant or unreasonable risk of illness or injury. In any proceeding under this paragraph, the United States shall have the burden of proof to show that a botanical is adulterated.

4. (Section 5) *Botanical Supplement Claims.* A publication, including an article, a chapter in a book, or an official abstract of a peer-reviewed scientific publication that appears in an article and

was prepared by the author or editors of the publication, which is reprinted in its entirety, shall not be defined as labeling when used in connection with the sale of botanicals to consumers under the following conditions:

a. It is not false or misleading.

b. It does not promote a particular manufacturer or brand of botanical.

c. It is displayed or presented with other items on the same subject matter so as to present a balanced view of the available scientific information on a botanical.

d. If displayed in an establishment, it is physically separate from the botanical and does not have appended to it any information by sticker or other method. This provision shall not apply to or restrict retailers of botanicals from selling books or publications as a part of their business.

5. (Section 6) A statement for a botanical may be made if the following conditions are met:

a. The statement describes the role of a botanical intended to affect the structure or function in humans, characterizes the documented mechanism by which a botanical acts to maintain such structure or function, or describes general well-being from consumption of a botanical.

b. The manufacturer of the botanical has substantiation that such a statement is truthful and nonmisleading.

c. The statement contains, prominently displayed and in bold-faced type, the following: "This statement has not been evaluated by the Food and Drug Administration. This product is not intended to diagnose, treat, cure or prevent any disease." Such statements cannot claim to diagnose, mitigate, treat, cure, or prevent any disease. The manufacturer of a botanical making such a statement shall notify the secretary (of the FDA) within thirty days after first marketing such a statement.

6. Botanical dietary supplements are misbranded if the following situations exist:

a. It is a botanical dietary supplement and the label or labeling of the botanical fails to list the name of each ingredient, the quantity of such ingredients, or, if a proprietary blend, the total quantity of all ingredients.

b. The label or labeling of the botanical fails to identify the product by the term *dietary supplement.*

c. The label or labeling of the botanical fails to identify any part of the plant from which the ingredient is derived.

d. The botanical
   • is covered by the specifications of an official compendium;
   • is represented as conforming to such official compendium and fails to do so;
   • is not covered by an official compendium and fails to have the identity and strength that it represents to have; or
   • fails to meet the quality, purity, or compositional specifications, based on validated assays or other appropriate methods, that it is represented to meet.

7. (Section 8) A botanical shall be deemed adulterated unless the following requirements are met:

a. The product contains only botanicals that have been present in the food supply as an article used for food in a form in which the food has not been chemically altered.

b. A history of use or other evidence of safety establishes that a new botanical (one not marketed in the United States before October 15, 1994), when used under conditions recommended in the labeling, will reasonably be expected to be safe. This should be shown at least seventy-five days before introduction into commerce to provide the secretary with the information on which the manufacturer has concluded that the botanical can reasonably be expected to be safe.

8. (Section 9) *Good Manufacturing Practices.* A botanical is unsafe if it is prepared, packed, or held under conditions that do not meet current good manufacturing practices (GMPs). The secretary may, through regulation, prescribe good manufacturing practices for botanicals that shall be modeled after current GMPs for food and may not impose standards for which there is no current and generally available analytical methodology.

9. (Section 10) A botanical is not a drug solely because its label or labeling contains a statement of nutritional support. Also, a botanical shall not be deemed misbranded if its label or labeling contains directions or conditions of use or warnings.

10. (Section 12) *Commission on Dietary Supplement Labels.* A commission shall conduct a study on, and provide recommendations for, the regulation of label claims and statements for botanicals, including the use of literature in connection with the sale of botanicals and procedures for evaluation of such claims. The commission shall evaluate how best to provide truthful, scientifically valid, and nonmisleading information to consumers.

11. (Section 13) *Office of Dietary Supplements.* The secretary shall establish an Office of Dietary Supplements (ODS) within the National Institutes of Health (NIH). The purposes of the office are as follows:

    a. To explore the potential role of botanicals to improve health care.

    b. To promote scientific study of the benefits of botanicals in maintaining health and preventing chronic disease.

The director of the ODS shall perform the following functions:

    a. Conduct and coordinate scientific research relating to botanicals that can limit or reduce the risk of diseases such as heart disease, cancer, birth defects, osteoporosis, cataracts, or prostatism.

    b. Collect results of scientific research related to botanicals and compile a database.

    c. Serve as a principle advisor to the NIH, the Centers for Disease Control and Prevention (CDCP), and the commissioner of the FDA on issues relating to botanicals, including botanical regulations, the safety of botanicals, and scientific issues arising in connection with the labeling and composition of botanicals.

The FDA's Proposed Regulation of Section 6

The most important (and controversial) change created by DSHEA is Section 6, which authorizes a new class of claims known as statements of nutritional support, more commonly referred to as structure/function claims (SFCs). As noted previously, such claims may describe the role of a botanical that is intended to affect the structure or function of the body, characterize the documented mechanism by which a botanical acts to maintain a bodily structure or function, or describe general well-being from consuming a (legal) botanical.

Section 6 claims are a hybrid between permissible but vague food benefit claims, such as "calcium builds strong bones," and frank drug claims. In an effort to distinguish SFCs from drug claims, Congress included the requirement that a disclaimer appear in conjunction with structure/function claims. The disclaimer makes it clear that the FDA has not evaluated these statements, and the SFC is not intended to diagnose, treat, cure, or prevent any disease. To date, the FDA has received over 3,000 notices of SFCs from industry, of which a very significant percentage are for botanicals. Typical claims resemble the following:

Ginkgo Biloba

- Promotes mental sharpness
- Improves circulation
- Improves memory and concentration

St. John's Wort

- Helps support healthy emotional balance
- Helps maintain positive attitude

Garlic

- Helps maintain healthy cholesterol levels

Valerian

- Supports restful sleep

Ginger

- Promotes healthy digestion

Saw Palmetto

- Helps maintain proper urine flow

Cranberry

- Helps support/maintain a healthy urinary tract

Echinacea

- Helps support a healthy immune system

On April 28, 1998, the FDA published a proposed rule defining the types of statements that can be made concerning the effect of a dietary supplement on the structure or function of the body. This rule also established criteria for determining when a statement about a dietary supplement is a claim to diagnose, cure, mitigate, treat, or prevent disease (Federal Register, 1998). The FDA's rationale for this rule was to give guidance to industry on the difference between allowable (to the FDA) SFCs and drug claims. To establish a line between these two classes of claims, FDA decided a new definition of disease was necessary:

> A disease is any deviation from, impairment of, or interruption of the normal structure or function of any part, organ, or system (or combination thereof) of the body that is manifested by a characteristic set of one or more signs or symptoms, including laboratory or clinical measurements that are characteristic of a disease. In determining whether a statement is a disease claim under these criteria, the FDA will consider the context in which the claim is presented. A statement claims to diagnose, mitigate, treat, cure, or prevent disease if it claims, explicitly or implicitly, that the product does any of the following:
>
> 1. Has an effect on a specific disease or class of diseases
> 2. Has an effect using scientific or lay terminology on one or more signs or symptoms that are recognizable to health care professionals or consumers as being characteristic of

a specific disease or a number of different specific diseases

3. Has an effect on a consequence of a natural state that presents a characteristic set of signs or symptoms recognizable to health care professionals or consumers as constituting an abnormality of the body
4. Has an effect on disease through one or more of the following factors:
   a. The name of the product
   b. A statement about the formulation of the product, including a claim that the product contains an ingredient that has been regulated by FDA as a drug and is well known to consumers for its use in preventing or treating a disease
   c. Citation of the title of a publication or reference, if the title refers to a disease use
   d. Use of the term "disease" or "diseased"
   e. Use of pictures, vignettes, symbols, or other means
5. Belongs to a class of products that is intended to diagnose, mitigate, treat, cure, or prevent a disease
6. Is a substitute for a product that is a therapy for a disease
7. Augments a particular therapy or drug action
8. Has a role in the body's response to a disease or to a vector of disease
9. Treats, prevents, or mitigates adverse events associated with a therapy for a disease and manifested by a characteristic set of signs or symptoms
10. Otherwise suggests an effect on a disease or diseases

This new definition is a dramatic departure and expansion over the existing definition of disease, or health-related condition, which reads as follows:

damage to an organ, part, structure, or system of the body such that it does not function properly (e.g., cardiovascular disease), or a state of health leading to such dysfunctioning (e.g., hypertension) . . ." (Federal Register, 1998, p. 23625)

In effect, should this proposal become final after notice and comment, a very important and broad class of conditions and natural states will become diseases. The consequences of this are far-reaching. First, many SFCs will become unapproved drug claims, since the definition of a drug follows the definition of disease. If natural states of aging such as menopause, poor digestion, or elevated cholesterol levels become diseases, the FDA will have effectively rewritten legislation by regulation. In passing DSHEA, Congress noted the following in its findings:

1. Dietary supplements have been shown to be useful in preventing chronic disease, and their appropriate use will help limit incidence of chronic disease and long-term health care costs.
2. Consumers should be empowered to make informed choices about preventative health care programs based on scientific studies relating to dietary supplements.

Clearly, Congress intends that dietary supplements be recognized for their health benefits, including prevention of the underlying causes of disease. It is expected that the millions of consumers who supported passage of DSHEA from 1992 to 1994 will express their strong objection to the FDA's attempt to undermine a key provision of DSHEA because this would have far-reaching potential effects on the practice of medicine, as well as payment and reimbursement for health care services, and would limit the ability of consumers to make important decisions about personal health.

DSHEA FIVE YEARS LATER:
HERBS ON THE RISE

The impact of DSHEA on the sale of herbs in the United States has been staggering. Table 2.1 lists the thirteen best-selling herbs in the mass market (food, drug, and mass merchandise stores but not health food stores) for the two-year period of 1997 and 1998 (compiled by Pharmavite). Significantly, of the top thirteen herbs in this

TABLE 2.1. Phytomedicinal Sales, 1997 and 1998

Herb	1998 Ranking	1997 Ranking	Retail Sales 1998 ($)	Retail Sales 1997 ($)	% Change 1997-1998
Ginkgo	1	1	150,859,328	90,421,640	66.8
St. John's Wort	2	5	140,358,560	48,446,328	189.7
Ginseng	3	2	95,871,544	86,216,928	11.2
Garlic	4	3	84,054,520	71,638,072	17.3
Echinacea/Goldenseal	5	4	69,702,144	49,245,168	41.5
Saw Palmetto	6	6	32,102,622	18,446,246	74.0
Kava-Kava	7	13	16,584,425	2,953,650	461.5
Pycnogenol®/ Grape Seed	8	7	12,113,555	9,973,348	21.5
Cranberry	9	9	10,378,810	6,188,689	67.7
Valerian root	10	10	8,650,521	6,112,876	41.5
Evening Primrose	11	8	8,552,860	7,308,980	17.0
Bilberry	12	11	6,441,501	4,560,067	41.3
Milk Thistle	13	12	4,966,170	3,038,425	63.4
Total (top 13 herbs)			**640,636,560**	**404,550,417**	**58.4**
Total herb sales			**688,352,192**	**442,928,512**	**55.4**

Source: Information Resources, Inc., Grocery, Drug, Mass Data, fifty-two weeks ending 12/27/98. Herbal Supplement Category as defined by Pharmavite. Private report, unpublished, from Pharmavite.

Note: This table lists the retail sales and the percent of increase in sales for the top thirteen herbs in food, drug, and mass merchandise (FDM) stores. The same herbs remained best-sellers from 1997 to 1998. These herb totals make up 91 percent of the total retail sales for all herbs in FDM retail outlets combined and do not constitute health/natural food stores, multilevel marketing (MLM) companies, mail order, professional sales, or Internet sales.

survey, four—ginkgo, St. John's wort, kava-kava, and valerian—are used specifically for their effects on mood, emotions, and mental state. Taking into account the growth rates for these four botanicals, one quickly recognizes the American public's interest in the natural products that affect state of mind. This comes as no surprise to those who lived through the 1960s but is indeed a telling indicator of social and cultural trends in present-day United States. Add to this the sales of ephedra, thought to exceed $1 billion a year in 1999, and the "psychoactive botanicals" represent the largest and most quickly growing sector of the commercial herb industry.

THE FUTURE OF HERBS IN AMERICA

Although DSHEA granted most herbs unrestricted market access and a generous claim structure, should herbs be dietary supplements in all cases? At least four regulatory classifications are possible for botanicals in the United States: (1) dietary supplement, (2) traditional medicine, (3) OTC drug, and (4) prescription (Rx) drug. Currently, the marketplace is driven by DSHEA. Yet, over the past ten years, much attention has been given to recognizing botanicals as traditional medicines, OTC drugs, or even prescription drugs.

In 1992, a consortium of European and American phytomedicine companies, known as the European American Phytomedicine Coalition (EAPC), formally petitioned the FDA to accept data as to the safety and effectiveness of phytomedicines sold for a "material time" and to a "material extent" in foreign countries. The FDA's long-standing position held that only OTC drug ingredients sold in the United States could be candidates for continued OTC drug status under the monograph review process.

Thus, many well-known and widely used herbal drugs in Europe, such as valerian, saw palmetto, hops, chamomile, and ginger, could not be reviewed as old drugs within the 1972 OTC drug review program. In 1994, two additional citizens' petitions were filed by the EAPC, formally requesting that valerian and ginger be recognized as old OTC drug ingredients and considered safe and effective for use as nighttime sleep aids and digestive aids, respectively. The agency issued a response to these petitions nearly six years later, hedgingly stating its willingness to accept such data, but only under very stringent conditions. Essentially, the OTC drug door remains shut to phytomedicines in the United States.

A presidential commission mandated by DSHEA examined the question of alternative regulatory recognition for herbs and strongly recommended that an expert advisory panel be established to thoroughly address this issue. According to the commission's report, serious consideration should be given to recognizing botanicals as traditional medicines and to removing obstacles to recognizing botanicals as OTC drugs.

Numerous experts agree that a select number of botanicals are proper candidates for OTC drug status. Although this would mean that some plant extracts would be available both as dietary supplements and OTC drugs, it is likely that many American consumers who currently would not use a certain herb as a dietary supplement would accept and use that same herb if it were offered as a drug that has received tacit government approval. Likewise, physicians, pharmacists, and other health care providers would be far more inclined to recommend, or at least not discourage, the use of an herbal OTC drug. The reasons are clear. OTC drugs are manufactured under stricter good manufacturing practices, and they have mandatory labeling that includes dosage recommendations, cautions, and warnings. Unfortunately, it does not appear that the FDA is prepared to actively develop an OTC pathway for botanicals, absent a legislative directive.

Throughout the developed world, botanicals are often sold as traditional medicines, in recognition of their long historical use and broad cultural acceptance. Germany, France, Switzerland, the United Kingdom, and other countries recognize many botanicals as traditional medicines. This approach is also supported by the World Health Organization and has received considerable attention by regulators on every continent in recent years. The United States, lacking such a cultural tradition, has not created a sanctuary for botanicals in the form of traditional medicines.

Traditional medicines create a useful bridge between the more formal OTC drug review process and the less formal dietary supplement regime that is a unique feature of the United States. Again, the FDA has not indicated its intention to explore further a traditional medicine model, but it is hoped that in coming years a more integrated structure will emerge that will accommodate botanicals as

prescription drugs, over-the-counter medicines, and traditional medicines, as well as dietary supplements.

In the meantime, herbs will continue to be used by millions of
Americans for a wide range of purposes, as more consumers become
familiar with the exotic names and strange descriptors that typify the
herbal marketplace. We will see botanicals become an increasingly
valued and important part of the emerging self-care marketplace. Un-
doubtedly, the pharmacologically and physiologically active plants,
such as ginkgo, St. John's wort, ephedra, kava, valerian, and others,
will lead the way, given their therapeutic significance and broad historical and commercial use worldwide. What regulatory scheme will
emerge to accommodate these varied uses remains unclear but prom-
ises to be an interesting and lively process, at the very least.

Chapter 3

Research Methodology: Probability, Statistics, and Psychometric Tests Employed in Herbal Medicine Studies

Robert Velin

INTRODUCTION

Throughout the ages, humanity has attempted to find ways to improve quality of life and effect positive change within the external environment and the human organism. To do so, it is essential to determine whether a given intervention or prescribed change results in the hypothesized or expected outcome. This requires us, as observers of behavior and as scientists, to formulate hypotheses, clearly identify problems, ask unambiguous questions, and observe data of interest in a standardized and reproducible fashion.

The objective of all research, regardless of specific scientific discipline, is to use the powers of observation as the basis for answering our questions of interest. These observations must be made systematically. Since the raw, unclassified observations frequently do not lend themselves well to direct interpretation, we utilize various statistical techniques to translate these into more manageable forms. Thus, the researcher must not only ascertain that the correct items of interest are being observed but also that the correct techniques are utilized to obtain these data and manage them subsequently. The purpose of this chapter is to examine two sets of factors paramount in the process: (1) factors related to *research design* and (2) factors specific to *statistical analysis*.

VALIDITY AND RELIABILITY OF MEASURES

To make appropriate observations, scientists routinely utilize standardized measures that allow them to gather pertinent data in a manner that is both valid and reliable. That is, they use instruments which will validly measure a specific factor, such as anxiety, depression, or blood pressure, and which are also reliable in measuring the factor reproducibly in subsequent trials. Both of these issues, validity and reliability, are essential in the context of scientific research.

Consider, for example, if one utilized a sphygmomanometer to measure blood pressure, but the instrument was so unreliable that it gave wildly different readings over time, even though the true reading remained relatively stable. As one can easily deduce, the quality of the measure utilized directly relates to the quality of the data obtained. Alternatively, imagine that a clinician used a technique to ascertain bone density, but the instrument instead measured tissue thickness. The technique may reliably provide the same result for a given patient time after time but is not validly measuring the construct of interest. Thus, one must remain cognizant of the underlying properties of a particular instrument. More specifically, if considering behavioral or psychological measures, the psychometric properties of these measures are essential to determining whether one may feel confident in drawing conclusions based on the observational data.

Although this text certainly cannot provide a comprehensive listing of the innumerable measures used in formal research, it is helpful to review some of the more common instruments employed in cognitive, behavioral, and psychological studies. This will allow more adequate interpretation of the herbal scientific literature presented in subsequent chapters.

GENERAL PSYCHOLOGICAL MEASURES

Perhaps the most widely used general psychological instruments in human studies are the Minnesota Multiphasic Personality Inventory, Second Edition (MMPI-2), and its predecessor, the Minnesota Multiphasic Personality Inventory (MMPI). The original MMPI was published by Hathaway and McKinley in 1943 and was then revised by Hathaway and colleagues in 1989, with an updated set of norms. The MMPI-2 is a self-administered test consisting of 567 true-or-false questions that measure a variety of emotional and personality characteristics. Although administration and scoring are relatively easy, especially with computer scoring programs, interpretation of the MMPI-2 requires considerable training and reasonable familiarity with the research literature. Computer interpretations obviously must be used very cautiously. Fortunately, from a research perspective, the validity of the old MMPI has been very well studied, and, increasingly of late, current literature is available on the MMPI-2 itself. Although the specific validity figures vary from scale to scale, diagnostic accuracy of the MMPI-2 profile is generally quite acceptable. For example, Patrick and his colleagues (Patrick, 1988) noted that the MMPI-2 revealed good validity for diagnosed schizophrenia, major depression, and paranoid disorders, as defined by the *Diagnostic and Statistical Manual of Mental Disorders* (American Psychiatric Association, 1994) (see the following diagnostic classifications section, p. 45). In short, the MMPI-2 is an excellent overall measure of various psychological characteristics, with reliability and validity generally in the acceptable ranges.

Often, rather than desiring a general measure of various psychological states, research is more specifically focused on a single emotional characteristic, such as anxiety or depression. In these instances, the Hamilton Rating Scale for Anxiety (HAMA) (Hamilton, 1959) and Hamilton Rating Scale for Depression (HAMD) (Hamilton, 1960) are very frequently used, especially in human studies of those disorders in the herbal literature. These instruments have some specific advantages over broader measures in terms of both their ease of administration (much shorter) and the specific nature of their intent. Their questionnaires combine adequate validity and reliability and provide relatively quick measures of levels of anxiety and depression in individual subjects. In addition, rather than relying on self-reporting of symptoms, they are based on the objective assessment of an observer. This serves to increase their accuracy and provides a corroboration of self-reported symptoms. Cut-off scores are available for each of the measures, allowing users to differentiate between unaffected and affected populations.

Generally, for clinical studies, values above 20 for both the HAMA and HAMD indicate severe anxiety and depression, respectively. A decrease of 10 points, or to a value of 10 or less after treatment, has been considered a significant result.

Another frequently used example of a symptom-specific instrument is the Beck Depression Inventory (BDI). This self-administered questionnaire consists of only twenty-one four-choice statements presented on a single page (Beck, 1967). This screening measure for depressive symptoms is thus much easier to administer and score than the MMPI-2, and its test/retest reliability has been acceptably demonstrated. In addition, as with the Hamilton scales, changes in scores tend to significantly parallel changes in depth of depression for individual patients (Beck, 1970).

One significant disadvantage for the symptom-specific, self-report instruments (such as the BDI) is that the items have fairly obvious face validity. That is, the individual taking the test can determine relatively easily what the instrument is attempting to measure, thus increasing the possibility of intentional manipulation of the score. Ultimately, these shorter self-report measures are best used when one is seeking screening measures possessing simplicity of administration, scoring, and interpretation, or when data can be corroborated by additional measures.

Another test of interest in the emotional realm is the Spielberger State-Trait Anxiety Scale Inventory (Spielberger, 1983). This instrument allows the measurement of what is referred to as trait anxiety (anxiety tendency of a given individual) and state anxiety (factors specific to a situational stressor). Thus, this instrument and its underlying theory allow for an interaction between person-specific and situational variables. This provides an examination of changes in anxiety at both levels, hopefully yielding additional information as a result of the multidimensional approach.

MEASURES OF BEHAVIOR
AND COGNITIVE FUNCTIONING

In addition to measures of emotional constructs, other general behavioral and cognitive characteristics may be objectively assessed. Within this realm, the various measures are simply too numerous to list in a comprehensive fashion, but some of particular interest that are frequently seen in the literature are described in this section.

In the area of attention-deficit hyperactivity disorder (ADHD), various aspects of children's functioning are observed. To organize these observations into a useful form, numerous rating scales have been designed. The Conner's Parent and Teacher Rating Scales, for example, are commonly used in this context and provide a way to measure, on a four-point scale, the frequency of various behaviors at home and in the classroom. For example, how frequently a given child is "off task" when in the course of an activity is rated by parents or teachers. These observations are then compared to a normative data set, thus allowing a determination of relevance. These particular measures, although prone to observer biases and variability across different observers, do provide an organized way to analyze ADHD behaviors, such as impulsiveness and off-task frequency.

The Clinical Global Impressions (CGI) scale (Guy, 1976) and the Clinical Global Impressions of Change (CGIC) (Schneider and Olin, 1996) are rating scales frequently used for a specific subject/patient in the study of dementia. Similar to the aforementioned Connor's scales, the CGI provides collection and organization of observations into a more useable form, but with the focus on a subject's overall clinical condition. The CGI has been used to estimate change in a person's condition over time, with two separate ratings used to form a "difference score." The CGIC represents a specific attempt to capture observations of change over time. Although both the CGI and CGIC are of some utility, concerns have been raised with respect to their validity and reliability (Schneider and Olin, 1996). In particular, the CGIC has failed to consistently detect the effects of treatment. Thus, research should employ additional measures to maximize the likelihood of detecting valid changes in clinical status.

Broad-based measures specifically assessing cerebral functions are also useful in this type of research. Within this realm, the Halstead-Reitan Neuropsychological Battery is frequently used. This battery consists of numerous individual tests that can be interpreted either individually or in terms of the overall data pattern. Specific summary indices and standardized T-scores (normalized score with a mean of 50 and a standard deviation of 10) are available that adjust for age, education, and gender (Heaton, Grant, and Matthews, 1991). It is beyond the scope of this chapter to address the specifics of the Halstead-Reitan Neuropsychological Battery. The interested reader is referred to the immense body of literature available elsewhere on this set of assessment procedures. It is useful to note, however, that, although very comprehensive and useful, one drawback of the Halstead-Reitan battery is the length of time necessary to administer and score it. Thus, other, shorter, measures of cerebral functioning frequently are utilized, particularly in the context of demented populations.

One specific instrument frequently employed with older patients or those with cognitive impairment is the Dementia Rating Scale (DRS) (Mattis, 1988). This tool is a brief instrument with relatively good validity and reliability, designed to assess cognitive efficiency. It is fairly easy to administer, requiring only ten to fifteen minutes in demented patients. The fact that it is designed specifically for use in the context of severe cognitive disorders results in its widespread utilization when other measures might be impractical, secondary to logistical concerns.

An additional measure of general cerebral functioning is the Bender-Gestalt Test and its several adaptations (Hutt, 1969). This is a primarily qualitative measure of visual-spatial functioning in which the subject/patient copies nine figures that are then scored along various dimensions. The results are used to infer the presence (or lack) of brain dysfunction as well to assess general brain efficiency. Various scoring systems are available for the Bender-Gestalt, making it difficult to compare across studies. Furthermore, the scoring, depending on the specific system used, can be somewhat subjective, raising the possibility of flawed interpretation. Nonetheless, it remains popular and can provide a brief screening measure of brain functioning.

Occasionally, specific measures of unitary motor abilities are desired, such as hand motor coordination or speed. The Purdue Pegboard Test or other equivalent tasks are used to measure finger dexterity or coordination. These are simple timed tasks in which individuals place pegs into keylike slots as rapidly as possible while their performance is timed. This allows for a measure of possible change across time or relative to other age-matched controls. The finger-tapping test similarly assesses simple motor speed in the hands. Comparisons can be made temporally as well as relative to other subjects.

DIAGNOSTIC CLASSIFICATIONS

Most human psychiatric research classifies individuals according to diagnostic categories. Diagnoses are made based on selective criteria. The two most common schemata are the *International Classification of Diseases* (ICD) (Practice Management Information Corporation, 1999), for medical disorders, and the *Diagnostic and Statistical Manual of Mental Disorders* (DSM) (American Psychiatric Association, 1994), for psychiatric and behavioral disturbances. Various versions of these manuals have been published over the years, with the ICD currently in its ninth edition (ICD-9) and the DSM in its fourth (DSM-IV). These two resource manuals are the basic bibles for diagnosis and provide a framework of consistency within which diagnoses can be made. Although psychological and psychiatric diagnoses remain subjective and require a clinician's judgment, these tools provide at least an element of standardization, improving validity and reliability of diagnosis. In short, these references provide an accepted set of diagnostic criteria as to what depression is or is not, for example. These templates generally do not provide particularly sensitive paradigms to measure severity of illness, except in the broadest terms. In rating disease burden, the more specific measures discussed previously are utilized.

RESEARCH DESIGN

Appropriate statistical analyses of research data are as essential as defined research methods, to ensure that no gross biases affect the manner of data acquisition.

For example, it is important, when a study medication is to be evaluated, that both the patient and the individuals obtaining observations remain unaware of whether a given subject is actually taking the medication (versus an inert placebo). In this way, neither party is as likely to inadvertently sway the results. When neither the observer nor the subject knows whether the subject is on placebo or actual medication, this is called a double-blind study, as both individuals are "blinded" as to the specific condition of the subject. Furthermore, subjects should generally be randomly assigned to a given treatment condition (true medication versus placebo or some other control group), so that researchers do not inadvertently "stack the deck" to favor a desired result. Similarly, the subjects' desire to be in the research project could produce a distorting impact. To minimize these concerns, subjects are randomly assigned to treatment modalities within a study, based on chance alone, once they have been accepted for inclusion.

Frequently, it is also necessary for a "crossover" to occur, whereby subjects who were previously on an inert placebo are changed to the active medication, while those receiving the active intervention are switched to placebo or some other control condition. The crossover design allows researchers to measure responses in all subjects as they make the transition from one modality to the other, thus increasing the confidence in the conclusions of the study.

A well-known phenomenon called the placebo effect may be operative in clinical drug studies. In essence, individuals in the research protocol may tend to get better simply because they believe they are receiving an intervention. This placebo effect is relatively universal and potentially quite strong, thus necessitating appropriate controls within the research design to address its presence. For example, if one examines individuals with complaints of headaches and provides them with sugar pills for relief, a certain percentage (often 30 percent) will vociferously report their headaches are much improved, even though they have not received any pharmacological treatment for their malady.

In appropriate research design, it is important to analyze the data properly once they have been collected. More specifically, it is important to determine whether the changes seen in the observations are above and beyond what would be expected by chance alone. Various tools are available in this assessment, such as the analysis of variance (ANOVA) procedure. This is a statistical method that examines a given measure and determines whether it is equivalent to, or different from, other observations. For example, one group of twenty subjects has a mean (average) weight of 100 pounds. Another group has been on a special diet for the past two months, with the hopes of losing weight, and has an average weight of ninety-eight pounds. However, when one considers the overall variability of weight within the two groups, it is very likely that this two-pound difference is relatively irrelevant. Thus, the analysis of variance procedure takes into account variability within the individual groups to allow researchers to come to more firm conclusions regarding differences between either individual subjects or groups of data.

The ANOVA procedure makes use of probability values, or what are commonly referred to as p values. These simply are the statistical shorthand that allows us to communicate the likelihood that a given difference could have occurred by chance alone rather than as the result of any specific intervention. Thus, when one reads that the p value is less than 0.05, this means that the probability of this difference existing by chance alone is less than 5 percent. Likewise, a p value less than or equal to 0.01 means that the probability of this score or difference occurring by chance alone is less than or equal to only 1 percent, obviously increasing confidence in the conclusions. Generally, any findings with a p value above 0.05 (5 percent) are regarded as scientifically insignificant, although they may give information regarding some basic trends in the data.

Occasionally, rather than directly evaluating a single group of subjects, researchers may analyze a cohort of studies to analyze a larger data set. Such an examination, commonly referred to as a "meta-analysis," can increase the ability to generalize a given conclusion by expanding the observations beyond smaller sets of data with very specific subject and research characteristics to larger sets that are likely more representative of the general population. In these instances, researchers are most often analyzing data from previously completed research rather than analyzing new data.

ANIMAL STUDIES

Frequently, research on herbal remedies or their chemical components is carried out on animals, such as mice or rats. In these instances, numerous paradigms are used that vary substantially from those utilized in human studies. For example, the elevated plus maze or some form of maze paradigm may be utilized to measure learning and memory in experimental animals. Animals are taught to navigate their way through a maze to obtain food. With increased practice, their progress through the maze tends to take less time. When the route of the maze is changed, they tend to negotiate the new route somewhat more quickly than animals that are new to the task. Various interventions, such as new medications, can be administered and the impact measured by observing the animals' performance in the maze environment.

Learned helplessness is another phenomenon observed in the animal literature. In this instance, one animal is paired with another in a learning paradigm. However, significant differences are devised in the control that these animals can exert over their environment. For example, two rodents are placed in boxes with electric grids on the floor and a small light on the side. At certain intervals, the light is turned on and, subsequently, an electronic impulse will be delivered to the grid on the floor, leading to a shock of the animal's feet. One of the animals may be able to press a lever placed on the wall of the box, thus preventing delivery of the shock. The other animal, however, continues to receive the shock without control over its occurrence. When placed into another paradigm with similar characteristics, the first rodent will readily learn to terminate the noxious stimulus, providing evidence that it has "learned" to exert some control over its environment. In contrast, the other animal will cower and ultimately show no behavioral response or attempt to avoid the noxious stimulus. Essentially, the animal has taken on a helpless posture, even though it may now have an available mechanism for avoiding the shock. This learned helplessness is frequently thought to be analogous to certain types of anxious behavior in humans.

CONCLUSIONS

When reviewing the scientific literature and interpreting studies, it is important to assess the quality and nature of the research design, as well as the underlying psychometric properties of the measures utilized. These considerations guide the degree of confidence that can be placed in the conclusions drawn.

In closing, scientific research is ideally based upon the analysis of observable data that are valid, reliable, and reproducible. It is only when others utilizing the same methods or design can replicate a given study's findings that we can be confident in the conclusions. If subsequent results occur in a similar study population, findings are deemed as having "passed the scientific test." Such methods have allowed us to more appropriately and accurately understand the world around us.

PART II:
PSYCHIATRIC CONDITIONS AND HERBS EMPLOYED IN THEIR TREATMENT

Chapter 4

Depression

On a basic personal level, almost everyone understands the concept of depression. It comes in many names and guises: "down in the dumps," "feeling the blues," "on a bummer." The cures for depression are legion as well and include "the talking cure," finding the "right" partner, a quart of chocolate ice cream, or even "tincture of time."

Biological or chemical depression must be distinguished from situational or exogenous depression. The latter is a temporary mood state motivated by specific external events. Endogenous depression, in contrast, is a biochemical recurrent disorder, often chronic, that tends to become more severe over time if left untreated. The contrast is clear in the title of Freud's famous essay of 1917, "Mourning and Melancholia." Mourning is a mood state of a certain expected duration, often culturally sanctioned. In the West, we might expect a person to reenter social interaction six to twelve months after the loss of a spouse. In some Native American cultures, a few days are allotted to family members to mourn, after which it is taboo to discuss the departed, for fear that the person's spirit will infect the living.

Melancholy, or depression, as we currently prefer, does not have a definite end point. Unfortunately, without intervention, it may become perpetual, rendering the person unhappy, unproductive, and unfit for pursuit of a livelihood or meaningful relationships.

Clinical depression is a very common disorder, affecting 3 to 5 percent of the population worldwide, according to the World Health Organization (WHO). Lifetime prevalence in the United States was estimated at 17 percent (Kessler et al., 1994). Economic costs are figured in the billions of dollars annually in the United States alone.

The natural products that historically have served to treat depression include cannabis, opium poppies, alcohol, belladonna, henbane, datura, and many others (Payk, 1994). Most provided temporary relief along the order of "drowning your sorrows." The modern era of psychopharmacology for depression has been beautifully reviewed in Kramer's book *Listening to Prozac* (Kramer, 1993). In essence, the first tricyclic antidepressant, imipramine, was introduced in 1957. Almost simultaneously, monoamine oxidase inhibitors (MAOI) appeared on the market. Both groups were believed to influence depression through effects of the biogenic amine theory of depression, meaning that depression is due to inadequate neurotransmitter levels in the brain, most often of norepinephrine and serotonin.

The tricyclics were known to boost norepinephrine levels early on, and, sometime later, it was discovered that serotonin levels were increased as well. MAOI drugs prevented the premature breakdown of these neurotransmitters by inhibiting the activity of a lytic or cleaving enzyme, monoamine oxidase. Although both classes of drugs are effective in the treatment of depression, about 70 percent of the time, they are similarly hampered by side effects. The tricyclic antidepressants (TCAs) frequently cause sedation, dry mouth, and constipation due to their anticholinergic tendencies. This has sometimes severely curtailed their acceptance by patients, particularly in long-term use. The MAOI drugs also have side effects and may be overtly dangerous in the presence of tyramine, an amino acid found in red wine, pickled herring, strong cheeses, nuts, and many other common foods. Ingestion of tyramine by the patient taking MAOIs may lead to dangerous blood pressure elevations, even hypertensive crisis or death. Patients who receive such drugs leave the physician's office with a long list of "do's and don'ts" that serve as a constant reminder that they have a condition, and a serious one, at that.

The antidepressant landscape was enriched with the advent of SSRI drugs, or selective serotonin reuptake inhibitors, in the late 1980s. These drugs include, in their order of introduction to the U.S. market: fluoxetine (Prozac), sertraline (Zoloft), paroxetine (Paxil), fluvoxamine (Luvox), and citalopram (Celexa). All are comparable to previous pharmaceuticals in terms of efficacy, but the true distinguishing feature has been their tolerability. The side effect ratio has been reversed: if 80 percent of patients complained of side effects on TCAs, only 20 percent have major objections to SSRIs. This level of acceptance has lead to societal questions, some not so satirical, as to whether SSRIs should merely be added to the collective water supply of our cities. That level of acceptance notwithstanding, SSRIs may still produce sedation, loss of libido, delayed or denied orgasm, and a variety of other complaints.

To complicate matters, it is apparent that disturbances in other neurotransmitter systems may precipitate depression. The antidepressant bupropion hydrochloride (Wellbutrin) is equally effective as the previously mentioned drugs but affects mainly the dopaminergic system. Theories implicating depression as due to decreased endorphins (endogenous morphine) such as methionine-enkephalin or leucine-enkephalin have been recently advanced (Morphy, Fava, and Sonino, 1993). The issue of cannabinoid receptor systems and their effect on mood remains to be explored (see section on cannabis in Chapter 9). As so nicely stated by Bennett and colleagues (1998, p. 1205), "the original monoamine hypothesis is gradually being expanded to a dysregulation hypothesis, which emphasizes the importance of proper balance in brain monoamine function and postulates that a disturbance at any point can lead to depression."

Even in the face of the best available drug management, 30 percent of depressed patients remain unimproved. The pharmacological search for relief continues and has opened the door to herbal alternatives.

ST. JOHN'S WORT:
Hypericum perforatum L. Hypericaceae
or Clusiaceae (Previously Guttifereae)

Synonyms

- St. John's wort
- Hypericum
- Klamath weed
- *Hyperici herba* (Latin)

- *Johanniskraut* (German)
- *Herbe de millepertuis* (French)

Botany

Hypericum perforatum, or St. John's wort (SJW), is a perennial, sometimes invasive weed, native to Eurasia and naturalized on most other continents. The genus contains almost 400 related species. This one reaches a height of 1 meter (m), and blooms from June to September in the Northern Hemisphere. The important medicinal portion consists of the aerial tops of the plants, with leaves, buds, and flowers. Preservation of biochemical activity requires quick drying and avoidance of light exposure.

Denke and colleagues performed a three-year cultivation trial of hypericum (Denke et al., 1999). They demonstrated that nitrogen fertilization increases green plant matter, but at the expense of production of secondary plant metabolites (flavonoids) that are essential to pharmacological activity. A similar scenario occurs with many herbs, which may flourish under adverse conditions.

Phytochemistry

This topic has proven to be extremely complex, and final answers as to the active ingredient(s) remain elusive. Fortunately, two excellent reviews have recently been offered (Nahrstedt and Butterweck, 1997; Upton, 1997).

The main constituents of dry extracts are phenylpropanes, flavonol glycosides, biflavones, and oligomeric proanthocyanidins, but additional components include phloroglucinols, xanthones, and naphthodianthrones. The phenylpropanes in hypericum include *p*-coumaric acid and caffeic acid. Chlorogenic acid is said to produce central nervous system stimulation (Nahrstedt and Butterweck, 1997).

Flavonol glycosides include quercetin, hyperoside, and rutin. One or another component exhibits MAO_A inhibition activity, but their concentration in the extracts is so low as to be felt irrelevant with respect to clinical efficacy as an antidepressant. Similarly, some flavonoids bind benzodiazepine receptors (Nahrstedt and Butterweck, 1997).

Biflavones may exhibit central nervous system depressant activity and bind benzodiazepine receptors, but no in vivo experimental activity has been apparent, suggesting that these components either fail to cross the blood brain barrier or are rapidly metabolized (Nahrstedt and Butterweck, 1997).

Tannins compose a fair percentage of hypericum extracts and may account for their prominent antibacterial and antiviral effects.

Xanthones again possess MAO_A inhibitory actions but are present in amounts too small to account for the antidepressant actions of hypericum (Nahrstedt and Butterweck, 1997).

The phloroglucinol fraction is the subject of increasing scrutiny. Hyperforin is the most important and is labile to heat and light. It is found only in the flowers and fruits, ranging from 2 to 4.5 percent content (Nahrstedt and Butterweck, 1997). The fact that it is a lipophilic molecule increases the likelihood that it penetrates the central nervous system (CNS). Hyperforin has proven to display important neurotransmitter inhibition and modulation effects, which will be discussed subsequently.

The essential oil of SJW contains mainly monoterpenes, such as pinene, myrcene, and limonene and sesquiterpenes, such as caryophyllene and humulene. It is said to have antifungal activity (Awang, 1991). Essential oil content varies form 0.1 to 0.35 percent (Bombardelli and Morazzoni, 1995). The components of the essential oil of hypericum, if not their proportions, are very similar to those of *Cannabis sativa*, except for the added presence of 2-methyl-octane (16.4 percent) (Upton, 1997).

A distinct component of the steam distillate is methylbutenol 17, which has sedative properties at high dosage, beyond those occurring in standardized extracts (Nahrstedt and Butterweck, 1997).

The crude extracts contain about 1 percent amino acids, including gamma-aminobutyric acid (GABA), an endogenous inhibitory neurotransmitter, but in a concentration too low to be active in their own right (Nahrstedt and Butterweck, 1997).

Naphthodianthrones, especially hypericin and pseudohypericin, are contained in the perforations in hypericum leaves and flowers. They account for the red color of SJW oil and attendant phototoxic reactions most commonly seen in grazing animals ("hypericism"). For many years, it was believed that the MAOI activity of hypericin accounted for the antidepressant effects of SJW. In 1984, Suzuki demonstrated this activity (Suzuki et al., 1984), but the extract he employed was only of 80 percent purity. Subsequently, Bladt and Wagner (1994) were unable to demonstrate MAOI activity with pure hypericin in rat brain homogenates. An inhibition of MAO was apparent with the whole-herb extract and certain fractions (mainly flavonoids), but only at a relatively high dosage. The authors said of the results, "In summary, none of the fractions of hypericum or their constituents tested in vitro in these experiments showed relevant MAO inhibition in relevant concentrations." They also stated, "Hence, the hypothesis of MAO inhibition as the mode of action of hypericum and its constituents may no longer have any real basis" (Bladt and Wagner, 1994, p. 559).

Similarly, Thiede and Walper (1994) showed MAOI activity of hypericin 100-fold less than that observed by Suzuki. They also posited that other components must account for MAO inhibition, and that hypericin concentrations in vivo would be insufficient to produce significant clinical effects.

Many current review articles and popular accounts about St. John's wort still refer to hypericin as the active ingredient, and the antidepressant action of hypericum as due to MAO inhibition. Given these recent research developments, this is a seemingly untenable proposition.

Nevertheless, in a new theory, Gruenwald (1997) has hypothesized that hypericin alters serotonin metabolism by absorbing long wave light, thus reducing depressive moods. The effects of raising melatonin levels and improving sleep were also claimed.

Thiele and colleagues proposed another mechanism of action for hypericum involving modulation of cytokines, inflammatory mediators (Thiele, Brink, and Ploch, 1994). This researcher examined blood of depressed patients treated with hypericum and demonstrated suppression of interleukin-6 release. It was hypothesized that this might influence depression through effects on corticotropin-releasing hormones.

Bombardelli and Morazzoni (1995) summarized the situation: "The active ingredient has to be considered the extract *in toto,* as the single constituents responsible for this activity are today still unknown" (p. 65).

History of Use

Hypericum was known to the ancient classical physicians and botanists and has primarily been employed for its wound-healing properties. The Latin generic name derives from terms meaning "above an icon," referring to its placement to ward off evil spirits. The species name refers to a spotted or perforated appearance when its leaves are held before the light. As to the common name, "wort" is a Middle English term for "plant."

Hypericum flowers initially bloom around June twenty-fourth in the Northern Hemisphere, the date of the feast of St. John. Similarly, the red spots in the leaves are said to be visible on August twenty-ninth, the date St. John was beheaded (Hobbs, 1988-1989).

Hypericum use for depression is documented for several hundred years. Turner said of it in the sixteenth century (Turner et al., 1995, p. 245), "If it be drunken with water and honey about the quantity of twenty ounces, it purgeth largely choleric humours. But it must be taken continually, till the patient be whole." Similarly, Culpeper (1994, p. 203) said, "A tincture of the flowers in spirit of wine, is commended against melancholy and madness."

Hypericum was approved by the German Commission E in 1984 for "Psychoautonomic disturbances, depression, anxiety and/or nervous unrest" (Schulz, Hänsel, and Tyler, 1998, p. 50). However, as clinical use and experimental trials progressed, the true role of this agent as an antidepressant, with a distinct mode of action, has become apparent. By 1994, German doctors had prescribed 66 million daily doses of hypericum (De Smet and Nolen, 1996).

Preparation of Extracts

The flowering tops of hypericum, including buds and blossoms, are collected and dried at a low temperature or lyophilized (freeze-dried) with liquid nitrogen. Upton and colleagues state, "Care should be taken to harvest only the middle to the top portion of the plant, approximately the top 30-60 cm (12-24 in). Harvesting the lower leaves will result in a significant lowering of constituent concentration" (Upton, 1997, p. 8).

Extracts are made with an aqueous/methanol mixture in darkness (Schulz, Hänsel, and Tyler, 1998). Most clinical trials have employed an extract labeled LI 160, but recently an extract called WS 5572 with a 5 percent hyperforin content has attracted attention. Previous commercial extracts have varied in hyperforin content from 1 to 5 percent (Schellenberg, Sauer, and Dimpfel, 1998).

Schempp and colleagues (1999) have recently suggested a photometric method of analyzing dry extracts with peroxidase-catalyzed indoleacetic acid oxidation as a quick, economical method of standardization of hypericum extracts. Hyperforin and various flavonoid components of hypericum affect peroxidase function, and an examination of standardized extracts showed parallels between enzyme activity and relative concentrations of catechols and quercetin glycosides.

Hyperforin may represent an important therapeutic component of hypericum. It accounts for 2 to 4 percent of the content of the dried herb but is quite prone to oxidation (Orth, Rentel, and Schmidt, 1999). The authors in this study found hyperforin to be optimally retained under a nitrogen atmosphere at $-70°C$. Fortunately, evidence suggests that hyperforin is more stable in hypericum extracts due to the presence of antioxidants in the plant cell matrix. In a manner of speaking, hypericum herb and extracts may serve as their own natural preservatives.

Studies of Cellular and Biochemical Mechanisms

In 1994, Müller and Rossol examined the effects of LI 160 on serotonin receptors in a neuroblastoma cell line over several hours of incubation. They observed a subsequent reduction in serotonin receptor expression that would serve to impair reuptake of serotonin into the cells. The authors postulated a similar mechanism to explain the antidepressant effects of hypericum (Müller and Rossol, 1994).

In 1995, Perovic and Müller examined LI 160 in rat synaptosomes, noting that it caused a 50 percent inhibition of serotonin reuptake. They stated, "therefore it is concluded, that the antidepressant activity of hypericum extract is due to an inhibition of serotonin uptake by postsynaptic receptors" (Perovic and Müller, 1995).

Cott employed a NovaScreen to demonstrate high affinity of the crude *Hypericum perforatum* extract to $GABA_A$ and adenosine receptors (Cott, 1995).

In 1997, Müller and colleagues assessed LI 160 antidepressant mechanisms in mice. They demonstrated that the extract inhibited synaptosomal uptake of serotonin, dopamine, and norepinephrine with similar affinities, about 2 micrograms (μg) per milliliter (ml) (Müller et al., 1997). A similar effect on three distinct neurotransmitter systems is unknown for any other substance. In addition, "subchronic treatment" in rats at extremely high doses, a down-regulation of beta-adrenoreceptor density was seen in the frontal cortex, along with an increase in serotonin 5-hydroxytryptamine, type 2 (5-HT-2) binding sites.

J. M. Cott (1997) examined the binding and enzyme inhibition effects of a crude hypericum extract in detail. Hypericin had affinity only for N-methyl-D-aspartate (NMDA) receptors, which, although not supporting its role as an antidepressant, may provide a rationale for its antiviral claims. Although the extract had significant affinity for adenosine, benzodiazepine, $MAO_{A,B}$, and $GABA_{A,B}$ receptors, the concentrations required in vitro were felt to be unattainable through oral dosing, except for the GABA activity. Cott noted the findings of previous researchers with respect to serotonin uptake and receptor expression but indicated, once more, that sufficient concentrations for these effects were unlikely in vivo. In contrast, the observed GABA receptor binding occurred at 6 nanograms (ng) per ml. Possible roles of the GABA system in enhancement of beta-adrenergic down-regulation and modulation of dopamine systems were offered as possible explanations of the antidepressant actions of hypericum.

In 1998, a new wrinkle appeared in hypericum research, with focus applied to a lipophilic component of the plant, hyperforin. Chatterjee and colleagues employed rat synaptosomal preparations and experiments in "behavioral despair" and "learned helplessness" to assess its role (Chatterjee, Bhattacharya, et al., 1998). Based on these experiments, they indicated that hyperforin is "a potent uptake inhibitor of serotonin (5-HT), dopamine (DA), GABA, and l-glutamate" (p. 499) and that the behavioral results correlated to hyperforin content. No relevant effect was seen on MAO function.

Neary and Yurong (Neary and Bu, 1999, p. 358) have recently examined the role of the LI 160 extract in inhibition of serotonin and norepinephrine uptake in astrocytes, which "surround synaptic terminals and regulate neurotransmission." Effects seen in cultured rat astrocytes included a 50 percent reduction in rate of transport of serotonin, and a 4.5-fold decrease in the affinity of norepinephrine for uptake sites. These effects disappeared when LI 160 was removed, thus ruling out a toxic effect of the hypericum extract. Results, if confirmed, would suggest that the actions of hypericum resemble those of venlafaxine (Effexor), an agent that affects both serotonin and norepinephrine uptake.

Kleber and colleagues (1999) demonstrated that a standardized alcohol extract of SJW inhibits the activity of dopamine beta-hydroxylase, whereas hypericin has a comparatively weak effect. Such activity might serve to increase dopamine levels in the CNS and provide partial explanation for antidepressant effects of the herb.

Denke and colleagues have demonstrated that hypericum extracts also inhibit myeloperoxidase-catalyzed dimerization of enkephalins (Denke, Schneider, and Elstner, 1999). The latter have been implicated in antidepressant mechanisms: depressed patients display lower baseline levels of plasma beta-endorphin, and its production slows with advancing age, mirroring an increase in incidence of depression. The authors suggested that the flavonoid components (hyperoside, isoquercitrin and quercitrin) inhibited the dimerization reaction.

Studies in Normals

Schulz and Jobert (1994) examined the effects of LI 160, 300 milligrams (mg) tid (three times a day), in twelve older healthy female volunteers over four weeks, in a double-blind, crossover, placebo-controlled study. Sleep polysomnography techniques were employed for assessment. Sleep onset was unchanged by hypericum and was interpreted by the authors as indication that SJW lacks sedative influences. The mean percentage of deep-sleep stages (3 to 4) increased from 1.5 to 6 percent under treatment. A slight reduction in REM (rapid eye movement, or dream) sleep latency of 10 minutes (min) was seen in the LI 160 group, but overall REM sleep was unchanged. This is distinct from effects of conventional antidepressants, which typically delay REM onset and reduce total REM time. The practical meaning of these results is still unclear.

Pharmacokinetic studies in 1994 with LI 160 in twelve healthy adults revealed a half-life for hypericin of about 24 hours (h) (Staffeldt et al., 1994). To some, this suggested the possibility of dosing hypericum once daily, as is common with tricyclic and selective serotonin reuptake inhibitor (SSRI) antidepressants. Unfortunately, this discovery of a long half-life for hypericin may have been rendered superfluous with respect to any antidepressant effect of that substance. Suggested dosing for hypericum extracts remains tid.

Sharpley and colleagues (1998) examined the effects of LI 160 on sleep polysomnograms in eleven normal volunteers in a placebo-controlled crossover design. Two different dosages increased latency to REM onset, as with other antidepressants, but without other effects on sleep architecture.

Biber and colleagues (1998) assessed oral bioavailability in six human volunteers. Two different extracts were employed, WS 5572, with 5 percent hyperforin content, and WS 5573, with 0.5 percent hyperforin. The extracts were said to be identical with respect to other hypericum components. Maximal plasma levels were attained in 3 to 3.5 h, "with a half-life of distribution and elimination half-life of 3h and 9h, respectively" (Biber et al., 1998, p. 36). They felt that in normal tid dosing of hypericum that effective plasma levels of 97 ng/ml could be attained. The authors contended that the higher potency hyperforin extract was active, whereas the one of lower potency was not.

The effects of these same extracts, at 900 mg taken daily for eight days, on quantitative electroencephalograms (qEEGs) in eighteen healthy young adults were recently assessed in a double-blind study (Schellenberg, Sauer, and Dimpfel, 1998). Placebo patients manifested no change, whereas high- and low-hyperforin groups showed peak effects between 4 to 8 h. By day eight, the 5 percent hyperforin group demonstrated increased qEEG power in delta, theta, and lower alpha frequencies (see Chapter 5). The authors concluded, "Accordingly, neuroelectrical measurements after oral administration of hypericum extracts lead to the hypothesis that this phytopharmacon acts neurochemically in the context of noradrenergic and serotonergic neurotransmission." They also suggested that "hypericum extracts with a high hyperforin content have a shielding effect on the central nervous system" (Schellenberg, Sauer, and Dimpfel, 1998, p. 52). These intriguing results await further developments.

Studies in Clinical Disease

In 1994, Harrer and Schulz reviewed twenty-five controlled studies of various hypericum extracts. There were 1,592 identified subjects, but dosing varied from 300 to 900 mg of extract per day, with a treatment duration of two to six weeks. Benefit on depression was demonstrated in three of four studies comparing hypericum to placebo, with rates comparable to those of synthetic antidepressants.

That same year, Hübner and colleagues examined the effects of LI 160, 300 mg tid, in a randomized, double-blind, placebo-controlled study of thirty-nine patients meeting ICD-9 criteria of neurotic depression (Hübner, Lande, and Podzuweit, 1994). The Hamilton Rating Scale for Depression (HAMD), the von Zerssen Health Complaint Survey, and Clinical Global Impressions (CGI) scales were employed. Respondents were defined as having a 50 percent reduction or a final score below 10 on the HAMD. At the end of four weeks, 70 percent of the LI 160 patients met these criteria, compared with only 47 percent of placebo controls.

Sommer and Harrer (1994) examined 105 adult outpatients with mild depression, as defined by ICD-9, in a four-week double-blind trial of LI 160, 300 mg tid, versus placebo. At the end of treatment, HAMD scores dropped, on average, from 15.8 to 7.2 (54 percent) in the hypericum extract group, compared to placebo values of 15.8 to 11.3 (29 percent). This difference was quite significant ($p < 0.01$). Overall, 67 percent of LI 160 patients responded versus 28 percent of controls (a figure that mirrors the frequent citation of a 30 percent placebo effect).

Hänsgen and colleagues pursued a similar study of seventy-two patients with LI 160 over six weeks but added a twist by switching the placebo group to "verum" (active drug) in the last two weeks (Hänsgen, Vesper, and Ploch, 1994). The hypericum group had improvements in four psychometric treatment measures, including somatic symptoms of depression, versus placebo ($p < 0.001$). In addition, the placebo group showed improvements in the final two weeks once on verum, while the LI 160 group continued to progress in symptom reduction.

Hypericum was compared favorably to light treatment (phototherapy) of seasonal affective disorder (SAD) (Martinez et al., 1994), but the small sample size of twenty patients makes further study advisable.

In 1994, Vorbach and colleagues assessed LI 160 at 900 mg per day versus 75 mg per day of imipramine in a double-blind study of 135 depressed patients, defined by DSM-III-R criteria, over six weeks (Vorbach, Hübner, and Arnoldt, 1994). HAMD scores fell from 20.2 to 8.8 in the LI 160 group (56 percent), while scores for imipramine patients fell from 19.4 to 10.7 (45 percent). CGI results were comparable. Side effects were noted by the hypericum patients at half the rate of those treated with imipramine, and to a lesser degree of severity.

Woelk and colleagues examined effects of LI 160 in four-week trials in 3,250 patients gleaned from 663 private practitioners (Woelk, Burkard, and Grünwald, 1994). Patients reported a 50 percent reduction in symptoms of depression, restlessness, and difficulty initiating and maintaining sleep, and in associated somatic symptoms. Posttreatment values of the von Zerssen Depression Scale were less than half of those prior to initiation of hypericum. Based on physician and patient assessment, 80 percent of patients were improved or symptom free after treatment, and only 15 percent failed to respond.

Harrer and colleagues compared LI 160 at 900 mg per day to 75 mg per day of maprotiline, a quadricyclic antidepressant, more popular in Germany than in the United States (Harrer, Hübner, and Podzuweit, 1994). The study involved 102 patients meeting ICD-10 criteria of depression who were examined over four weeks. HAMD scores dropped 50 percent in both treatment arms, with similar changes in von Zerssen Depression Scale and CGI, such that no significant differences were ascertained between hypericum and maprotiline. However, hypericum was favored, according to patients' characterizations. Of those calling themselves "very much improved," hypericum-treated patients outpolled the maprotiline patients 23:16, while it was touted by those "no longer ill," 22:12.

Of maprotiline patients, 22 percent noted fatigue versus 4 percent for hypericum patients.

In a landmark 1996 study, Linde and colleagues performed a meta-analysis of randomized clinical trials of hypericum in treatment of depression. Twenty-three studies with 1,757 patients were found. While admitting that many studies were not exemplary in their performance, the authors concluded that the data supported hypericum extracts to be significantly more effective in treating depression than placebo (observed side effects fewer than with TCAs), and that they were equally effective compared to synthetic antidepressants (which did not include SSRIs). The side effect profile of hypericum markedly favored them compared to TCAs (Linde et al., 1996).

In an editorial comment on this study in the *British Medical Journal,* De Smet and Nolen (1996) retained criticisms of hypericum as an antidepressant. They noted that despite the evidence against MAOI activity of hypericin, that component was still employed as the biochemical marker in the production of commercial SJW extracts: "Standardisation of hypericum extracts on hypericin content may therefore offer no guarantee of pharmacological equivalence" (De Smet and Nolen, 1996, p. 241). They also opined that studies lacked a certain degree of diagnostic precision and, for the most part, were of inadequate treatment length. They did not feel that existing studies supported usage of hypericum in major depression, according to European Union regulations, in part due to a dearth of data concerning patients with more severe disease.

Perhaps in response to such criticisms, Vorbach and colleagues examined LI 160 at 600 mg tid versus imipramine at 50 mg tid in 209 severely depressed patients, defined by ICD-10 criteria, over a six-week double-blind course (Vorbach, Arnoldt, and Hübner, 1997). Results indicated drops of about 50 percent in HAMD scores in both groups, with no significant differences between groups on von Zerssen Depression Scale, while CGI scores favored imipramine, with a trend of p = 0.079. Of imipramine patients, 41 percent noted adverse effects, compared to 23 percent in the hypericum group. The authors concluded that the use of LI 160 need not be limited to mild to moderate cases of depression, but more severely affected patients could be successfully treated with a dose of 1800 mg of hypericum per day, with fewer side effects than with TCAs.

In 1997, Volz reviewed available clinical studies of hypericum once more. Twelve studies met established criteria. All things considered, it was the author's conclusion that, among hypericum preparations, antidepressant efficacy was established solely for Jarsin 300, a German LI 160 preparation. Volz also stated, "hypericum extracts are not recommended in complicated depressive courses, including therapy resistance, suicidal tendencies, delusions and severe depression" (Volz, 1997, p. 76).

Wheatley (1997) compared LI 160 at 300 mg tid to amitriptyline at 25 mg tid in 165 mild to moderately depressed outpatients, according to DSM-IV criteria, in a double-blind study over the course of six weeks. HAMD scores were significantly improved in both groups, with a slight preference for amitriptyline by the end of the study interval. However, hypericum was significantly better tolerated, with 37 percent adverse events versus 64 percent for the TCA. The author stated, "the major advantage of the phytopharmacon consists in adequate antidepressant efficacy with a favourable side-effect profile . . . Additionally, the absence of sedation or interference with cognitive function renders LI 160 a valuable alternative to tricyclics" (Wheatley, 1997, p. 80).

In a 1997 review, the innately conservative *Medical Letter* was less convinced. Their conclusion, after citing actual review of only four studies, was, "Better, longer studies are needed to establish the effectiveness and safety of St. John's wort for treatment of depression. The active ingredients, the potency and the purity of the preparations sold in the USA are all unknown" (*Medical Letter,* 1997, p. 108). The latter statement is patently false, inasmuch as standardized hypericum preparations with excellent quality control are available even in this underregulated herbal backwater.

Contrast this with the statement of Jerry Cott, an actual researcher in the area, whose experience with the issues is extensive (Cott and Fugh-Berman, 1998, p. 500), "SJW has a significant therapeutic effect on depression and achieves this effect with fewer side effects than tricyclic antidepressants."

A long-awaited "head-to-head" comparison of hypericum to SSRI antidepressants is currently underway in the United States at the time of this writing but is expected to require three years for completion.

Recently, Ernst and colleagues reviewed a large variety of "complementary therapies" in the treatment of depression (Ernst, Rand, and Stevinson, 1998b). The only effective alternative modalities they cited as successful were aerobic activity and hypericum.

The hyperforin issue has been evaluated in 147 mildly to moderately depressed patients, by DSM-IV criteria, in a six-week study by Laakmann and colleagues (1998), employing WS 5572, with 5 percent hyperforin, versus WS 1573, with 0.5 percent hyperforin, versus placebo. Both groups received 300 mg tablets tid, said to be otherwise identical in hypericum component composition. HAMD, von Zerssen Depression Scale, and CGI were assessed. At the end of the treatment period, HAMD scores dropped an average of 10.3 points for the 5 percent hyperforin group, 8.5 points for the 0.5 percent hyperforin group, and 7.9 points for the controls. The latter two were not significantly different, while the WS 5572 was superior ($p = 0.004$). In the high-hyperforin group, 49 percent had 50 percent or greater reductions in HAMD scores, indicative of treatment success. Differences were also apparent for von Zerssen Depression Scale and CGI values. For the latter, 70 percent of the high-hyperforin group rated "much or very much improved," as compared to 55 percent of the low-hyperforin group and 47.9 percent of the placebo group. Interestingly, the incidence of reported side effects, which was low in any event, was lowest in the high-hyperforin treatment group. The authors concluded that (1) WS 5572 was effective in treatment of mild to moderate depression, (2) hyperforin is primarily responsible for the antidepressant effects of SJW, and (3) hyperforin content should be the standard for hypericum preparations, rather than hypericin content. Given the roller-coaster history of this agent, it is unclear to the author that pertinent developments have ceased, or that additional revelations as to hypericum components and their actions are not forthcoming.

In 1997, Upton noted, "The lack of a clearly definable pharmacologic mechanism is not unlike many other psychotherapeutic agents and is therefore not particularly problematic" (p. 25). Some may have issue with this statement. However, given the proven efficacy and safety of hypericum extracts, we are left with an intriguing mystery as to its action, but little debate as to its efficacy or safety, both of which are conclusively established.

The author's personal experience would support the statement that fully 90 percent of clinical treatment failures with hypericum in the United States occur in patients taking nonstandardized preparations in inadequate doses or for insufficient periods of time.

Toxicity and Side Effects

The U.S. Food and Drug Administration (FDA) declared hypericum unsafe in 1980, not due to any documented problems in humans, but rather on the basis of hypericism, a phototoxic reaction in some grazing animals (FDA, 1980).

In 1994, Harrer and Schulz reviewed treatment results in 3,250 patients following use of hypericum extracts in clinical trials (Harrer and Schulz, 1994). Only 2.5 percent had side effects, usually mild. No sedative effects were noted, nor were interactions with alcohol reported. In reviewing the same cohort, Woelk and colleagues noted a total incidence of side effects of 2.43 percent, including gastrointestinal complaints in 0.6 percent, allergies in 0.5 percent, fatigue in 0.4 percent, and agitation in 0.3 percent (Woelk, Burkard, and Grünwald, 1994).

An obscure report in 1981 indicated in vitro uterotonic effects in an animal model (Shiplochliev, 1981), which has led to the recommendation that hypericum be used cautiously in pregnancy. This issue should be revisited, especially in view of recent data supporting the relative safety of SSRI antidepressants in pregnancy.

The presence of hypericism in grazing animals has also led to warnings about possible phototoxicity in humans. Such reactions have been observed at high oral doses (1,800 mg per day), or after parenteral administration in viral studies of hypericin as an antiviral agent (Upton, 1997). Two earlier cases of phototoxicity in humans were noted, one untraceable reference in a person drinking hypericum tea, and another cited in a German article (Golsch et al., 1997). In analyzing data on this issue, Ernst and colleagues "estimated that it would require a dose of hypericum 30-50 times greater than the recommended daily dose taken at one time, to lead to severe phototoxic reactions in humans" (Ernst, Rand, and Stevinson, 1998a, p. 592).

In 1998, Bove reported a single case of hypersensitive feelings and pain in the hands and face, extending to the arms and legs after sun exposure. No pigmentary changes occurred, and no documented neurological deficits were found upon examination. Nevertheless, the author implicated a "subacute toxic neuropathy" attributed to St. John's wort, which resolved spontaneously. The patient had been taking "ground whole St. John's wort (500 mg/day) for mild depression" (Bove, 1998, p. 1121). This association, though interesting, must be considered speculative. The preparation employed was not a standardized extract.

Caution in sun exposure is advisable for patients taking SJW, but little practical danger seems apparent. Unfortunately, the phototoxicity issue continues to be trumpeted in superficial journal review articles (Winslow and Kroll, 1998), along with the baseless warnings of possible tyramine food reactions with hypericum usage.

No studies of human overdose cases are known in the literature.

In 1998, Hippius was able to state, "Overall, for a total of around 3.8 million patients treated during the period 1991 to 1996 with *Hypericum* extract LI 160 (Jarsin®, Jarsin® 300), there have been only 32 spontaneous reports of side effects recorded by the German reporting system" (p. 181).

Ernst and colleagues examined the adverse effects profile of hypericum in detail in a recent review (Ernst, Rand, and Stevinson, 1998a). The authors examined data from the WHO Collaborating Centre for International Drug Monitoring. In twenty years of data, to May 1998, among patients from Sweden, Ireland, Germany, and Bulgaria taking single hypericum preparations, a total of fifty-seven adverse reactions were reported. Among the complaints were: sixteen allergies or skin disorders; fifteen "psychiatric disorders"; five "central and peripheral nervous system disorders"; four respiratory system disorders; four platelet, bleeding, and clotting disorders; four liver and biliary system disorders; two gastrointestinal system disorders; two cases of edema; and one case each of bradycardia, cerebral hemorrhage, interstitial nephritis, "therapeutic response decrement," and conjunctivitis. No analytical data were collected as to other possible etiologies for these complaints.

From 1989 to 1997, the German *Bundesinstitut fur Atzneimittel und Medizinprodukte (BfArM)* (national drug safety body) noted eight reports of possible side effects, but six were from patients taking combination drug products of hypericum in parenteral forms, and all were on more than one medication (Ernst, Rand, and Stevinson, 1998a).

Similarly, in the United Kingdom, by March 1998, the Committee on Safety of Medicines (CSM) received no reports of any hypericum side effects (Ernst, Rand, and Stevinson, 1998a).

The authors considered restriction of tyramine-containing food by hypericum patients to be unnecessary. As to use in pregnancy and lactation, no significant data were available, and they suggested avoidance of hypericum in these conditions (Ernst, Rand, and Stevinson, 1998a).

An interesting feature of the previous spontaneous reports of side effects on hypericum is how rare they seem to be in contrast to studies comparing SJW to conventional antidepressants. Ernst and colleagues attributed this to patient expectation and stated that "this could suggest that some ADRs [adverse drug reactions] reported for hypericum should actually be viewed as nocebo [negative placebo] effects." They concluded that the "risk-benefit profile of hypericum could be considered to be superior to that of conventional antidepressant drugs" (Ernst, Rand, and Stevinson, 1998a, p. 599).

One case of suspected hypericum reaction occurred in a patient who was taking "St. John's wort in powdered form, in a dosage of 600 mg. per day" (Gordon, 1998, p. 950). Subsequently, the patient became "groggy and lethargic" after taking a single dose of 20 mg of paroxetine (Paxil). This was offered as a caveat to such combinations and as warning of toxic interactions.

A "potential metabolic interaction" of SJW with theophylline was recently reported (Nebel et al., 1999, p. 502). A woman taking the latter drug needed a marked increase in dose to maintain an adequate serum level two months after beginning on an SJW supplement, 300 mg daily (qd) that was said to be standardized to 0.3 percent hypericin. Discontinuation of SJW led, in turn, to higher theophylline serum levels. The authors hypothesized that the hypericin induced hepatic enzymes, such as CYP1A2, necessary for theophylline clearance. Given the low dose of the hypericum product employed, and lacking further analysis of its actual content, this author suggests that it is difficult to formulate a broader message from this anecdote.

There were no significant reports of drug interaction concerns with hypericum until very recently. In February 2000, the journal *Lancet* documented two areas of possible concern.

Piscitelli and colleagues (2000) noted that a hypericum preparation administered to eight healthy volunteers reduced the area under the curve of indinavir concentration by a mean of 57 percent. Indinavir is a protease inhibitor drug employed in HIV treatment. The research group obtained the St. John's wort from the Hypericum Buyers Club of Los Angeles. It was purportedly standardized to 0.3 percent hypericin. No additional assay was performed on it. The authors posited that this hypericum preparation affected indinavir by induction of the cytochrome P450 (CYP) enzyme system. Since protease inhibitors are substrates for part of that system, it was stated (p. 547), "induction by St. John's wort might have serious clinical implications." They added that the risk of antiretroviral resistance and treatment failure dictated that all patients on protease inhibitors should avoid hypericum treatment. Although this study was experimental, and no corresponding clinical reports of protease inhibitor treatment problems have been reported with standardized hypericum preparations, this caution is worth noting until additional data are available.

Ruschitzka and colleagues (2000) presented a second report of hypericum-drug interactions. They described symptoms or laboratory data in two cardiac transplant patients receiving cyclosporine (immunosuppressive therapy) supporting the development of acute rejection soon after beginning treatment with LI 160 hypericum, 300 mg tid. Both episodes of rejection were successfully abrogated, and no additional problems were noted after discontinuation of hypericum. The close temporal relationship was believed suggestive of hypericum as the cause of the episodes and thought to be a potential risk in transplant patients. Once again, induction of the cytochrome P450 complex was cited as the culprit.

However, what was not noted are observations of important kinetic interactions with other common drugs, or even food and drink. As observed by Brynne and colleagues (1999), fluoxetine (Prozac) and grapefruit juice (Jobst et al., 2000) potently *inhibit* cytochrome P450. These effects could *increase* serum levels of cyclosporine and indinavir.

At the current time, cautions do appear to be well advised with respect to hypericum use by transplant patients on cyclosporine and HIV patients on protease inhibitors. Only additional research will elucidate the degree of risk from hypericum and its context in relation to other drugs and dietary influences.

Cost

Monthly costs for SJW as LI 160 average $15 to $30 in the United States, whereas TCAs cost $10 as generics, $30 to $90 as brand names, and SSRIs are about $60 to $70 (*Medical Letter,* 1999a).

Panel and Regulatory Information

The European Scientific Cooperative on Phytotherapy, ESCOP, has recommended hypericum as standardized preparations in the treatment of mild to moderate depression (ESCOP, 1997). A discontinuation of treatment after four to six weeks was recommended in the absence of clinical response. No negative effects on ability to drive or perform on the job were noted.

The Commission E revised its original monograph on hypericum in 1990. In addition to external uses of hypericum oil in a variety of indications, internal use was approved for "psychovegetative disturbances, depressive moods, anxiety and/or nervous unrest" (Blumenthal et al., 1998, pp. 214-215). No contraindications or drug interactions were cited. See Table 4.1 for a summary of hypericum-related information.

5-HYDROXYTRYPTOPHAN:
Griffonia simplicifolia (Vahl ex DC.) Baill.
Fabaceae (Caesalpiniaceae)

Synonyms

- *Bandeiraea simplicifolia* Benth.
- 5-HTP
- 5-hydroxy-l-tryptophan
- 5-OH-Trp
- Oxitriptan

TABLE 4.1. St. John's Wort Summary

What it is:

Hypericum or SJW is an extract of the aerial tops, buds, and flowers of the *Hypericum perforatum* herb.

What it does:

Hypericum, when taken in a standardized extract, 300 mg tid, successfully treats mild to moderate depression in 60 to 70 percent of patients, with fewer side effects than synthetic antidepressants. Preliminary evidence supports doses of 600 mg tid in treatment of severe depression.

What it does not do:

Hypericum cannot change a person's life in isolation and does not replace lifestyle adjustments such as maintenance of aerobic fitness or counseling as helpful modalities in the holistic treatment of depression.

What to look for:

The author recommends preparations standardized to 0.3 percent hypericin content at the aforementioned dosage, corresponding to the LI 160 extract. Another standardized extract, WS 5572, with 5 percent hyperforin content, may also be clinically effective. New standardization schemes may be recommended in the near future.

Cautions:

Until additional studies are undertaken, hypericum should be used with caution, if at all, in women who are pregnant or breast-feeding. People taking hypericum should be careful of ultraviolet (UV) light exposure, particularly if fair-skinned or on higher dosage regimens.

HIV/AIDS patients on protease inhibitor drugs and transplant patients on cyclosporine should consult their physicians before using hypericum.

Recommendations:

Hypericum is a safe and effective herbal alternative in the treatment of depression when taken at 300 to 600 mg tid of a standardized extract corresponding to LI 160 and, perhaps, WS 5572.

Botany

Griffonia simplicifolia is the botanical source of the phytopharmaceutical (but not, strictly speaking, botanical product), 5-hydroxytryptophan, or 5-HTP.

Griffonia simplicifolia is a leguminous tree found on West African savannas and coastal plains, but it also may be found as a liana (woody vine) in secondary forests (Dwuma-Badu et al., 1976) from Liberia to Gabon (Irvine, 1961).

Ethnobotanical information on the species reveals that the leaf is used for diarrhea, as a purgative, as an aphrodisiac, and to kill lice in henhouses. Furthermore, the stems and twigs are variously employed to treat soft chancre, vomiting and diarrhea, and as an aphrodisiac (Ayensu, 1978; Irvine, 1961; Iwu, 1986).

Phytochemistry

Bell and Fellows (1966) showed that *Griffonia simplicifolia* contained free 5-hydroxytryptophan in its seed. The amino acid had previously been identified in bacteria and tissue slices of watermelon, but in much smaller amounts.

Subsequently, quantitative assays demonstrated a yield of 5-HTP of some 6 to 10 percent fresh weight in the mature seed (Fellows and Bell, 1970), where it was the only remaining indole. Levels of tryptophan hydroxylase in *Griffonia* varied seasonally. Seedpods also contained 5-HTP, along with serotonin, but in concentrations of 0.1 to 0.2 percent dry weight. The authors indicated that this species is the only one known in which 5-HTP represents the principal metabolic end product.

In addition to 5-HTP, *Griffonia simplicifolia* yields indole derivatives such as indole-3-acetylaspartic acid, 5-hydroxy indole-3-acetic acid, the glucoside griffonin, and an algycone, griffolide (Dwuma-Badu et al., 1976).

The pertinent chemistry here revolves around 5-HTP itself. The commercial product is designed to be a pure isolate of that compound.

History of Use

Therapeutic use of 5-HTP is a relatively recent event. This agent has been studied in Europe for about three decades, but has been widely available in the United States only since 1998.

In the late 1980s, another serotonin precursor, L-tryptophan, was a popular supplement in the treatment of depression, anxiety, and insomnia. In 1990, a minor epidemic of a serious, and sometimes fatal, disorder called eosinophilia-myalgia syndrome developed in some L-tryptophan patients. Virtually all cases were subsequently attributed to a contaminant in a product produced by one manufacturer, Showa Denko of Japan. However, the FDA chose to ban all

L-tryptophan products as a result of this event, and they remain available only by physician prescription, or for veterinary use.

The use of 5-HTP differs from other agents in this book, in that its metabolic effects are quite well known. Its intake increases the levels of the cerebral neurotransmitter serotonin, or 5-hydroxytryptamine. The natural pathway is quite simple: dietary tryptophan → 5-hydroxytryptophan (5-HTP) → 5-hydroxytryptamine (serotonin). Dietary tryptophan is not converted solely to 5-HTP and may be diverted to other uses. Its absorption from the gastrointestinal (GI) tract is limited, and it is subject to hepatic metabolism (Byerley et al., 1987). It must also compete for transport across the blood brain barrier with other amino acids. In contrast, 70 percent of 5-HTP is absorbed from the gut (Birdsall, 1998). 5-HTP is only one metabolic step from serotonin and thus, is more likely to boost levels of that neurotransmitter. At higher doses, 5-HTP is also taken up by noradrenergic and dopaminergic neurons, possibly modulating their activity (Byerley et al., 1987). One commercial producer of 5-HTP claims that it is 50 times more potent in its clinical application than equivalent doses of tryptophan.

Preparation of Extracts

5-HTP is isolated from seeds of *Griffonia simplicifolia*.

Studies in Clinical Disease

The various clinical applications of 5-HTP, including treatment of depression, anxiety, insomnia, and migraine, have been nicely summarized in an inexpensive booklet (Morgenthaler and Lenard, 1998).

Byerley and colleagues (1987) reviewed earlier studies of 5-HTP in depression in detail, and examination of their findings provides a suitable point of departure. An aggregate of clinical studies revealed that 59 percent of 251 patients treated with 5-HTP had favorable responses over three to four weeks. They identified seven double-blind controlled studies of six or more weeks' duration that supported antidepressant efficacy. Some prior studies employed simultaneous administration of carbidopa (a prescription pharmaceutical that antagonizes the peripheral decarboxylation of 5-HTP). Most modern studies do not perpetuate this practice.

Kahn and colleagues (1987), in the Netherlands, compared the effectiveness of 5-HTP with carbidopa in doses up to 150 mg qd versus placebo and clomipramine at 150 mg (a TCA antidepressant) in double-blind fashion in treatment of forty-five patients with DSM-III-defined anxiety over eight weeks. Hamilton anxiety and depression scales were combined with a present-state examination (PSE) and a ninety-item symptom checklist (SCL) to assess efficacy. At treatment end, PSE measures improved with clomipramine ($p < 0.05$), with little baseline change observed for placebo and 5-HTP ($p < 0.05$). Some specific subtest measures were improved by 5-HTP. Furthermore, state anxiety levels, as measured by the Spielberger State-Trait Anxiety Scale Inventory, were improved with clomipramine and 5-HTP over placebo ($p < 0.01$). Overall, eleven of fifteen clomipramine patients, five of fifteen 5-HTP patients, and one of fifteen placebo patients demonstrated drops of 50 percent in the HAMA. It was noted that the improved patients were almost totally relieved of panic symptoms. Overall, the examiners rated the results of the drugs on anxiety as highly effective for clomipramine and moderately effective for 5-HTP. The latter had no significant effect on depression symptoms in this trial.

In a French review of various 5-HTP indications (Uldry and Regli, 1987), the authors noted that 5-HTP restored sleep-wake cycles in patients with insomnia, with prolongation of REM (rapid eye movement) sleep or dreaming, without effects on slow-wave sleep.

In a German study (van Praag and Kahn, 1988), the authors recommended that treatment of anxiety or depression with 5-HTP should commence with doses of 25 mg qd and be raised incrementally over two weeks to 200 mg qd or more. Therapeutic effects were to be expected in five to twenty days.

Pöldinger and colleagues compared the effects of 5-HTP at 100 mg with fluvoxamine (an SSRI) at 50 mg a day in a double-blind, double-dummy study over six weeks in sixty-nine patients with the Hamilton Rating Scale for Depression and a self-assessment scale (Pöldinger, Calanchini, and Schwarz, 1991). By treatment end, reductions in the Hamilton scale were essentially equivalent in the two groups, demonstrating equal efficacy and high significance ($p < 0.0001$). Seasonal affective disorder (SAD) scores were similarly improved on each regimen ($p < 0.0001$). The number of treatment failures was 17.2 percent for fluvoxamine and 5.9 percent for 5-HTP. Side effects were similar in the two groups with respect to the types of complaints, but when severity factors were examined, 5-HTP patients had primarily mild effects, with fluvoxamine producing moderate to severe complaints (p < 0.001). Overall, 94.5 percent rated tolerability of 5-HTP as good to very good, versus 84.8 percent for fluvoxamine. The authors assessed the two agents as equally efficacious, but with greater tolerability and safety for 5-HTP. A therapeutic response in depressed patients that responded to treatment was seen in four to seven days for fluvoxamine and three to five days for 5-HTP.

In conclusion, the authors had a strong statement to make (Pöldinger, Calanchini, and Schwarz, 1991, p. 68):

> With all due deference to scientific scepticism, the reluctance shown by some authors of recent textbooks on the subject and by others to concede 5-HTP its place among acknowledged pharmacotherapeutics routinely applied against depression does not seem warranted.

They added, "the outcome of the present trial should warrant 5-HTP being admitted to the core group of routinely applied antidepressive drugs," and "the physiological nature of this serotonin precursor may afford a certain psychological advantage over non-physiological compounds" (Pöldinger, Calanchini, and Schwarz, 1991, p. 76).

To date, SSRIs, such as fluvoxamine, have not been compared head to head in published studies with other botanical agents in treatment of depression and anxiety.

Toxicity and Side Effects

In their extensive review, Byerley and colleagues (1987) noted the most common side effects of 5-HTP to be gastrointestinal complaints such as cramping, nausea, and diarrhea. Most are self-limited and brief. Some manufacturers provide enteric coating to reduce this risk. Less frequently, treated patients may complain of palpitations, insomnia, or headache. Mania or hypomania has also been reported.

The force of current events requires the inclusion of another alleged danger of 5-HTP, although the author finds it far from convincing. In 1998, Mayo Clinic researchers claimed to have identified a "Peak X" (6-hydroxy-1,2,3,4,4a,9a-hexahydro-beta-carboline-3-carboxylic acid) on an HPLC (high-performance liquid chromatography) plate of samples of 5-HTP, which they relate to two prior cases of eosinophilia-myalgia syndrome (EMS) occurring in 1980 and 1991 (Williamson et al., 1998). In truth, the association of EMS with 5-HTP in those cases was never conclusively established. In addition, the relative amount of Peak X in six commercial samples was only 2.9 to 14.1 percent of that in the "case-implicated" 5-HTP. Despite this poorly proven link, the authors chose to beat a drum of paranoia with respect to 5-HTP and the natural products market, in general.

Rather, this author recommends that concerned consumers query the manufacturer of their prospective 5-HTP supplement as to whether it contains Peak X. Reputable companies will gladly answer the question and hopefully allay undue fears of the ravages of EMS.

The author believes that cautious optimism should apply to use of 5-HTP, particularly for depression. For those inclined toward natural medicine, its choice will have certain appeal.

Cost

In the United States, the novelty of this agent has led to elevated price structures. One manufacturer sells 100 5-HTP 50 mg units for $25 at wholesale. Thus, for higher dosages, this agent is currently (unnecessarily) expensive.

Panel and Regulatory Information

None is available.

LICORICE:
Glycyrrhiza glabra L. Fabaceae

Dr. James Duke (1997) has posited an antidepressant effect for licorice based on its content of eight monoamine oxidase inhibitory compounds. There is no traditional ethnobotanical usage of licorice in this manner, and no clinical data are available. Long-term use of licorice may produce mineralocorticoid stimulation, producing water and sodium retention, hypertension, edema, and other changes (Blumenthal et al., 1998).

ESSENTIAL FATTY ACIDS (EFAs)

The author would like to introduce this entry with three separate threads of information. Although this may result in a prolonged digression from the topic of psychotropic herbs, the convergence, and hopefully the integration, of these concepts provides a likely explanation and possible solution to one of the great mysteries of modern medicine—why is depression so prevalent in modern society?

Robert Burton's Anatomy of Melancholy

In 1621, the life's work of scholar Robert Burton, *The Anatomy of Melancholy,* was printed (Burton, 1907). Its subject was depression, seemingly one without mass appeal, before our modern age of rampant mental illness and self-absorption (and resultant self-help guides). Despite that, Samuel Johnson, author of *A Dictionary of the English Language* (1755), called it a "valuable book" of "great spirit and great power." According to Johnson's biographer (Boswell, 1960, p. 389), "Burton's *Anatomy of Melancholy,* he said, was the only book that ever took him out of bed two hours sooner than he wished to rise."

Burton's (1907) treatise examined the subject of depression exhaustively and suggested legion cures. Paramount among them were herbs, such as cannabis (see Chapter 9) and specific foods. He suggested a diet rich in brains as one cure for depression, but also servings of fish and borage:

> In this catalogue, borage and bugloss [another boraginaceous plant] may challenge the chiefest place, whether in substance, juice, root, seeds, flowers, leaves, decoctions, distilled waters, extracts, oils, &c., for such kind of herbs be diversely varied. (p. 565)

Shortly before this, in 1597, Gerard had also endorsed the herb as worthy (Gerard, 1931, p. 166):

> Borage is called in shops *Borago: Pliny* calleth it *Euphrosinum,* because it makes a man merry and joyfull: which thing also the old verse concerning Borage doth testifie:
>
> > *Ego Borago gaudia semper ago.*
> > I Borage bring alwaies courage.
>
> Those of our time do use the floures in sallads, to exhilerate and make the minde glad. There be also many things made of them, used for the comfort of the heart, to drive away sorrow, & increase the joy of the minde.
>
> The leaves and floures of Borrage put into wine make men and women glad and merry, driving away all sadnesse, dulnesse, and melancholy.
>
> Syrrup made of the floures of Borrage comforteth the heart, purgeth melancholy, and quieteth the phrenticke or lunaticke person.

Culpeper (1994, p. 57) also endorsed borage and bugloss as "great strengtheners of nature." He stated of borage, "The leaves, flowers, and seed, all or any of them, are good to expel pensiveness and melancholy."

Grieve added additional endorsements (Grieve, 1971), attributing to borage the "absolute forgetfulness" of Nepenthe. John Evelyn noted, at the end of the seventeenth century, "Sprigs of Borage are of known virtue to revive the hypochrondriac [sic] and cheer the hard student" (cited in Grieve, 1971, p. 120). Bacon indicated that it "hath an excellent spirit to repress the fuliginous vapour of dusky melancholie" (cited in Grieve, 1971, p. 120).

What is the secret then of this almost forgotten herb, so precious to our forebears?

The Changing Incidence of Depression

In 1930, near the end of his career, Sigmund Freud wrote a disparaging tome titled *Civilization and Its Discontents* (Freud,

1930), in which he expounded on the deterioration he had observed in the mental health of society over two generations. He placed the bulk of the blame on the demands of modern life, its preoccupation with technology, and similar factors.

Although the etiology of depression in modern times may prove otherwise, Freud was certainly correct about its increasing incidence and prevalence. Modern research has confirmed the trend in a striking fashion.

Klerman and Weissman (1989) reviewed a variety of epidemiological studies and demonstrated an increased prevalence of depression in children and young adults, along with greater rates of alcoholism, other drug abuse, and suicide attempts and completions. Average age of incidence of depression has declined in this century, while the incidence has progressively risen. Using one point on a curve of graphed data, the cumulative probability of developing an affective disorder for a thirty-year-old was calculated as about 4 percent for a person born before 1915, but 40 percent for those born between 1945 and 1955, a tenfold difference. The authors examined a multitude of factors that might explain an ascertainment bias: differential mortality or institutionalization, selective migration, changing diagnostic criteria, changes in attitude of physicians and psychologists, liberalization in societal opinions on depression, reporting bias, and memory problems in older patients. All of these were subsequently rejected as accounting for the rise in the prevalence of depression. In addition, they posited eight environmental factors that might contribute to the trend, but it now seems likely that none of these are etiologically linked.

This study was subsequently expanded to examine a worldwide population by the Cross-National Collaborative Group (1992). The results were similarly compelling. An increase in cumulative lifetime rates of major depression was seen in successive generations in the twentieth century in every country examined.

The Paleolithic Diet

Eaton and his colleagues have examined in detailed fashion the manner in which early humans lived, in a book titled *The Paleolithic Prescription* (Eaton, Shostak, and Konner, 1988), and in a series of articles with similar themes (Eaton 1990; Eaton, Eaton, and Konner,

1997; Eaton et al., 1998; Eaton and Konner, 1985). In essence, our forebears were an extremely aerobically active bunch of hunter-gatherers whose diet bore little resemblance to that of modern humans, with our reliance on complex carbohydrates, sugar, and saturated and hydrogenated fats. Rather, ancient humans ate game meat in large quantities, along with a wide variety of seeds, nuts, and berries. At a certain point, the skills of fishing were acquired, and, seasonally, huge stores of salmon, herring, and other anadromous fish were collected. Fossil records indicate that, although our forebears suffered the ravages of infectious disease, they were as tall as modern humans. They had thick, healthy bones, lacked dental caries, and seemed to be in top-notch general condition. The modern scourges of arteriosclerosis, hypertension, diabetes, and many cancers remain rare in such populations, as they were in industrialized Western cultures before the last century. Based on surveys of contemporary vestiges of hunter-gatherer cultures pursuing similar lifestyles, their mental health was probably excellent as well.

Although culinary mores and nutritional content have changed over the ages, our genetic attributes have not. One may postulate that our genes today reflect the same basic design for living as those of our Paleolithic ancestors, including our dietary requirements. For them, caloric intake was about equally divided between plant and game sources. Their meat was five times richer in polyunsaturated fat than modern supplies, especially in eicosapentanoic and docosahexanoic acids, which are essentially absent in contemporary beef supplies (Eaton and Konner, 1985). Before the agricultural revolution, grains and starch were scarce commodities, and vegetables in the Paleolithic diet were relatively richer in protein and, especially, polyunsaturated fatty acids (PUFAs).

The balance of those fatty acids has also changed remarkably. The PUFAs are named by their chain length in carbon atoms, the number and location of their double bonds, and the distance of the bonds from the terminal methyl group. Thus, arachidonic acid is labeled C20:4n-6 because it has twenty carbon atoms and four double bonds, with the last of those being six carbon atoms away from the methyl group. Two major divisions of PUFAs are recognized, the n-3 and n-6, or omega-3 and omega-6, fatty acids. Their metabolic pathways are outlined in Figure 4.1.

FIGURE 4.1. Central Fatty Pathways

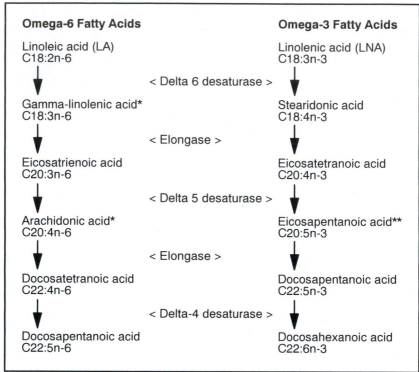

Omega-6 Fatty Acids		Omega-3 Fatty Acids
Linoleic acid (LA) C18:2n-6		Linolenic acid (LNA) C18:3n-3
	< Delta 6 desaturase >	
Gamma-linolenic acid* C18:3n-6		Stearidonic acid C18:4n-3
	< Elongase >	
Eicosatrienoic acid C20:3n-6		Eicosatetranoic acid C20:4n-3
	< Delta 5 desaturase >	
Arachidonic acid* C20:4n-6		Eicosapentanoic acid** C20:5n-3
	< Elongase >	
Docosatetranoic acid C22:4n-6		Docosapentanoic acid C22:5n-3
	< Delta-4 desaturase >	
Docosapentanoic acid C22:5n-6		Docosahexanoic acid C22:6n-3

Source: Modified and adapted from Borkman et al., 1993, p. 240.

*AA → Inflammatory eicosanoids. Platelet aggregation increased.
**GLA/EPA → Anti-inflammatory eicosanoids. Platelet aggregation decreased.

Linoleic acid (LA), and linolenic acid (LNA) (sometimes labeled alpha-linolenic acid [ALA]) are *essential fatty acids* because humans are not able to synthesize them from other precursors.

Arachidonic acid (AA) and eicosapentanoic acid (EPA) in cellular membranes are substrates for conversion via lipooxygenase (LO) and cyclooxygenase to form eicosanoids. These include leukotrienes, prostaglandins, and thromboxane, which possess crucial physiological effects. Eicosanoids from AA are stimulators of inflammation and platelet aggregation, while those from EPA have anti-inflammatory and platelet inhibitory effects (Mantzioris et al., 1995). It is widely held that modern humans exhibit far too much inflammatory tendency and require stimulation of the alternative pathways.

Synaptic membranes are composed of up to 45 percent EFAs, especially arachidonic acid and docosahexanoic acid (DHA). Mammals are incapable of interconverting n-3 and n-6 series fatty acids (Hibbeln and Salem, 1995).

Whereas the modern diet with its reliance on corn and peanut oil provides a balance of n-6 to n-3 PUFAs of some 50:1 in some individuals, estimates are that the Paleolithic diet yielded a ratio much lower, even approximating 1:1. Our current dietary status certainly seems to be out of synch with our nutritional history and, likely, is highly incompatible with our genetic requirements.

EFAs: A Review of Studies of Pertinence to Their Role in Human Mood

Mantzioris and colleagues (1994) demonstrated experimentally that flaxseed (linseed) oil, the richest known source of the n-3 EFA linoleic acid, when added to the diet, increased levels of eicosapentanoic acid significantly. This result is important because, although EPA is a component of fish and game meats, it is not present in vegetable matter. EPA promotes formation of anti-inflammatory prostaglandins, while inhibiting AA formation and subsequent inflammatory prostaglandin E-2 synthesis (Wagner and Nootbaar-Wagner, 1997) (see Figure 4.1).

Smith (1991) advanced a theory that excessive secretion of monokines by macrophages is a, or the, cause of human depression. This might explain the association of depression with coronary disease, rheumatoid arthritis, and other diseases. It was posited that the low incidence of depression in Japan relates to suppressive effects on macrophages of EPA in the fish-rich diet of that country.

Schubert and Foliart (1993) demonstrated an increased morbidity of depression in multiple sclerosis patients that cannot be accounted for by their disease burden, as compared to that associated with other chronic degenerative neurological conditions.

Insulin resistance has been offered as an explanation for treatment-resistant obesity, depression, and other disorders. Borkman and colleagues (1993) demonstrated that insulin sensitivity was associated with concentrations of PUFAs in muscle phospholipids.

Increased dietary intake of n-3 fatty acids increased membrane fluidity and number of insulin receptors. These actions might modulate insulin activity with resultant importance with respect to depression, due to effects on glucose metabolism.

Docosahexanoic acid is widely acknowledged as being essential to proper development of the retina and brain, where it is a key component of neuronal membranes. When DHA is unavailable in deficiency states, it is replaced by n-3 components (Hibbeln and Salem, 1995).

DHA is found, once again, in generous amounts in fish and game, and in eggs to a modest degree (Sanders and Reddy, 1994). It can be generated by humans de novo from linolenic acid (LNA) but is competitively inhibited by linoleic acid (LA), as the two compete for enzyme systems (see Figure 4.1) (Sanders and Reddy, 1994). The authors recommended that vegetarians preferentially employ soy or canola (rapeseed) oil in their diets in place of corn, sunflower, or safflower oil to lower ratios of LA to LNA intake.

Mantzioris and colleagues (1995) confirmed experimentally that vegans, vegetarians who strictly eschew animal and fish products, could increase EPA and DHA content in their bodies with flaxseed supplementation, especially if LA intake was limited.

In healthy adults, the efficiency of conversion of LNA to DHA is estimated at about 5 percent (Conquer and Holub, 1996). Strict vegans who wish to supplement their DHA intake may do so with commercially available algal sources. However, this is a very expensive proposition, some $50 for a month's supply of a commercial preparation providing 1,500 mg of DHA per day.

Hansen (1994) indicated that the endogenous cannabinoid anandamide (arachidonylethanolamide) may be synthesized from n-3 fatty acid precursors, especially AA. Anandamide is a neuromodulator with presumed activity on anxiety, memory, and pain mechanisms in the CNS (see Chapter 9). It was recently demonstrated that anandamide and tetrahydrocannabinol (THC) inhibit tumor necrosis factor (TNF), a mediator of inflammation (Cabral et al., 1995). Caughey and colleagues (1996) were able to demonstrate that flaxseed oil supplementation also inhibited TNF.

Salem and Niebylski (1995) have hypothesized that phospholipids such as phosphatidylserine must contain DHA for optimal

CNS function, and that AA and other n-6 fatty acids do not adequately substitute for that component in their synthesis.

Stevens and colleagues (1995) demonstrated a significantly lower complement of AA, EPA, and DHA in plasma and blood cell lipids in fifty-three boys with attention-deficit hyperactivity disorder (ADHD) compared to normal controls. The following year, the same team demonstrated a greater incidence of behavioral problems on Conner's rating scales in boys with lower total n-3 fatty acid concentrations (Stevens et al., 1996). These studies certainly point out a putative nutritional factor in ADHD, and possible therapeutic approaches worthy of consideration on an individual case basis.

Hibbeln and Salem (1995) reviewed the subject of PUFAs and depression in detail, noting many salient features. As mentioned, inadequate n-3 fatty acid intake has been implicated as etiologic for both coronary disease and depression. It follows that the two might be comorbid conditions. In fact, this is the case, and to a remarkable degree ($p < 0.0000001$).

Alcoholism and depression are similarly comorbid: 58 percent of alcoholics are depressed, whereas only 32 percent of opiate addicts and 28 percent of schizophrenics are so affected (Hibbeln and Salem, 1995). The authors noted an effect of alcohol on promotion of lipid peroxidation of DHA, with resultant depletion of neuronal cell membranes of n-3 fatty acids. Fish oil supplementation was suggested to stimulate recovery. Spontaneous improvement in the depressive symptoms of alcoholics is frequently observed about four to six weeks after they become abstinent. Certainly, improved nutrition has an important role in recovery.

Returning to the issue of multiple sclerosis (MS), the authors cited the finding of depletions of AA and DHA in brain areas unaffected by demyelinating plaques of that disorder. Supplementation with oils from fish, evening primrose, black currant, and borage seed have all been reported to have modest beneficial effects on relapses in MS, with more demonstrable benefit in subjective measures of well-being (Hibbeln and Salem, 1995).

Pregnancy, especially multiple pregnancies, may lead to a depletion of maternal DHA, which is shunted to the developing fetus.

This provides a compelling explanation for postpartum depression (Hibbeln and Salem, 1995).

The authors also posited a role of EFAs of CNS membranes in a variety of neurotransmitter functions, especially serotonin and nora-drenergic systems, exemplified by their greater concentration in animals supplemented with DHA-rich phosphatidylserine (from brain), compared to those receiving DHA-poor supplements (from soybean) (Hibbeln and Salem, 1995).

Experimental evidence from rats suggests that prolonged stress inhibits activity of delta-5 and delta-6 desaturase enzymes neces-sary for conversion of LNA to DHA (Hibbeln and Salem, 1995). This supports a chemical explanation for the clinical observation of persistent depression in humans following stressful events.

Mahadik and colleagues (1996) demonstrated depressed levels of delta-4 desaturase activity in fibroblasts from schizophrenic pa-tients, even in initial psychotic episodes. Fibroblasts are effective mirrors of many CNS biochemical functions, and this result pro-vides an intriguing insight into the possible role of DHA deficiency in the pathophysiology of schizophrenia.

Adams and colleagues (1996) examined the correlation between phospholipid levels of n-3 and n-6 in plasma and red blood cells of twenty moderately to severely depressed patients. A significant association was seen between erythrocyte AA to EPA ratios and severity of depression, as measured by the Hamilton depression scale ($p < 0.05$) and a linear rating scale ($p < 0.01$). On this basis, the authors suggested clinical trials of nutritional approaches that would lower the AA:EPA ratio.

In a similar vein, Maes and colleagues (1996) examined AA:EPA ratios, finding these elevated in fifty depressed patients as compared to twenty-four control subjects ($p = 0.0018$).

Hamazaki and colleagues (1996) in Japan used DHA supple-mentation for three months to assess its effects on aggressive ten-dencies of students facing the stresses of final examinations. Whereas "extraggression" increased in the control group under stress ($p = 0.018$), measures were unchanged in the DHA subjects, whose DHA concentrations doubled during the trial.

Hibbeln and colleagues (1997) addressed an unintended conse-quence of some cholesterol-lowering drugs: they alter PUFA levels and may actually increase depressive symptoms. They also examined DHA as a treatment for depression and hostility. Forty-five healthy subjects had cerebrospinal fluid (CSF) levels of 5-hydroxy-indole acetic acid (5-HIAA) (a serotonin metabolite) and homovanillic acid (HVA) (a norepinephrine metabolite) measured in relation to total PUFAs in blood samples. PUFA levels predicted CSF 5-HIAA ($p < 0.005$) and CSF HVA levels ($p < 0.001$).

In the event that the previous evidence of a correlation between EPA and DHA and depression is not sufficiently compelling or etiological, Hibbeln (1998) provided a graphic representation of how incidence of the disorder varies some sixtyfold across countries. Thus, a prevalence of depression of 0.12 percent is seen in Japan, where annual fish consumption is about 70 kilograms (kg) per capita, versus the situation in New Zealand, where depression affects 5.8 percent of the populace, who average, per capita, only about 20 kg of fish consumption annually.

Edwards and colleagues (1998) examined n-3 levels of ten DSM-IV-depressed patients on antidepressant medication versus fourteen normal controls. The n-6 levels showed no correlation to depression, but DHA levels were lower in depressed patients ($p < 0.02$). Red blood cell (RBC) (erythrocyte) membrane levels of LNA in the depressed patients were a predictor for Beck Depression Inventory (BDI) scores ($p = 0.008$). Correlations were noted in dietary content of n-3 fatty acids: depression was less severe in those with higher n-3 intake. In addition, in depressed subjects, LNA intake significantly correlated with tissue EPA and DHA measures. This implied that no metabolic derangements were present in depressed subjects, and that supplementation of n-3 or EPA or DHA may be valuable in the treatment of depression.

Peet and colleagues (1998) also examined RBC membrane levels of depressed patients, and demonstrated depletion, compared to controls, of n-3 ($p = 0.02$) and DHA ($p = 0.009$). In addition, oleic acid (18:1n9), a monosaturated fatty acid, was increased in depressed patients ($p = 0.001$). Interestingly, this study demonstrated that antidepressant treatment, which was usually disallowed in other experiments, did not serve to alter observed metabolic deficiencies of n-3 fatty acids in depressed patients. Furthermore, an increase was observed in oxidative damage to RBC membranes in depressed subjects, suggesting abnormal defense mechanisms. Once more, membrane fluidity was cited as a key factor in serotonin transport of neurons.

Hibbeln and colleagues (1998) examined CSF neurotransmitter metabolites versus plasma DHA in controls and violent, impulsive subjects. The violent group had significantly lower concentrations of CSF 5-HIAA. Again, low DHA levels correlated with decreased 5-HIAA values (p < 0.005). The authors suggested a treatment role for DHA in impulsive, violent patients.

Practical Considerations

It is clear from the previous discussion that a compelling argument can be made that modern diets are deficient in n-3 PUFAs. It is certainly arguable that this is *the reason* for the explosive incidence of depression in modern cultures. Certainly, an increase in fish intake would be advisable, particularly if coupled with reductions of n-6 intake. The FAO (Food and Agriculture Organization)/WHO Expert Consultation on Fats and Oils in Human Nutrition in 1994 recommended an n-6:n-3 ratio of 6:1 to 4:1 (Galli and Marangoni, 1997). This certainly represents an improvement upon current societal norms, but other authorities would recommend a ratio of 3:1 (Erasmus, 1993), while the Paleolithic norm might even be 1:1.

Unfortunately, fish stocks around the world are already depleted, through a combination of overfishing, wasteful netting techniques, and industrial pollution. Aquaculture may represent a partial solution, although environmental concerns remain apparent in that industry. Few modern people will rely on game meat to supply their missing n-3 fatty acids, but buffalo ranching could be a viable alternative, as long as grazing is the norm, and not grain supplementation in feedlots.

More germane to this volume would be the issue of whether an herbal nutritional solution to depression treatment is possible. We know that flaxseed contains about 58 percent LNA, and at a conversion rate to DHA of 5 percent in healthy individuals, 15 grams (g) of daily intake would provide a net of 435 mg of DHA. The experiments cited earlier employed dosages of DHA from 1,000 to 1,600 mg, with effective increases seen in tissue measures in three weeks. It is certainly possible that these lower levels of LNA intake would lead to significant elevation of tissue DHA levels over time, and amelioration of depression.

Flaxseed oil is extremely perishable once it is pressed and is considered unpalatable by many (Conrad, 1997; Wirtshafter, 1997). Cognoscenti of flaxseed supplementation frequently recommend that the fresh seed be ground before each use, or the purchased flaxseed oil be kept frozen.

Other alternatives exist. Hemp seeds have been human fodder since ancient times and were one of the seven basic grains of the early Chinese culture (Li, 1974). Hemp seed represents the single most complete food on the planet, with its 35 percent content of highly digestible protein and 35 percent oil content. The latter is the most highly unsaturated of the world's known vegetable oils, and almost exactly fits the 3:1 ratio of n-6:n-3 fatty acids. Up to 25 percent of hemp oil is LNA, and up to 9 percent is GLA, which has also been advocated in treatment of inflammatory conditions (rheumatoid arthritis, MS). Gamma-linolenic acid (GLA) inhibits formation of pro-inflammatory compounds from AA (Wagner and Nootbaar-Wagner, 1997).

Compared to flax, hemp seed and its oil are quite palatable, and 100 g of hemp seeds provides 8,750 mg of LNA, which might provide 435 mg of DHA. Similarly, 15 g of hemp seed oil might lead to 188 mg of accumulated DHA.

Hemp seeds are illegal in many countries, although THC content is negligible. Some cases of positive drug tests for THC metabolites have occurred in individuals eating the seeds (Callaway et al., 1997). On this basis, some have called for prohibition of hemp seeds in the United States, where importation of sterilized hemp seed is still legal. Sterilization prevents seed sprouting, which not only disallows the possibility of hemp cultivation but also the provision of an additional beneficial protein and EFA source.

For the more politically cautious, pumpkin seed may represent an alternative to hemp seed nutrition. Oil content is 50 percent, with high vitamin E content (Murkovic et al., 1996). 15 percent of the oil is LNA, with about 42 percent LA. As an added bonus, pumpkin seed is a rich source of magnesium, a mineral that is a cofactor in the enzymatic pathways leading to serotonin synthesis, and a substance of purported antidepressant activity in its own right. Similarly, pumpkin seed is rich in tryptophan, and this was advanced as a primary factor in a case study in which depression was successfully treated with pumpkin seed supplementation (Eagles, 1990).

Ultimately, we return to borage. Its seed oil is the richest known source of GLA, some 19 percent. Since GLA inhibits conversion of AA to proinflammatory substances, it may support hypothetical claims of efficacy in nutritional prophylaxis of depression. Although legitimate safety concerns have been raised due to the presence of hepatotoxic pyrrolizidine alkaloids in fresh borage seed (Foster and Tyler, 1999), these have not been detected in most commercial sources of borage seed oil supplements. Appropriately wary customers may inquire of their supplements' manufacturer in this regard, and they should receive a reassuring response or look elsewhere.

Perhaps Burton had wise solutions in mind when he recommended brains, fish, and borage as dietary remedies for melancholy.

Chapter 5

Insomnia

"I can't sleep!" Who among us has not had to utter these words at some point in our lives? Similar to depression, which presents as an episodic or chronic complaint, insomnia varies markedly in its severity but is rampant in modern industrial societies. It can refer to difficulty falling asleep (greater than 30 min latency) or staying asleep (due to frequent or early morning awakenings). Insomnia is a very frequent presenting complaint of patients in doctors' offices, including its attributed loss of work efficiency, accidents, and a decrease in general quality of life. It exacts a staggering economic toll, estimated at $100 billion annually (Wagner, Wagner, and Hening, 1998).

Insomnia incidence is very high. Episodic problems occur in about one-third of Americans in a given year, and 10 to 15 percent suffer on a chronic basis (Wagner, Wagner, and Hening 1998). Incidence increases with age, as women must endure the snoring of their spouses, only to arouse them and hear, "How could I be snoring? I was awake!"

Interestingly, 69 percent of patients with insomnia have never visited their doctor for attempted treatment of the complaint (Wagner, Wagner, and Hening, 1998). The reservoir of potential patients is huge, and many are contemplating herbal alternatives.

The treatment of insomnia has involved one potion or another since the dawn of humankind. Whether herbal or chemical, treatment seeks to balance on a fine line between production of restful sleep and the pitfalls of hangovers, dependency, and tachyphylaxis. No ideal hypnotic or soporific has emerged to date.

Judgment of treatment trials in insomnia has been hampered by the fact that subjective assessments by patients of the amount of time that they actually slept are notoriously unreliable. This has been rectified, to a degree, by the advent of sleep polysomnography measures. This technique employs a combination of EEG, or electroencephalogram, measures with monitors of eye movement, nasal airflow, electromyogram (EMG, or muscle activity), chest and abdominal expansion, electrocardiogram (EKG), and other measures to assess states of wakefulness and sleep.

"Sleep staging" examines these measures to judge sleep duration, quality, and pathology. In brief, wakefulness in the adult patient is marked in the EEG by posterior alpha activity (8 to 12 hertz [Hz]), along with some degree of EMG activity, particularly in temporal areas. Stage 1 of sleep, or drowsiness, is marked by wandering eye movements and desynchronization of the EEG, with the appearance of theta brain waves slowing (4 to 7 Hz). In stage 2, or early sleep, sleep spindles, K complexes, and slow waves are coupled with cessation or marked reduction of muscle activity. Stages 3 and 4 are often considered together as deep or slow-wave sleep, in which fewer spindles are observed and EEG activity consists of high-voltage slowing in the delta range (0.5 to 3 Hz). Finally, dreaming, or REM (rapid eye movement) sleep, occurs sporadically during the night, most often after an initial latency of 90 min. The polysomnographic correlates are a "paradoxical" activation of EEG activity in the faster ranges, coupled with a total elimination of peripheral muscle activity, while eye movements increase markedly. Both slow-wave and REM sleep are felt to have importance in restorative qualities of sleep.

Unfortunately, the hardware necessary for polysomnographic sleep studies produces its own inhibiting effects on restful sleep, to some degree. Nevertheless, careful research designs allow accumulation of useful correlates in drug studies of insomnia. However, although EEG studies may increase the scientific objective data acquired in clinical studies, to quote Schulz and colleagues (Schulz, Hänsel, and Tyler, 1998, p. 78), "In themselves, drug-induced EEG changes do not prove therapeutic efficacy."

Thus, hardware notwithstanding, an effective hypnotic must satisfy the patient's desire to sleep well. As stated by Leathwood and Chauffard, 1985, p. 147), "whatever the results of objective studies, if the patient does not feel that he or she slept better, the hypnotic is useless."

VALERIAN:
Valeriana officinalis L.
Valerianaceae

Synonyms

- Valerian
- Setwall
- *Valerianae radix* (Latin)
- *Phu* (Greek)

Botany

Valerian is a perennial herb native to Eurasia but naturalized in temperate wet or swampy locales around the globe, reaching 0.5 to 1.5 m in height. It has terminal cymes of white or pink flowers with an intoxicating scent. The medicinal portions are the roots, rhizomes, and stolons, which, when dried, have a characteristic pungent odor.

The genus contains over 200 species. *Valeriana edulis, wallachi,* and others have been similarly used medicinally. In 1996, Capasso and colleagues (1996) demonstrated sedative effects of the Andean species, *Valeriana adscendens,* and believed them to be qualitatively similar to those of *V. officinalis.* Apparently, great potential exists for the study of therapeutic effects of other members of the genus.

Phytochemistry

Attention has long focused on the importance of the essential oil fraction of valerian root, which varies from 0.1 to 2 percent in composition and contains bornyl acetate, isovalerate, valerenic acid, hydrovalerenic acid, acetoxyvalerenic acid, valerenal, valeranone, and elemol. Valerenic acids are unique to *Valeriana officinalis* and serve as a marker for that particular species. For better or worse, the essential oil content and clinical efficacy of extracts do not correlate in previous studies.

Other important components, common to other *Valeriana* species are the valepotriates. These represent 1.2 percent of dried *V. offi-*

cinalis but reach much higher levels in other species. Important breakdown products include baldrinal, homobaldrinal, and valtroxal (Morazzoni and Bombardelli, 1995). Valepotriates have demonstrated sedative and muscle relaxant effects in some experiments but are rapidly metabolized (Morazzoni and Bombardelli, 1995). Similarly, although cytotoxic effects of valepotriates have been noted, intestinal inactivation is likely, inasmuch as they are hydrolyzed by moisture and heat (Wagner, Wagner, and Hening, 1998). Glucuronidation is another likely method of metabolism (Schulz, Hänsel, and Tyler, 1998). High doses did not produce teratogenic effects in rats (Tufik et al., 1994).

Both valerenic acids and valerenal and their derivatives have demonstrated sedative activities. Valerenic acid was also believed to inhibit enzymatic degradation of GABA (Morazzoni and Bombardelli, 1995).

Interestingly, the alkaloids of valerian, valeranine, and actinidine are said to have excitatory effects in vitro and in vivo (Morazzoni and Bombardelli, 1995).

Bos and colleagues carefully documented seasonal variations in cultivated valerian constituents in Holland (Bos, Woerdenbag, et al., 1998). The highest content of essential oil in roots occurred in the September after planting and varied from 1.2 to 2.1 percent. Valerenic acid, its derivatives, and valepotriates peaked the following March. Through refinement of techniques, it was concluded that plants should be harvested in September of the year sown, with resultant essential oil content of 0.9 percent and valerenic acid fraction of 0.5 percent.

History of Use

The classical authors Dioscorides and Galen recognized valerian, sometimes called *phu,* perhaps an onomatopoeic rendition of the utterances issuing from those having smelled the dried root. The genus name *Valeriana* may derive from the Latin *valere,* referring to well-being. Most modern peoples liken the odor to that of sweaty socks. The author recommends against the home brewing of the raw dried herb due to the likelihood that the aspiring herbalist will likely improve his or her sleep by virtue of being left alone in the domicile except, perhaps, for the cats. The odor of the dried root is said to be attractive to felines, and their assessment may provide a reliable method of qualitative bioassay (Foster 1996f).

However, tastes change, and the odor of valerian has appealed quite distinctly to different societies. Turner said of it (Turner et al., 1995, p. 765), "Some lay the root amongst clothes to make them smell sweet."

Culpeper (1994, p. 378) described the medicinal use of the wild plant, which was considered stronger than the cultivated form: "The root has a strong and disagreeable smell, warm to the taste, bitter, and a little acrid. . . . It is excellent against nervous affections, such as headaches, trembling, palpitations, vapours, and hysteric complaints."

Valerian enjoyed a reputation as an anticonvulsant for a time. Interestingly, in the nineteenth century, the valerian herb was considered a *stimulant* (Pereira and Carson, 1852, pp. 611-612): "Valerian excites the cerebro-spinal system. Large doses cause headache, mental excitement, visual illusions (scintillation, flashes of light, etc.), giddiness, restlessness, agitation, and even spasmodic movements. . . . Valerian may be employed as a nervous excitant, and where stimulants are admissible, as an antispasmodic."

American herbalist Jethro Kloss (1975, p. 322) stated, "Excellent nerve tonic—very quieting and soothing. Useful in hysterics. . . . Excellent for children in measles, scarlet fever, and restlessness."

Grieve (1974, p. 828) cited it as an effective agent to treat extreme stress: "During the recent War [World War II], when air raids were a serious strain on the overwrought nerves of civilian men and women, Valerian, prescribed with other simple ingredients, taken in a single dose, or repeated according to the need, proved wonderfully efficacious, preventing or minimizing serious results."

Valerian was included in the *National Formulary* of the United States until 1940, when it was dropped due to the popularity of barbiturates (Wagner, Wagner, and Hening, 1998). It is an interesting commentary that those agents are rarely employed in medical practice today, except as anticonvulsants and operative anesthetics, due to their addictive potential, residual sedation, and adverse effects on cognition and learning.

Preparation of Extracts

Despite being one of the most recognized medicinal herbs in the world, standardization of valerian extracts is not highly developed. Roots are usually collected in September in the Northern Hemisphere and dried below 40°C (Medical Economics Company, 1998). It is only then that the characteristic smell of isovaleric acid becomes apparent (Morazzoni and Bombardelli, 1995). This odor may be eliminated by hand washing with sodium bicarbonate (Houghton, 1994).

Both aqueous and ethanolic extracts (usually 70 percent ethanol with herb-to-extract ratio of 4 to 7:1) have been employed in recent medical studies (Schulz, Hänsel, and Tyler, 1998).

Bokstaller and Schmidt (1997) examined HPLC patterns of valerian and suggested methods of phytopharmaceutical standardization based on content of flavonoids and sesquiterpenes.

Biochemical and Animal Studies

Hendriks and colleagues (1981) examined the effects of various components of valerian essential oil—valerenal, valerenic acid, valeranone, and isoeugenyl-isovalerate—by intraperitoneal (ip) injection in mice. Valerenal and valerenic acid produced sedative activity at 50 mg/kg, as compared to the higher doses necessary for the essential oil itself and its other components.

Houghton (1988) reviewed the biological activity of valerian, confirming a sedative effect of an alcoholic extract of fresh valerian roots. This was attributed to valepotriate content, and the author advised caution in chronic use due to possible cytotoxic effects. He also cited sesquiterpenes in the essential oil as having sedative properties.

In 1989, Holzl and Godau demonstrated binding of valerian to benzodiazepine receptors in vitro. Similarly, Mennini and Bernasconi (1993) noted binding of valerian to GABA receptors in vitro. The authors postulated a combination of ingredients cumulatively affecting GABA receptors to produce sedative effects.

Santos and colleagues (1994) examined the effects of an aqueous valerian extract on transport of gamma-aminobutyric acid (GABA) in rat synaptosomes. GABA is believed to be a primary inhibitory neurotransmitter in the central nervous system. GABA is normally conserved through reuptake into presynaptic terminals. Low concentrations of the extract inhibited this activity by 50 percent, as well as inducing the calcium ion-dependent release of GABA from synaptosomes. The authors indicated that the results support the concept that valerian increases the available supplies of GABA in the synaptic cleft, and this would possibly explain the effect of the herb in reducing sleep latency. It requires emphasis that this study employed an extract rather than isolated components, so that a synergistic effect of different compounds is distinctly possible.

Cavadas and colleagues (1995) employed aqueous and hydroalcoholic extracts of valerian standardized to valerenic acid content to assess, once again, effects on rat GABA receptor activity, which they interpreted as being the primary mediator of sedation in the CNS. Both types of extracts displaced tritiated muscimol in its bindings to crude synaptic membranes with similar potencies. Valerenic acid in isolation did not have this action. They also examined the role of amino acid constituents of valerian. Glutamate had a mild inhibitory effect on muscimol binding but was present only in the aqueous extract. GABA itself was present in both extracts and had a similar inhibitory effect, but it does not cross the blood brain barrier efficiently and could not account for the sedative effects of valerian observed clinically.

Cott (1995) employed a NovaScreen to demonstrate high affinity of the crude *Valeriana officinalis* extract to $GABA_B$, AMPA (quisqualate), kainate, NMDA, and CCK_A (cholecystokinin) receptors.

Hiller and Zetler (1996, p. 145) examined the effects on mice of ethanol extracts of valerian. They prefaced their study with the statement that "the evidence that valerian is sedative in man has been equivocal for many decades." Their extract was determined to be free of valepotriates. An ethanolic extract had no visible effect on maternal behavior or pain thresholds of temperature in mice, whereas diazepam had clear sedative effects on all activities. They indicated a lack of support for valerian's possessing the antianxiety effects of benzodiazepines.

Both preparations prolonged anesthesia with thiopental. Diazepam diminished convulsant effects of picrotoxin and harmane, whereas the valerian extract reduced seizures only to picrotoxin. This failure to affect harmane-induced seizures was taken as evidence against actions of valerian on benzodiazepine receptors.

The authors posited "a positive interaction of valerian at the barbiturate binding site of the $GABA_A$-benzodiazepine receptor complex." They further stated, "One may conclude that valerenic acid contributes to the pharmacological efficacy of our valerian extracts" (Hiller and Zetler, 1996, p. 149).

The pharmacokinetics of valerian extracts and components in human clinical usage have not been adequately studied.

Studies in Normals

In 1982, Leathwood and colleagues examined the effects of two different aqueous extracts of valerian versus placebo in 128 people. Unfortunately, only subjective measures of sleep, via a questionnaire, were employed in the assessment. Valerian produced a reported decrease in sleep latency and improvement in sleep quality, particularly in those who rated themselves as having previous difficulties. Spontaneous waking episodes, recall of dreams, and morning "hangover" symptoms were apparently unaffected in comparison to placebo.

Balderer and Borbély (1985) studied aqueous valerian extracts in ten normal patients at home and eight in the sleep laboratory with a combination of questionnaires, self-rating, and polysomnographic monitoring. Doses of 450 and 900 mg of valerian, prepared as for Leathwood's studies, and said to contain no valepotriates on thin-layer chromatography (TLC), were employed in double-blind crossover fashion. The extracts reduced subjective assessment of sleep latency and time awake once having fallen asleep. Sleep latency was reduced 50 percent at the higher dose of valerian ($p < 0.01$). Wakening episodes were said to be "declining," but this did not attain statistical significance. However, no clear changes were seen in sleep stages based on EEG parameters when comparing valerian to placebo. The authors assessed the aqueous valerian extract as having mild hypnotic activity and postulated that components other than valepotriates must be responsible.

In 1989, another double-blind study of a valerian extract containing primarily sesquiterpenes was carried out in Sweden (Lindahl and Lindwall, 1989). A highly significant benefit was said to occur in poor sleep, with 44 percent of subjects reporting "perfect sleep," while 89 percent noted "improved sleep" without side effects.

In 1996, Gerhard and colleagues compared valerian to flunitrazepam with respect to vigilance measures in normal volunteers taking single oral doses. Various tests of cognitive performance and questionnaires were combined. Interestingly, the only objective impairments occurred in the benzodiazepine group, with confirmation by subjective complaints. All medicated groups reported improved sleep quality over placebo. In the valerian group, no hangover was noted, and, in fact, patients maintained that they were better rested, more alert after sleep, and felt better overall.

Studies in Clinical Disease

Valerian, for all its popularity and worldwide name recognition, has been studied only superficially in comparison to some other phytopharmaceuticals in this book. Numbers are further reduced by virtue of the fact that some existing studies have included combination herbal sleep preparations, which will not herein be considered. Results are equivocal and occasionally contradictory. To summarize one view (Foster, 1996f, p. 4), "Long-standing clinical experience has provided ample evidence of the value of valerian as a sedative. Discrepancies in results are due to variations in dosage, as well as quality of commercial preparations." He went on to indicate that large doses, along the order of 5 ml, are necessary when employing tinctures.

In 1985, Leathwood and Chauffard employed aqueous extracts of valerian, 450 or 900 mg, versus placebo in a double-blind manner to examine the effects in eight mildly affected insomniacs over five nights. In this instance, subjective assessments were combined with activity meters worn on the wrists. Sleep onset was defined as occurring when a patient went 5 min without motion. Sleep latency with the 450 mg dose was about 9 min, as compared to 15.8 minutes with placebo. This compares favorably with the results of treatment with benzodiazepine hypnotics. The higher dose of valerian failed to produce additional reductions in time to sleep onset. No carryover effect of valerian from one night to another was noted, and total sleep time was apparently unaffected. It was judged that valerian produced more stable sleep patterns in the initial hours of sleep. Some hangover was noted subjectively by study patients on the 900 mg dose, but not with the 450 mg one.

Schulz and colleagues employed a commercial aqueous valerian extract, 405 mg given tid with meals, to assess fourteen elderly poor sleepers in a double-blind placebo-controlled study with polysomnographic techniques (Schulz, Stolz, and Müller, 1994). No statistically significant changes were seen.

The most convincing study of valerian, to date, was published in German in 1996 by Vorbach, Görtelmayer, and Bruning. Their study employed 600 mg of a standardized 70 percent ethanol extract of valerian in 121 patients with significant sleep disturbances. Patients with depression or taking other hypnotics were excluded. A physician-rated sleep scale, Görtelmayer sleep questionnaire, von Zerssen mood scale (BF-S), and Clinical Global Impressions (CGI) scales were studied at baseline and twice during the one-month trial. Although early changes in sleep and other parameters were modest, by the end of the study, significant improvements were seen in three of four scales in the valerian group compared to placebo. Due to a marked placebo effect, the SRA scale showed no significant differences.

The CGI results in this study were the most striking compared to placebo ($p < 0.001$). Schulz and colleagues interpreted the results as follows (Schulz, Hänsel, and Tyler, 1998, p. 80): "valerian preparations probably do not produce immediate effects like those of a typical sleep aid, and . . . 2-4 weeks' therapy is needed to achieve significant improvement, especially in daily mood." They continued by explaining that in chronic insomnia, this delayed effect should not be a hindrance, inasmuch as the acute effects of benzodiazepines and other hypnotics may produce dependency and other liabilities. In summary, they noted (Schulz, Hänsel, and Tyler, 1998, p. 81), "valerian is not a suitable agent for the acute treatment of insomnia. Its essential value may lie in its ability to promote natural sleep after several weeks of use, with no risk of dependence or adverse health effects."

In a 1998 review of hypnotic medications, the authors attributed to valerian (1) a decrease in sleep latency, (2) no change to an increase in total sleep time, (3) an increase in delta (slow-wave) sleep, (4) no effect on REM (dreaming) sleep, and (5) an increase in sleep quality, with no reports of tolerance or abuse. While citing the difficulty in comparing studies with different preparations, the authors concluded, "limited studies provide evidence for the mild hypnotic activity of valerian" (Wagner, Wagner, and Hening, 1998, p. 687).

Although valerian has often been cited as efficacious in the treatment of attention-deficit hyperactivity disorder (ADHD) (Valpiani, 1995), no controlled studies were found in the world's literature. After a generation of work in clinical child neurology, the author has not seen a case of attention-deficit disorder convincingly treated with this herb, much to his disappointment.

Toxicity and Side Effects

In 1995, a well-studied case of overdose with a popular American valerian preparation was published (Willey et al., 1995). To summarize, an eighteen-year-old presented to an emergency room 3 h after ingesting an estimated 20 g of powdered valerian root extract. Symptoms included fatigue, abdominal pain, chest tightness, tremor, and lightheadedness. Vital signs remained stable, and physical examination merely demonstrated hand tremor and pupillary dilation (mydriasis). An EKG, complete blood count (CBC), and chemistry panel tests indicative of electrolyte balance, hepatic function, and renal function were unaffected. A urine toxicology screen showed only THC metabolites, attributed by the patient to cannabis use two weeks previously. The patient received activated charcoal orally as the sole treatment. All symptoms were gone within twenty-four hours.

This result demonstrates the relatively benign nature of a dosage some twenty times greater than that recommended for therapeutic valerian usage. The study did not mention how well the patient slept after the ordeal.

Bos and colleagues evaluated the cytotoxicity of valerian components in vitro (Bos, Hendriks, et al., 1998). In essence, valepotriates displayed the greatest cytotoxicity due to alkylating effects, in the range of IC 50 values of 1 to 6 micromolar (μM), whereas baldrinal was ten- to thirtyfold less potent, and valerenic acids had low toxicity. Despite experimental and clinical data supporting the relative safety of valepotriates taken orally in low dosages, the authors stated, "Nevertheless, more and more preference is given to valerian preparations that are devoid of these potentially hazardous constituents" (p. 224). They observed that tinctures stored for one to two months were likely safer.

In a poorly documented letter, results of overdosage were reported in twenty-four patients taking valerian in Hong Kong. It was stated that "[t]he clinical problems were mainly central nervous system depression and anticholinergic poisoning" (Chan, 1998, p. 569). Not surprisingly, this was due to the fact that the preparation employed was a valerian dry extract of low dosage, but also containing hyoscine (an atropine relative) and cyproheptadine (a sedating H-1 type antihistamine). No documentation was made as to treatment duration. In any event, no hepatic toxicity was observed. Whether appropriate or not, the letter was labeled as pertaining to "valerian overdose" and may be offered by the less discriminating critic as evidence of the dangers of this herbal agent.

Although better documented, another dubious case of "valerian root withdrawal" was reported in 1998 (Garges, Varia, and Doraiswamy, 1998). To briefly summarize, a fifty-eight-year-old male with preexisting coronary disease, hypertension, and congestive heart failure on a variety of medicines had been taking large doses of a valerian extract multiple times a day as a sedative. This patient subsequently developed "high-output cardiac failure." Because he improved when placed on a benzodiazepine, once deprived of his customary medicine, an implication of causation was made. The authors cited similarities in valerian effects on GABA and benzodiazepine mechanisms as evidence that "it can be hypothesized that valerian root also may produce a benzodiazepinelike withdrawal syndrome" (pp. 1566-1567). This is a difficult allegation to make, let alone prove, given 2,000 years of previous usage without a similar report. The authors did state, "Since this patient was taking multiple medications and had undergone a surgical procedure, we cannot causally link valerian root to his symptoms." Unfortunately, the *Journal of the American Medical Association* has validated this unsupported allegation by virtue of its publication.

Similarly, the *Archives of Internal Medicine* has published false characterization of valerian as "hallucinogenic" (Winslow and Kroll, 1998, p. 2196).

Cost

One standardized valerian preparation costs about $7.50 monthly as a hypnotic. In comparison, the benzodiazepine agents, generic flurazepam (Dalmane) and triazolam (Halcion) cost $18 and $26 per month, respectively. The antidepressant trazodone (Desyrel), as a hypnotic agent, costs $10 per month as a generic, and $25 to $50 as a brand name (*Medical Letter,* 1999a). Finally, diphenhydramine (Benadryl) is the agent most frequently employed in OTC hypnotic sleep aids in the United States, at a cost of $3 or less per month.

Panel and Regulatory Information

Valerian is an approved food in the United States, on the GRAS list (generally recognized as safe).

In 1998, the *United States Pharmacopeia* (USP) failed to certify valerian as effective, but the composition of the advisory panel and its review techniques have been widely criticized among herbal cognoscenti.

ESCOP (1997) has recommended tea infusions or tinctures of valerian for restlessness or difficulty falling asleep. No restriction was placed on duration of use, but valerian was not recommended for those under age three. No drug interactions were noted, and no data were cited on use during pregnancy or lactation. Caution while driving or operating machinery was advised while under the influence of valerian.

Valerian was approved by the German Commission E in 1985, with a revision in 1990 (Blumenthal et al., 1998), for restlessness and sleep disorders due to nervous conditions. Again, no contraindications of note, drug interactions, or side effects were cited. See Table 5.1 for a summary of valerian-related information.

TABLE 5.1. Valerian Summary

What it is:

Dried root for infusion (tea), tincture, or extract of *Valeriana officinalis.*

What it does:

Tinctures of fresh root may effectively treat acute sleep difficulties. Ethanol extracts safely treat chronic insomnia over a period of four weeks, with reported improvement in other parameters of well-being.

What it does not do:

Valerian does not guarantee a full night's sleep, acutely. It has no proven efficacy in treatment of ADHD.

What to look for:

Root or fresh tincture from a reliable source or, preferably, a standardized 70 percent ethanol extract.

Cautions:

Valeriana officinalis is generally quite safe. Preparations of alternative species may contain high levels of valepotriates and probably should be avoided. Use of valerian with alcohol or other sedative drugs should be pursued cautiously, if at all.

Recommendations:

Data on valerian are incomplete, but the most reliable data favor use of the standardized 70 percent ethanol extract, with dosage of 600 mg to be taken 2 h before bedtime for at least four weeks.

PASSION FLOWER:
Passiflora incarnata L.
Passifloraceae

Synonyms

- Maypop
- Passion vine
- Apricot Vine
- *Passiflorae herba* (Latin)
- *Passionsblumenkraut* (German)
- *Herbe de passiflore* (French)

Botany

Passiflora incarnata is a relatively hardy climbing vine of the southeastern United States and Caribbean Basin. The genus contains more than 450 mostly tender tropical species (Griffiths, 1994; Vanderplank, 1996). The vine may sprawl and attain a length of 10 m. Its beautiful, delicate flowers reach 7.5 centimeters (cm) in diameter and vary from white to pink to purple, lasting only one day. Especially after hand pollination, tart-sweet fruits follow. The plant may die back to the ground in colder climates and reemerge from its underground roots the following spring.

The juice of the maypop is rich in vitamin C, at some 22.1 percent (Svanidze et al., 1974).

Brasseur and Angenot (1984) published a detailed monograph in French on botanical features of this species. They cited a range as mentioned previously but claimed Brazil and Peru as the probable countries of origin. The latest authorities indicate that this species is not found in Peru (Brako and Zarucchi, 1993).

The French have been effusive in their praise of this species. Leclerc (1920, p. 548) observed, "Passionflowers . . . present themselves to us, dressed in the richest and most varied tints that the ingenious palette of nature has ever decorated a plant [translation E.B.R.]."

Phytochemistry

The aerial parts contain up to 2.5 percent flavonoids, including vitexin, saponarin, orientin, and others; 0.05 percent maltol; small amounts of cyanogenic glycosides (gynocardin) (occasionally reported); an essential oil with 150 components; and, variably, beta-carboline alkaloids (harmane), usually at undetectable levels (Bisset and Wichtl, 1994; ESCOP, 1996-1997). Brasseur and Angenot (1984) noted a total alkaloid content of only 0.032 percent.

Rahman and colleagues (1997) recently isolated isoscoparin-2″-*O*-glucoside from *Passiflora incarnata,* along with eleven other known flavonoids.

Bokstaller and Schmidt (1997) examined HPLC patterns of *Passiflora incarnata* and suggested methods of phytopharmaceutical standardization based on content of flavonoids and sesquiterpenes.

History of Use

Although *Passiflora incarnata* was known to Native Americans as a fruit, its employment as a medicine was apparently quite limited (Moerman, 1998). The only practices that suggest psychotropic usage are that of the Houma employing the root infusion as a blood tonic and of the Cherokee for assistance in weaning infants.

Svanidze and colleagues (1974) indicate that the species was discovered by the first Spanish missionaries in the New World and was brought to Europe by Jac Boccio in 1610. Naturally, some debate exists. Leclerc (1920) indicates that *Passiflora incarnata* was the first known species in the genus and was described as *Grenadille* by Nicolas Monard at the end of the sixteenth century. He likened it to ivy and observed that "[i]ts flower strongly resembles a white rose, with leaves of which one sees certain features imprinted with the Passion of Jesus Christ" (p. 549). Leclerc expounded (1920):

> Our ancestors, whose imagination was not their least attribute, had no difficulty in recognizing in the passion flower all the instruments of the Passion: the leaves terminated in three points represented the lance, the borer, the whip, the three styles the nails, the stigma the sponge, the filaments of the receptacle the crown of thorns, the central column the shaft on which they attached Christ during the flagellation. (p. 549) [translation E. B. R.]

Subsequently, many authors have drawn parallels between the botanical features of this genus and aspects of early Christian history. Reportedly, it served as an early teaching aid for the missionaries in their conversion of the Native American population.

Tyler indicates that passion flower was introduced to American medicine by Dr. L. Phares of Mississippi, in 1840, and popularized by Professor I. J. M. Goss of Atlanta, Georgia, in the latter part of the nineteenth century (Foster and Tyler, 1999). In 1867, Phares noted *Passiflora incarnata* as a treatment for tetanus in a young child.

In 1897, Bullington noted a role in epilepsy and "other neuroses":

> Insomnia has been treated by me in many cases, . . . and I fail to recall a case where used, in which I did not see beneficial results.

> Hysteria and neurasthenia have improved by its use in my hands. I use it extensively in the fretful and nervous condition in children as a substitute for the very unpleasant bromides. A case of night terrors, with somnambulistic manifestations, has been most happily controlled by passion flower alone. (p. 108)

Felter and Lloyd (1900) observed the following of *Passiflora incarnata:*

> It is specially useful to allay *restlessness* and overcome *wakefulness,* when these are the result of exhaustion, or the nervous excitement of debility. It proves specially useful in the *insomnia* of infants and old people. It gives sleep to those who are laboring under effects of mental worry or from mental overwork. It relieves the nervous symptoms due to reflex sexual or menstrual disturbances, and the *nervous irritability* resulting from prolonged illness. (p. 440)

Stapleton (1904) promoted tincture of *Passiflora incarnata* for a variety of indications:

> I have used the drug with great success in insomnia, hysteria, neurasthenia, neuralgia, nervous and physical prostration and alcoholism.
> . . . in those cases in which there is mental unrest, agitation, worry and exhaustion, . . . you will find in passiflora incarnata an excellent remedy.
> . . . In the nervousness and sleeplessness accompanying acute or chronic alcoholism, passiflora offtimes acts like a marvel.
> . . . There is also another condition, which for the lack of a better name is called "nerves." . . . Here is another case in which passiflora has acted better in my hands than either opi-

um, bromides or chloral, and I use it without fear of forming a drug habit, causing constipation, biliousness or any one of the other after-effects of the above mentioned drugs. (pp. 17-18)

Leclerc (1920) cited an early American user of the herb, Dr. Lindsay, who denied a narcotic or stupefying effect. Reportedly, the person treated with the herb was easily awakened and could speak reasonably, but "leave him for a moment and he will soon be off to the Elysian field again" (p. 551). Leclerc also reported on his own trials of passion flower. He preferred a fresh tincture of the herb, collected in May:

It presents the great advantage of provoking a sleep that approximates that of the normal individual and to bring about no effect of nervous depression, no obnubilation of the sense of the spirit; sick people who make usage of it awaken as alert as they were at the moment of retiring, conserving all their lucidity, all their faculties of thought, of speech and action. (p. 552)

Passion flower was included in the *National Formulary* from 1916 to 1936, before falling into disuse (Foster and Tyler, 1999). Due to a dearth of supportive data, the U.S. Food and Drug Administration withdrew recognition of its safety and efficacy in 1978.

Passiflora incarnata has retained a folk usage as a "nervine," hypnotic, sedative, and spasmolytic, especially in children. It was used in homeopathy in France before World War I, when it was said to have a favorable action on the "anguish of the war [translation E. B. R.]" (Brasseur and Angenot, 1984, p. 19).

Despite widespread folk and clinical use in Europe, *Passiflora incarnata* has been little investigated in formal human trials.

Siegel (1976, p. 476) claimed usage as "[s]moke, tea, or capsules as marihuana substitute" with reported effects of "[m]ild stimulant."

Preparation of Extracts

The herb is most often made as a tea, usually as 2 g of passion flower infused and strained after 10 min. A 1:8 tincture is available, with dosage of 1 to 4 ml taken qid, or at bedtime. The botanical preparation includes all aerial parts (Brasseur and Angenot, 1984). Extracts are popular in Europe, usually as one component of mixed commercial products.

Basic Science and Animal Studies

Great controversy has arisen due to the putative presence of beta-carboline alkaloids in some cultivars of *Passiflora incarnata*. These include harmane, harmaline, and others. In physiological doses, these are monoamine oxidase inhibitors (MAOIs). Literature has even supported the use of maypop, ingested or smoked, as an *"ayahuasca* analogue" that serves as the MAOI which permits oral activity of DMT (dimethyltryptamine)-containing plants (e.g., *Banisteriopsis caapi, Phalaris,* etc.) (Ott, 1994, 1996). However, such alkaloids are trace elements in select maypop samples, while most commercial preparations are devoid of these components (ESCOP, 1996-1997). No hypertensive crises or other clinical sequelae have been reported in relation to such activity after use of *Passiflora incarnata.* Interestingly, most experimenters taking such alkaloids in isolation have reported mild levels of sedation, and no antidepressant or stimulatory effect (Ott, 1994).

In 1974, a group of Japanese researchers demonstrated the presence of maltol, a pyrone derivative, in the plant, with sedative properties in mice when injected subcutaneously. A 75 mg/kg dose reduced spontaneous motor activity 50 percent and prolonged hexobarbital sleeping time after much higher oral doses (Aoyagi, Kimura, and Murata, 1974). However, the doses of maltol employed far exceed those which could be derived from the use of herbal passion flower. The authors conceded that action of maltol alone would not explain the observed sedative effects of *Passiflora incarnata* extract.

A 1988 Italian study employed an ethanolic extract of *Passiflora incarnata* in rats (Speroni and Minghetti, 1988). Some analgesic effects were observed, and on ip injection, pentobarbital sleeping time was increased in two extract fractions, and locomotor activity reduced in three. Harman was barely detectable in their herbal material. The authors attributed these activities to two compounds, one lipophilic and one polar. Unfortunately, neither was positively isolated or identified.

In 1990, another Italian team examined the effects of an oral hydroethanolic extract given to rats over three weeks in doses corresponding to 5 g/kg. No changes were seen in animal weight, pain responses, or coordination. Some reduction was observed in general activity in maze tests, but no surface or deep EEG changes were observed (Sopranzi et al., 1990).

Subsequently, a variety of other European studies have produced similar supportive and occasional negative findings in rodent testing. Wolfman and colleagues (1994) were able to demonstrate in mice anxiolytic effects of the compound chrysin, derived from the related species *Passiflora caerulea*. That agent binds to benzodiazepine receptors without reported sedative or muscle relaxant effects.

Cott employed a NovaScreen to demonstrate high affinity of the crude *Passiflora incarnata* extract to $GABA_A$ and $_{-B}$, AMPA (quisqualate), glycine, NMDA (N-methyl-D-aspartate), and chloride ion channel receptors (Cott, 1995).

A French study has recently examined *Passiflora incarnata* extracts and components in mice (Soulimani et al., 1997). A hydroalcoholic extract at 400 mg/kg injected intraperitoneally reduced measures of anxiety in the mice, as evidenced by an increase in rearing and climbing in a staircase test and time spent in the light part of a light/dark box choice test (all $p < 0.05$). Similarly, an aqueous extract injected ip at the same dose displayed sedative effects with a reduction in "rears" ($p < 0.001$), steps climbed ($p < 0.01$), and locomotion in a free exploratory test ($p < 0.01$). The aqueous extract also potentiated the hypnotic effect of low-dose pentobarbital.

Administration of flumazenil (a benzodiazepine receptor antagonist) did not affect sedative influences of the aqueous extract. Interestingly, addition of pure harmane alkaloids, maltol, and mixed flavonoids failed to alter any observed behavioral parameters. The authors determined that the latter could not account for the observed pharmacological effects (Soulimani et al., 1997).

Apparently, this study further muddies the waters by demonstrating anxiolytic effects with one extract and sedation with another, and by providing additional negative data in support of putative active compounds.

Studies in Normals

Virtually no formal studies have been pursued in humans with this agent.

Maluf and colleagues (1991) were able to demonstrate some nonspecific sedative effects in mice and human volunteers with *Passiflora edulis* in Brazil, but laboratory parameters indicated signs of hepatic and pancreatic toxicity.

Studies in Clinical Disease

Virtually no formal studies have been pursued in humans with this agent.

As is the case with valerian, *Passiflora incarnata* is frequently recommended as effective in treatment of attention-deficit hyperactivity disorder (ADHD) in children. No modern clinical data whatsoever are available to support this claim.

Toxicity and Side Effects

An early report of possible *Passiflora* toxicity was published at the end of the nineteenth century (Harnsberger, 1898). A young woman with complex symptomatology experienced dizziness and blindness for about one day after taking a mixture of fluidextract of passion flower in combination with potassium bromide during the prior week. The documentation of this paper does not support clear evidence of an etiological association of *Passiflora* to this malady, which may well have been a spontaneous migraine, in this author's estimation.

A case of vasculitis (inflammation of blood vessels) was reported after exposure to an herbal mixture containing *Passiflora* extract (Smith, Chalmers, and Nuki, 1993). Close examination revealed that the resulting cutaneous eruption in this patient, who had an autoimmune disease, occurred in areas in which he employed a nonsteroidal anti-inflammatory gel. Although the authors implicated the *Passiflora* extract as the sensitizing agent, many may find their logic highly questionable.

ESCOP (1996-1997) reports no contraindications, special warnings, drug interactions, or toxic effects in overdose. Due to possible drowsiness, caution in driving or operating machinery was advised. No data are available regarding use in pregnancy and lactation, so avoidance is suggested. Hypersensitivity reactions were said to be rare.

The German Commission E suggested that harmane alkaloid content should be less than 0.01 percent (Blumenthal et al., 1998). Contraindications, side effects, and interaction with other drugs were all labeled as "none known."

Comparison to Existing Pharmaceuticals

Insufficient scientific data exist to hazard observations as to the appropriate role of *Passiflora incarnata* as a stand-alone agent in clinical treatment of insomnia or anxiety.

Benefits

A long history of safe use seems to ensure that *Passiflora incarnata* is relatively benign in routine use at appropriate dosages. Some patients report benefit. Certainly, it deserves further examination in controlled trials.

Cost

Passiflora incarnata is infrequently seen as a single-ingredient preparation in the United States. It is relatively inexpensive. One source sells it for about $5 to $7 for 100 330 mg capsules.

Panel and Regulatory Information

ESCOP (1996-1997, p. 1) recommends *Passiflorae herba* for "tenseness, restlessness and irritability with difficulty in falling asleep."

The German Commission E approved passion flower herb initially in 1985 and revised the monograph in 1990 (Blumenthal et al., 1998). It is approved for use in "nervous restlessness." See Table 5.2 for a summary of information on passion flower.

TABLE 5.2. Passion Flower Summary

What it is:

Dried aerial parts or extract of *Passiflora incarnata.*

What it does:

Purportedly, safely treats insomnia and anxiety, but reported clinical results vary.

What it does not do:

Demonstrate an extensive record of scientific verification of clinical efficacy.

What to look for:

A high-quality herbal preparation, tincture, or single-agent extract.

Cautions:

Do not use in pregnancy or lactation, while driving or operating machinery, or in combination with alcohol or other sedative agents.

Recommendations:

Although seemingly safe, insufficient quality data currently exist for this agent to recommend widespread clinical use.

GERMAN CHAMOMILE:
Matricaria recutita L. Asteraceae

Synonyms

- True chamomile
- *Chamomilla recutita*
- *Matricaria chamomilla*
- *Flos chamomillae vulgaris* (Latin)
- *Fleur de camomile* (French)
- *Kamillenblüten* (German)

Botany

German chamomile is the familiar daisylike annual with white ray flowers and a yellow center, attaining a height of 60 cm. The name derives from the Greek terms *chamos,* or ground, and *melos,* or apple, referring to its apple scent when trod upon or brushed

(Foster, 1996c). It is indigenous to Europe and Western Asia but has been naturalized widely.

The plant is closely related, botanically, chemically, and in herbal practice, to *Chamaemelum nobile (Anthemis nobilis)* or Roman (English) chamomile, which is considered in a separate section.

Phytochemistry

The plant contains a wide variety of essential oil components (bisabolol, chamazulene, and others), flavonoids (apigenin, rutin, quercetin, etc.), sesquiterpene lactones, and coumarins (Bisset and Wichtl 1994; Medical Economics Company, 1998). Essential oil content was measured as 0.25 percent dry weight of the flowers, with a specific gravity of 0.923 (Ahmad and Misra, 1997).

Some have claimed a higher apigenin content in South American cultivars (Viola et al., 1995).

Herniarin, a coumarin recently isolated from *Matricaria chamomilla* flowers, has anticonvulsant and spasmolytic properties (Ahmad and Misra, 1997).

History of Use

This herb is of ancient usage, and legion claims have been made for its anti-inflammatory, gastrointestinal, and dermatological benefits. We will merely refer in this context to its sedative uses. Traditionally, this herb is employed as a soothing infusion. Tyler indicates that only 10 to 15 percent of the essential oils are extracted in steeping a cup of German chamomile tea (Foster and Tyler, 1999).

Preparation of Extracts

The tea is usually composed solely of flowers. Some European extracts have a standardized apigenin content (1.2 percent).

Basic Science and Animal Studies

Fundaro and Cassone (1980) in Italy investigated the essential oil of chamomile and demonstrated a depressive effect on rats, but only at a dosage they considered toxic. At lower doses, its effect was dubious.

Cott employed a NovaScreen to demonstrate high affinity of the crude *Matricaria chamomilla* extract to $GABA_A$ and $GABA_B$, AMPA (quisqualate), kainate, glycine, NMDA (N-methyl-D-aspartate), CCK_A (cholecystokinin), and chloride ion channel receptors (Cott, 1995).

In recent times, increasing scrutiny of apigenin has revealed it to be possibly responsible for the sedative properties of German chamomile. Viola and colleagues (1995) isolated several fractions of the herb with affinity for benzodiazepine receptors. Apigenin, or 5,7,4′-trihydroxyflavone, was detected in one of them (Viola et al., 1995). Apigenin competitively inhibited flunitrazepam binding (a benzodiazepine) but had no effect on tested adrenergic, cholinergic, or GABA systems. In animal experiments, statistically significant anxiolytic effects were observed in mice in the elevated-plus maze (3 mg/kg ip), without notable sedative or muscle relaxant effects. Sedation was observed only with tenfold dosage increases.

Although the anxiolytic effects without significant sedation at lower doses are intriguing, the authors pointed out that the results did not support apigenin as the sole agent responsible for sedative effects of chamomile tea, unless it represented 50 percent of its content (Viola et al., 1995).

In a follow-up study, another South American team of investigators was able to demonstrate that apigenin achieved its anxiolytic effects in rats without deleterious effects on memory acquisition (Salgueiro et al., 1997). In addition, RO 15-1788, a specific benzodiazepine receptor blocker, negated the anxiolytic effects of apigenin, supporting the concept that it is a partial agonist at that site. A related flavonoid, quercetin, lacked anxiolytic and benzodiazepine-binding activity. The authors called for clinical trials of apigenin as a nonsedating agent for anxiety, without effects on memory or muscle tone.

Studies in Normals

No studies in humans were noted.

Studies in Clinical Disease

No studies in humans were noted.

Toxicity and Side Effects

This herb is quite safe for general usage. Rare allergic reactions have been observed. One unusually well-documented case of ana- phylaxis and stillbirth was recently reported (Jensen-Jarolim et al., 1998), but this occurred after the application of an enema of an oily extract of chamomile. A homologue of the birch pollen allergen Bet v 1 was isolated in this case. The rectal route of drug administration may be suspect in this instance, as it allows absorption of food and drug components that may be inactivated by oral intake and diges- tion.

Panel and Regulatory Information

The German Commission E approved chamomile flowers in 1984 and revised the monograph in 1990 for dermatological and gastrointestinal indications only (Blumenthal et al., 1998). (Blu- menthal has indicated that he believes that recent research might change that recommendation to include psychotropic indications, if it were considered.) No contraindications, side effects, or drug interactions were listed.

This author believes that German chamomile is a very safe, time- honored herb that may serve many well as a relaxing tea or a safe phytomedicinal for stress and tension. Further experimentation is needed to establish the role of apigenin as a stand-alone agent in human trials.

ROMAN (ENGLISH) CHAMOMILE:
Chamaemelum nobile (L.) Allioni Asteraceae

Synonyms

- *Anthemis nobilis*
- *Chamomillae romanae flos*
- *Römische Lamillenblüten* (German)

- *Fleur de camomille romaine* (French)
- Sweet chamomile

Botany

Roman chamomile is a perennial composite herb reaching 30 cm in height (Griffiths, 1994). It is indigenous to Southern Europe and North Africa but has been naturalized widely (Medical Economics Company, 1998). Its flowers, which appear from June to September, have a strong odor and bitter taste (Pereira and Carson, 1852).

Phytochemistry

Roman chamomile contains a variety of essential oils, flavonoids, (including apigenin), and sesquiterpene lactones (Bisset and Wichtl, 1994; Medical Economics Company, 1998). Pereira and Carson (1852) assigned stimulant and antispasmodic values to the essential oil.

History of Use

Roman chamomile has largely ridden the herbal coattails of its similarly named cousin. The two are used fairly interchangeably, but documentation of effects for this species has been quite scarce. Its primary use has been in teas for gastrointestinal complaints.

Basic Science and Animal Studies

By implication of its components in common with *Matricaria recutita,* Roman chamomile may have mild sedative or anxiolytic properties. Corresponding documentation is notably lacking.

Rossi and colleagues (1988) examined the effects of the essential oil of two cultivars in rats. The high dose of 350 mg/kg administered ip significantly reduced motility, but over a time course of approximately 30 min.

Studies in Normals

None were discovered.

Studies in Clinical Disease

None were discovered.

Toxicity and Side Effects

No side effects or toxicity are reported beyond possible allergic reactions and anaphylaxis.

Panel and Regulatory Information

The German Commission E evaluated Roman chamomile in 1993 for gastrointestinal and other uses (Blumenthal et al., 1998). It was not approved, inasmuch as the effectiveness of claimed indications were not supported by the literature.

CALIFORNIA POPPY:
Eschscholzia californica Cham. Papaveraceae

Synonyms

• *Kalifornischer Goldmohn* (German)

Botany

California poppy, an annual or short-lived perennial of the Southwest United States and northern Mexico, has golden orange blooms and attains a height of 60 cm (Griffiths, 1994). It prefers sandy, dry soil (Rolland et al., 1991). It is the state flower of California, and a protected species.

Phytochemistry

The aerial parts of the plant contain isoquinolone alkaloids—californidin, eschscholzine, protopine, alpha-allocryptine, and beta-allocryptine—as well as cyanogenic glycosides (in the fresh state)

(Medical Economics Company, 1998). Flowers contain 5 percent rutin (Schäfer et al. 1995), while the alkaloid content of the roots and in the herb is 2.7 percent and 0.06 to 0.29 percent, respectively. The latter authors noted twenty-three alkaloids in six different classes.

In a recent investigation, six flavonol 3-*O*-glycosides were isolated from *Eschscholzia californica,* including two new compounds, quercetin 3-*O*-[alpha-rhamnopyranosyl-(1-4)-alpha-rhamnopyrano-syl-(1-6)-beta-glucopyranoside and isorhamnetin 3-*O*-[alpha-rham-nopyranosyl-(1-4)-alpha-rhamnopyranosyl-(1-6)-beta-glucopyranoside (Beck and Haberlein, 1999).

History of Use

The California poppy has a traditional use by Native Americans of the Southwest (Moerman, 1998). However, employment as a sedative was not extensive. Costanoans claimed that the flowers placed under a child's bed aided sleep. Perhaps they considered it too strong, since a flower decoction was also used to kill head lice. More pertinent, perhaps, was its use by the Mendocino tribe. Reportedly, for them, the root had a stupefying effect.

In France, the herb has been used as a treatment for insomnia and pharmaceutical drug dependency (Schäfer et al., 1995).

Somehow, California poppy has taken on a reputation as a recreational drug and is even smoked. Siegel (Siegel, 1976) noted a usage as a marijuana substitute, with a reported mild euphoriant effect. However, this alleged activity seems to be undeserved. Michael Moore notes (Moore, 1979, p. 50), "The tea is functional, not fun." Similarly, Gregory Tilford observes (Tilford, 1997, p. 26), "For any devious readers seeking recreational plant exploits, forget it. You won't find any satisfaction in the abuse of this plant."

Preparation of Extracts

California poppy is prepared as a tea or may be an ingredient in combination herbal sedatives. Schäfer and colleagues (1995) indicate that only aqueous or alcoholic extractions performed at high temperature show significant effects.

Basic Science and Animal Studies

These are relatively recent and few in number. In 1988, an Italian team examined a whole-plant tincture and cyclohexane extract given ip to mice in a dose corresponding to 130 mg/kg of crude drug (Vincieri et al., 1988). Both preparations reduced locomotor activity and pentobarbital sleeping time, more so for the tincture (p = 0.0001) versus the cyclohexane extract (p = 0.001). They asserted that the biological activity resided primarily, but not exclusively, in the alkaloid fraction, due to protopine.

In 1991, a French team of researchers tested an aqueous extract in mice (Rolland et al., 1991). A variety of behavioral measures suggested a sedative effect at 100 to 200 mg/kg. They also observed anxiolytic effects at 25 mg/kg, as the extract produced an increase in scores on the staircase test and time spent in the lit part of a box. No toxic effects were observed. The authors felt that these results supported the traditional herbal usage.

Kleber and colleagues (1995) demonstrated an inhibition of enzymatic degradation of catecholamines through an inhibition of dopamine beta-hydroxylase and MAO_B by an aqueous alcoholic extract of *Eschscholzia californica*. The authors posited that a preservation of high catecholamine levels would explain antidepressive actions, but also sedative and hypnotic actions. The latter appears pharmacologically contradictory.

Reimeier and colleagues (1995) demonstrated an inhibition on peroxidase-catalyzed met-enkephalin dimerization by extracts of California poppy. This action might serve to modulate analgesic and antidepressant effects.

Schäfer and colleagues (1995) cited evidence that protopine alkaloids increase GABA binding to its receptor, comparably to diazepam, and displace flurazepam from benzodiazepine receptors.

Studies in Normals

None were discovered.

Studies in Clinical Disease

None were discovered.

Toxicity and Side Effects

These have not been properly established.

Panel and Regulatory Information

The German Commission E assessed California poppy in 1991. It recommended avoidance in pregnancy and lactation. Their evaluation was negative: "Medical and/or clinical reports and other material of empirical medicine concerning the phytotherapeutic application of California Poppy is not available. Since the effectiveness for the claimed uses is not documented, a therapeutic application cannot be recommended" (Blumenthal et al., 1998, p. 389).

HOPS:
Humulus lupulus L. Cannabinaceae

Synonyms

- *Lupuli strobulus* (Latin)
- *Hopfenzapfen* (German)

Botany

Hops species belong to a genus in the Cannabinaceae family, as do *Cannabis* spp. The hop plant is a twining, hardy herbaceous perennial, indigenous to Europe, whose strobiles are best known as the bittering agent for beer and ale.

Phytochemistry

Hops contain unstable polyphenolics, humulone, and lupulone that provide the bitter principles, along with an essential oil that yields sesquiterpenes: myrcene, linalool, caryophyllene, and others (Bisset and Wichtl, 1994; Foster and Tyler, 1999). 2-methyl-3-butene-2-ol appears as a breakdown product on storage, at a concentration of 0.15 percent (Foster and Tyler, 1999).

History of Use

Hops have been known since early times. Hildegard von Bingen, the twelfth-century German visionary, abbess, herbalist, and composer, did not consider it highly, however (Hildegard, 1998, p. 36): "It is not much use for a human being, since it causes his melancholy to increase, gives him a sad mind, and makes his intestines heavy."

Culpeper (1994) cited uses as a detoxifying agent, for headache, and legion complaints.

Robert Burton (1907, p. 566), in his seventeenth-century tome, *The Anatomy of Melancholy,* stated, "Lupulus, hop, is a sovereign remedy . . . it purges all choler, and purifies the blood."

American herbalist Jethro Kloss (1975, p. 248) commended it vigorously: "An excellent nervine. Will produce sleep when nothing else will. Two or three cups should be taken hot. Valuable in delirium tremens [Author's note: Is this a bit of the "hair of the dog"?] . . . good for excessive sexual desires."

Hops are frequently used in Europe as a bitter tonic to stimulate appetite. Hop pillows are a traditional remedy for insomnia that seems to have little physiological basis.

In a final twist, Siegel (1976, p. 474) noted another use of hops: "Smoke or tea as marihuana substitute" but with reported effects of "None."

Preparation of Extracts

Hops are used medicinally as a tea or dry extract, often in combination with other sedative agents.

Basic Science and Animal Studies

A group in Spain examined tranquilizing effects of hops in rats (Bravo et al., 1974). They demonstrated that a 10 percent aqueous extract of hops injected ip at a dose of 1 ml per 20 g of weight produced a significant reduction in spontaneous activity for about 30 min. An alcoholic extract was less potent, and an ether extract even weaker.

In 1980, the soporific activity of the hops breakdown product, 2-methyl-3-butene-2-ol, was tested in mice (Hänsel, Wohlfart, and Coper, 1980). In animals given ip doses at 800 mg/kg, an 8 h narcotic effect was observed.

Cott employed a NovaScreen to demonstrate high affinity of the crude *Humulus lupulus* extract to $GABA_A$ and $GABA_B$, AMPA (quisqualate), kainate, glycine, NMDA (N-methyl-D-aspartate), CCK_A and CCK_B (cholecystokinin), and chloride ion channel receptors (Cott, 1995).

Studies in Normals

None were identified.

Studies in Clinical Disease

None were identified.

Toxicity and Side Effects

No contraindications, drug interactions, toxicity, or other dangers are reported (Blumenthal et al., 1998; ESCOP, 1996-1997).

Panel and Regulatory Information

ESCOP (1996-1997, p. 1) endorsed the use of hops for "Tenseness, restlessness and difficulty in falling asleep," as an infusion or 1:5 tincture, 1 to 2 ml up to tid.

The German Commission E evaluated hops in 1984 and revised the monograph in 1990. They approved uses for "mood disturbances such as restlessness and anxiety, sleep disturbances" (Blumenthal et al., 1998, p. 147).

LEMON BALM:
Melissa officinalis L. Lamiaceae

Synonyms

- Balm
- Sweet balm
- Melissa
- Honey plant

- *Melissae folium* (Latin)
- *Melissenblätter* (German)
- *Feuilles de mélisse* (French)

Botany

Melissa, a deciduous, hardy perennial herb, is a member of the mint family. It is native to the Eastern Mediterranean and Western Asia, but it is cultivated and has been naturalized widely. Plants attain a height of 90 cm and have a pleasant lemon scent (Griffiths, 1994; Medical Economics Company, 1998).

Phytochemistry

Melissa contains an essential oil (0.05 percent or more) primarily derived from citronellal, citral a and b (geranial and neral), beta-caryophyllene, linalool, geraniol, and others. It also contains eugenol glycoside; rasmaric acid; flavonoids, including cynaroside, cosmosiin, rhamnocitrin, and isoquercitrin; glycosides of luteolin, quercetin, apigenin, and kaempferol (Mulkens and Kapetanidis, 1987); and volatile triterpene acids, such as ursolic acid (Bisset and Wichtl, 1994; Medical Economics Company, 1998; ESCOP, 1996-1997).

History of Use

Melissa was described by Theophrastus, the Greek philosopher of the fourth to third centuries B.C.E., but without a medical context (Theophrastus, 1948). The genus name derives from the Greek word for "bee," while the species name, *officinalis,* denotes a medical usage. Balm is short for "balsam," referring to a fragrant or resinous substance.

Tyler indicates (1993, pp. 33-34), "The plant is familiar to bee keepers all over the world because the odor of its essential oil resembles that of the pheromone produced by bees which consequently find the plant very attractive."

In the sixteenth century, Gerard (1931, pp. 164-165) extolled its virtues: "Bawme drunke in wine is good against the bitings of venomous beasts, comforts the heart, and driveth away all melancholy and sadness." He added, "Bawme makes the heart merry and joyfull, and strengtheneth the vitall spirits."

Culpeper added his assent (1994, pp. 36-37): "it causeth the mind and heart to become merry . . . and driveth away all troublesome cares and thoughts out of the mind, arising from melancholy and black choler: which Avicen [Avicenna, ibn Sīnā] also confirmeth."

Robert Burton, in the early seventeenth century, had much to say of its benefits (Burton, 1907, p. 565):

> Honeyleaf balm hath an admirable virtue to alter melancholy, be it steeped in our ordinary drink, extracted, or otherwise taken. . . . It heats and dries, saith Heurnius, in the second degree, with a wonderful virtue comforts the heart, and purgeth all melancholy vapors from the spirits, Matthiol. *in lib. 3. Cap. 10. in Dioscoridem.* Besides they ascribe other virtues to it, "as to help concoction, to cleanse the brain, expel all careful thoughts, and anxious imaginations:"

Grieve cited two cases of longevity attributed to melissa (Grieve, 1971, p. 77): "John Hussey, of Sydenham, who lived to the age of 116, breakfasted for fifty years on Balm tea sweetened with honey, and herb teas were the usual breakfasts of Llewelyn, Prince of Glamorgan, who died in his 108th year."

This herb has been extensively employed for its wound-healing properties, including instances of herpetic cold sores (Tyler, 1993).

Preparation of Extracts

The herb is usually collected near the time of flowering and dried at a low temperature. True melissa essential oil is a very rare commodity, and often an adulterated product of synthetic or blended source is misrepresented.

Alcoholic extracts may be employed in combination sedative preparations or, less often, on their own. However, the dried herb is most commonly infused as a tea.

Basic Science and Animal Studies

Soulimani and colleagues (1991) studied the effects on mice of a hydroalcoholic extract made from the cryogrinding of fresh leaves and the essential oil of melissa. After ip administration, melissa extract produced a reduction in "rearings" in the two-compartment test ($p < 0.005$) and a decrease in locomotor activity in a dose-dependent manner. In the staircase test, melissa also decreased rearings, but with maximum effect at a lower dose of 25 mg/kg ($p < 0.001$). The essential oil of melissa did not affect behavioral observations in the staircase test.

The melissa extract significantly decreased time of sleep induction under low-dose pentobarbital while increasing sleep time after higher dosing ($p < 0.01$). The essential oil was "inefficient" in sleep induction. The authors believed that their results supported sedative effects of the leaf extract, while refuting activity of the essential oil, which had been accepted traditionally as the responsible fraction.

Studies in Normals

None were identified.

Studies in Clinical Disease

None were identified.

Toxicity and Side Effects

None were identified in the review of many sources, including ESCOP and Commission E monographs.

Benefits

Melissa seems to be a pleasant, refreshing, inexpensive herbal tea with relaxing properties. One brand sells for $5 to $8 for 100 350 mg capsules of the herb. Melissa essential oil costs $50 for 2 ml.

Panel and Regulatory Information

ESCOP (1996-1997, p. 1) cites melissa leaf as indicated for "Tenseness, restlessness and irritability; symptomatic treatment of digestive disorders such as minor spasms."

The German Commission E (Blumenthal et al., 1998) evaluated the herb in 1984 and revised the monograph in 1990. They approved fresh or dried melissa leaf for nervous sleeping disorders and functional gastrointestinal complaints.

LINDEN:
Tilia spp. Tiliaceae

Synonyms

- Basswood
- Lime tree
- *Tiliae flos* (Latin)
- *Lindenblüten* (German)
- *Fleur de tilleul* (French)

Botany

Lindens are hardy deciduous trees of the Old and New World, attaining a height of up to 30 m. The flowers, which bloom in the spring, spreading a heavenly honey scent, are the medicinal portions of interest. *Tilia cordata* and *T. platyphyllos* are the species most frequently employed.

Phytochemistry

The flowers contain 1 percent flavonoids, including hyperoside, rutin, quercitrin, and isoquercitrin; hydroxycoumarins, including calycanthoside and aesculin; the caffeic acid derivative chlogenic acid; mucilages; and about 0.2 percent essential oil, with paraffins, citral, citronellal, limonene, nerol, 2-phenylethyl alcohol and its esters, feranil, eugenol, and farnesol (Bernasconi and Gebistorf, 1968; Bisset and Wichtl, 1994; Duke, 1985; Medical Economics Company, 1998).

History of Use

Theophrastus (1948) described the tree botanically but cited no medicinal usage. The tea has a traditional use as a diaphoretic (agent that induces perspiration).

Gerard (1931, p. 92) stated, "The floures are commended by divers against paines of the head proceeding of a cold cause, against dissinesse, the Apoplexie, and also the falling sicknesse [epilepsy]."

Culpeper (1994, p. 216) noted, "The flowers are the only parts used, and are a good cephalic and nervine, excellent for apoplexy, epilepsy, vertigo, and palpitations of the heart."

Although the flowers remain widely employed for sedative purposes in Europe, Moerman (1998) cites use of a shoot infusion of *Tilia americana* L. Tiliaceae by the Iroquois "when feeling worn out" (p. 562). Also interesting is its suggested use for developmental delay: "Decoction of the branches used as wash for babies that do not walk but should."

Preparation of Extracts

Flowers are shade dried and subsequently protected from moisture and light (Bisset and Wichtl, 1994; Foster and Tyler, 1999). Linden is a component of some mixed sedative preparations.

Basic Science and Animal Studies

Buchbauer and colleagues examined the effects of inhaled linden essential oil and its components in mice (Buchbauer, Jirovetz, and Jager, 1992). In the inhalation tests, mouse motor activity was significantly reduced by the essential oil, less by benzyl alcohol alone, and slightly more (55 percent of control) by the benzaldehyde component. After ip caffeine injection, the mice showed little change in motor activity with the essential oil, but the two components still caused a significant decrement in motor activity. Presence of the chemicals was demonstrated in blood samples by GC-MS.

Viola and colleagues (1994) studied the effects of *Tilia tomentosa* Moench Tiliaceae flowers on benzodiazepine receptors. The authors employed an ethanol/water extract in mice via ip injection. Several benzodiazepine receptor-binding ligands, including flavonoids apigenin and chrysin (as in previous examples of *Matricaria recutita* and *Passiflora coerulea* respectively), were identified. Kaempferol inhibited flunitrazepem binding but did not demonstrate anxiolytic effects in the elevated-plus maze. One fraction, which remained unidentified, did produce anxiolytic effects ($p < 0.05$), without signs of sedation. This fraction was believed by the authors to exert its effects in a synergistic fashion.

Studies in Normals

None were identified.

Studies in Clinical Disease

None were identified.

Toxicity and Side Effects

Grieve (1974, p. 486) states that old flowers induce "narcotic intoxication," but this is not otherwise substantiated in the literature.

No other precautions or side effects were noted upon examination of numerous sources.

Benefits

The tea of linden flowers is a pleasant beverage that may have mild sedative properties.

The essential oil, although difficult to find, may have therapeutic applications based on the previous information (see Chapter 9).

Cost

Linden flower tinctures are about $7 to $10 for 30 ml. Linden essential oil costs about $25 for 2 ml.

Panel and Regulatory Information

The German Commission E approved linden flowers in 1990 as a tea for cough and colds (Blumenthal et al., 1998) but did not comment on sedative indications.

SCULLCAP:
Scutellaria lateriflora L. Lamiaceae

Synonyms

- Blue skullcap
- Mad-dog weed
- Helmet flower

Botany

Scullcap, a perennial herb attaining 60 cm in height, flowers in the summer. It is indigenous to the United States but cultivated in Europe (Medical Economics Company, 1998).

Phytochemistry

The plant contains several monoterpenes, scutellarin, and other flavonoids, as well as essential and other oils. It is said to have sedative, anti-inflammatory, and lipid peroxidation inhibitory effects (Medical Economics Company, 1998).

History of Use

Kloss (1975, p. 313) spoke of scullcap as follows: "Is one of the best nerve tonics, often combined with others. Very quieting and soothing to the nerves of people who are easily excited. In delirium tremens will produce sleep. . . . Splendid to suppress undue sexual desire."

Grieve (1974) seems also to have been an active proponent of this herb, but the underpinnings of her enthusiasm are unclear to the author. She called it "one of the finest nervines ever discovered" (p. 724). The "mad-dog" appellation derives from "having the reputation of being a certain cure for hydrophobia" (p. 724). Tyler indicates that a Lawrence Van Derveer introduced the herb for this usage in 1773 (Foster and Tyler, 1999). Foster elaborated on this topic (Foster 1996d), indicating that 400 cases were treated over forty years with only two alleged deaths. Surely this is wishful thinking. Less than a handful of rabies survivors have ever been documented, and these have been due to fortune rather than any medical intervention. Many bites, even by rabid dogs, fail to break the skin more than superficially or to inoculate pathogenic microbes.

Despite Van Derveer's reported success, scullcap had fallen into disuse and was considered a "quack remedy" by 1820. It did enjoy a resurgence as a nervine and was included in the USP from 1863 to 1916 and in the *National Formulary* until 1947 (Foster and Tyler, 1999).

The herb remains popular in some modern circles as a tea for headache and sedation. However, as a plant native to the United States, one would expect support by indigenous authorities. Moerman (1998) does cite gastrointestinal and gynecological indications by Native Americans for *Scutellaria lateriflora,* but none that support CNS activity.

Foster (1996d, p. 16) has said of it, "scullcap is one American medicinal plant about which we know virtually nothing."

Preparation of Extracts

The three- to four-year-old herb is pulverized in June (Medical Economics Company, 1998) and used as a tea, powder, or liquid extract.

Basic Science and Animal Studies

These are quite sparse and usually relate to other species. No pertinent citations were identified.

Studies in Normals

None were identified.

Studies in Clinical Disease

None were identified.

Toxicity and Side Effects

PDR for Herbal Medicines indicates (Medical Economics Company, 1998, p. 1129), "No health hazards or side effects are known in conjunction with the proper administration of designated therapeutic dosages." However, Foster and Tyler (1999) note several cases of possible hepatotoxicity and adulteration with germander and other herbs. Quality control being lacking in the American market, extreme caution certainly seems warranted.

Benefits

Foster and Tyler (1999, pp. 350-351) provided a concise assessment: "a nearly worthless and essentially inactive plant material. . . . Deficiencies in activity, safety and quality all make scullcap a good herb to avoid." This author has no useful information that would refute this statement.

Cost

One brand sells for $7 to $10 for 100 425 mg capsules.

Panel and Regulatory Information

Neither ESCOP nor the German Commission E has deigned to evaluate this herb.

OATS:
Avena sativa L. Poaceae

Synonyms

- Wild oats
- Green oats
- *Avenae herba (recens)* (Latin)
- *Grüner Hafer* (German)
- *Herbe d'avoine* (French)

Botany

This herb is derived from the green tops of the familiar oats plant, an annual grass family member. It is native to Eurasia and North Africa. *Avena* is Latin for "oats," while *sativa* signifies "cultivated" or "sown."

Phytochemistry

The herb contains silicon dioxide, esters of silicic acid, with polyphenols and mono- and oligosaccharides, flavones, manganese, zinc, and triterpenoid saponins (Medical Economics Company, 1998).

History of Use

Oats were one of the early, domesticated grains, cultivated in northern climes since the second century B.C.E. (Bisset and Wichtl, 1994). Most of the early herbalists are mute with regard to psychotropic effects of oats. However, Hildegard von Bingen offered this account (Hildegard, 1998, p. 112): "Oats are a happy and healthy food for people who are well, furnishing them a cheerful mind and a pure, clear intellect." She added, "One who is *virgichtiget,* and from it has been made a bit mad, with a divided mind and crazy thoughts, should take a sauna bath. He should pour the water in which oats have been cooked over the hot rocks. If he does this often, he will become himself and regain his health."

Oat herb tea has taken on a folk usage as a sedative for nervous states and insomnia, without corresponding scientific verification (Bisset and Wichtl, 1994).

Preparation of Extracts

The herb consists of the fresh or dried aerial parts of the plant, including ripe, dried fruits, collected during the flowering season (Bisset and Wichtl, 1994; Medical Economics Company, 1998).

Basic Science and Animal Studies

None were noted.

Studies in Normals

None were noted.

Studies in Clinical Disease

None were noted.

Toxicity and Side Effects

Various sources confirm a lack of known side effects, aside from rare allergic reactions (Bisset and Wichtl, 1994; Blumenthal et al., 1998; Medical Economics Company, 1998).

Benefits

These are unclear based on limited available data.

Panel and Regulatory Information

The German Commission E assessed oat herb in 1987, citing uses for "acute and chronic anxiety, stress and excitation, neurasthenic and pseudoneurasthenic syndromes." However, the analysis resulted in this statement: "The effectiveness for the claimed applications is not documented." Ultimately, they asserted, "Since the effectiveness of oat herb preparations is not documented, the therapeutic administration cannot be recommended" (Blumenthal et al., 1998, pp. 355-356).

Chapter 6

Dementia and Cognitive Impairment

Dementia is an extremely common and important disorder in our aging societies. The term derives from the Latin *dementare*, "to deprive of mind," which aptly describes the attendant loss of memory, personality, and cognitive function that accompanies this process.

The herbal literature pertaining to dementia is hampered by a lack of diagnostic precision. Most earlier European articles refer to dementia as "cerebral insufficiency," a term that includes symptoms as diverse as memory loss, headache, tinnitus (ringing in the ears), senile depression, fatigue, decreased physical prowess, and other concomitants of advanced age. It might include diagnoses of Alzheimer's disease or multi-infarct dementia (MID), or, as it is currently labeled, vascular dementia. The latter are considered pathologically distinct diagnoses in the United States.

To better define these terms, vascular dementia occurs in any situation in which stroke (CVA, or cerebrovascular accident) has destroyed 100 ml, or cubic centimeters, of cerebral tissue in both hemispheres. It is actually relatively uncommon compared to the higher incidence of Alzheimer's disease.

Everyone suffers some degree of memory loss with age. If this merely consists of forgetting a word here and there, or repeating one's self from time to time, it is most likely "benign senile forgetfulness," which occurs as a function of mild cerebral atrophy (shrinkage) and milder involutional biochemical and structural changes.

When such changes are more pronounced and threaten the patient's independence and basic cognitive abilities, the more formal diagnosis of senile dementia, Alzheimer's type (SDAT) is warranted. However, this is a diagnosis of exclusion. In other words, all treatable causes of dementia must first be eliminated diagnostically. Often, this requires a complete examination by a neurologist, cerebral imaging, electroencephalography (EEG, or brain wave testing), neuropsychological test battery, and extensive blood chemistry analysis to rule out thyroid disease, syphilis, hepatic or renal disease, human immunodeficiency virus (HIV), hypovitaminosis of B_{12} or folate, and a variety of other causes.

In practice, positive results that lead to benefits on these tests are relatively rare. The author recalls one case in which a kindly old gentleman was suffering loss of mental faculties and interest in his ranch work. In the course of evaluation, we discovered low vitamin B_{12} and thyroid values in his blood tests. Both parameters were treated medically, but with no functional improvement in his status. Lacking evidence for other causes, most senile dementias prove to be secondary to SDAT.

Currently, no reliable blood tests for SDAT are available, although some are on the horizon. Alzheimer's remains a pathological diagnosis, meaning it can only be truly defined on the basis of microscopic analysis of brain tissue. Such examination reveals neurofibrillary tangles, or plaques, and deposition of amyloid, a collection of abnormal protein.

About 25 percent of cases of SDAT are familial, and certain gene markers of interest have been identified. However, the basic pathological processes are still unknown. Treatment of this ever more common scourge has been equally difficult, and even the best pharmaceutical agents work in only a small proportion of cases, and then incompletely and temporarily. Early identification and preventive treatments would seem to be high priorities, in an attempt to intervene prior to irreversible deterioration.

With this introduction aside, we can now turn to an examination of *Ginkgo biloba*, arguably the most fascinating, complex, and potentially useful herbal agent in this book.

GINKGO:
Ginkgo biloba L. Ginkgoaceae

Synonyms

- Ginkgo
- Maidenhair tree
- *Salisburia adiantifolia* (obsolete/invalid)

- *Salisburia macrophylla* (obsolete/invalid)
- *Ya chio* (Chinese)
- *Yin hsing* (Chinese)
- *Kung sun shu* (Chinese)
- *Pei-kuo* (Chinese)
- *Icho* (Japanese)
- *Ginnan* (Japanese)
- *Yin-kuo* (Japanese)

Botany

Ginkgo biloba is a deciduous, dioecious tree (one having male and female flowering structures on separate trees) reaching 40 m in height. The trees do not blossom before twenty to thirty years of age. Female trees bear fruits (technically fleshy seeds) with a pungent smell that may cause contact dermatitis reactions in sensitive individuals. The fruits harbor nuts that are edible after roasting or boiling.

The medicinal portion of importance is the leaf, which is shaped like a fan. It is botanically unique in that it lacks central ribs and cross-venation. In addition, ovules of the plant are fertilized by motile sperm cells, a feature usually seen in lower plants such as the ferns and cycads (Hirase, 1895).

Phytochemistry

On commercial plantations, ginkgo is harvested in the late spring, dried, and extracted in acetone/water with no subsequent additions. Standardized extracts are known under the names EGb 761 and LI 1370. Both represent 50:1 extracts of leaf containing 24 percent flavonoid glycosides (quercetin, kaempferol, and isorhamnetin), 6 percent terpene lactones (with 3 percent ginkgolides A, B, and C), 3 percent bilobalide (a trilactonic sesquiterpene), and ginkgolic acids less than 5 parts per million (ppm) (Medical Economics Company, 1998; Schulz, Hänsel, and Tyler, 1998).

To quote Schulz, Hänsel, and Tyler (1998, p. 41), "As with other phytomedicines, all the constituents of ginkgo extracts are assumed to contribute in their totality to the therapeutic effect." However, specific actions are known for ginkgo fractions. The flavonoids are preeminent free-radical scavengers, in that they tend to reduce oxidative reactions in cortical cell membrane lipids that are one key to age-related cerebral function deterioration. Rutin components reduce blood seepage secondary to capillary fragility (Schulz, Hänsel, and Tyler, 1998).

Zhu and colleagues (1997) have demonstrated that a *Ginkgo biloba* extract and the component ginkgolide B protected against neuronal cell death in mice in tests of glutamate-induced neurotoxicity, preventing induced elevations in calcium ion levels. Such activity would provide important neuroprotection against brain injury of diverse causes.

The ginkgolides, which have been found nowhere else in nature, inhibit platelet-activating factor (PAF). PAF is a cell membrane component that has been implicated in numerous pathological conditions. It promotes platelet aggregation and helps mediate allergic inflammation (Braquet, 1997). PAF receptors occur in brain cells, and platelet aggregation under conditions of ischemia (oxygen deficit) is mediated by that agent (Schulz, Hänsel, and Tyler, 1998).

Bilobalide reportedly protects the trees from bacterial attack (Itil and Martorano, 1995).

The flavonoid fractions reduce oxidation in cerebral neurons (Oyama et al., 1994). Another mechanism pertains to the reported ability of ginkgo extracts to affect dopaminergic function (Ramassamy et al., 1992). This group indicated that EGb 761 reduced neurotoxic effects of 1-methyl-4-phenyl-1,2,3,6-tetrahydropyridine (MPTP), an agent that induces parkinsonian degeneration in the midbrain.

Cott (1995) employed a NovaScreen to demonstrate high affinity of the crude *Ginkgo biloba* extract to $GABA_A$ and $GABA_B$, AMPA (quisqualate), kainate, and CCK_A (cholecystokinin) receptors (Cott, 1995).

Zhu and colleagues (1997) examined mechanisms of a standardized ginkgo extract, ginkgolide B, and quercetin on neurotoxicity in mice. All these components showed statistically significant activity in promotion of neuronal viability in the face of glutamate-induced injury and calcium ion toxicity. A synergism of the flavonoid quercetin with ginkgolide B was also observed.

Sasaki and colleagues (1999) have recently demonstrated an anti-convulsant effect of bilobalide by modulation of GABA neuronal transmission in mice. Oral treatment with 30 mg/kg daily for 4 days significantly boosted levels of GABA and glutamic acid decarboxy-lase, the enzyme responsible for GABA's production from gluta-mate. Observed increases in GABA function in the hippocampus may support neuroprotective effects of *Ginkgo biloba* on memory function in dementia treatment.

Winter and Timineri have suggested an effect of ginkgo on sero-tonergic systems (Winter and Timineri, 1999). In their experiment, EGb 761 was administered ip to rats in a dose of 10 mg/kg shortly before an operant conditioning task. Performance of the rats was impaired by administration of WAY-100635, a selective 5-HT1A antagonist. Results of this type lend strong credence to the concept of *Ginkgo biloba* as a multipronged tonic for various types of CNS dysfunction.

Pierre and colleagues (1999) demonstrated a neuroprotective ef-fect of EGb 761 in mice through a completed abolishment of a reduction in sodium, potassium (Na,K)-ATPase activity induced by ischemia. This mechanism would serve to prevent lipoperoxidation and other sequelae of circulatory or respiratory compromise.

History of Use

The history of ginkgo is extremely interesting, but not without controversy. Many sources claim an ancient medical lineage for this agent, but careful analysis reveals clear usage for the past 1,000 years (Li, 1956). The tree itself is truly a botanical dinosaur, or living fossil, having been present on earth for 200 million years, during which time it has remained virtually unchanged morphologi-cally. Although 200 species may have existed in the *Ginkgo* genus in the Jurassic period (Pang, Pan, and He, 1996), *Ginkgo biloba* is the sole remaining species today. Fossils of gingko occur through-out the world outside tropical areas. In the United States, one such site is the Ginkgo Petrified Forest State Park in central Washington State, near Vantage, in the Columbia River Gorge.

Ginkgo biloba also has the botanical distinction of being the only member of its own family. Quite appropriately, it provokes effusive prose, as in this quote of Albert Seward: "It appeals to the historic soul: we see it as an emblem of changelessness, a heritage from worlds too remote for our human intelligence to grasp, a tree which has in its keeping the secrets of the immeasureable past" (Seward, 1938, p. 440).

Li (1956) documented that the tree became isolated to a small reserve in the Tien Mu Shan mountains of eastern China, in the southern Anhui, in the Ningkuo and Suancheng regions. Here, it somehow escaped the ravages of the ice age that removed all other Ginkgoaceae from the Northern and Southern Hemispheres. Pang, Pan, and He (1996) indicate that several ginkgo trees estimated to exceed 3,000 years of age can be found in Shandong, Anhui, Hunan, and Sichuan provinces. However, they counted fewer than 100 trees that surpass one millennium.

The first clear appearance of ginkgo in Chinese literature was in the eleventh century in the Sung Dynasty, a time when the area south of the Yangtze River became developed. In the city of Kai-feng, ginkgo was known for its fleshy seeds, samples of which were sent to the emperor, leading to its eventual cultivation and dissemination. Its early name was *ya chio,* or duck's foot, referring to the shape of the leaves. As the seeds became popular, the name *yin hsing,* or silver apricot, came into prominence.

The first unequivocal herbal citations of ginkgo occurred in *Shih Wu Pen Ts'ao* (Edible herbal) by Li Tung-wan, and *Jih Jung Pen Ts'ao* (Herbal for daily usage) by Wu Jui, around 1289 to 1368 (Li, 1956). These pertained to the edible seed, which in excessive quantities could be toxic, especially to children. The seeds remain part of Chinese cuisine and are "believed to aid digestion and to diminish the intoxicating effects of wine" (Huh and Staba, 1990, p. 92).

Another name, *Kung Sun Shu,* or grandfather-grandson tree, points out the investment of time necessary between planting and harvest of this venerable botanical.

The famous herbal, *Pen Ts'ao Kang Mu* (Herbal of Kang Mu) by Li Shih-chen, in the sixteenth century, included ginkgo.

Ginkgo trees were probably introduced into Japan about the same time that they were spreading through China. Japanese names are *icho,* for the tree, and *ginnan,* for the fleshy seed.

The ginkgo tree was brought to Europe by Engelbert Kaempfer, a German physician, scientist, and adventurer, who first encountered it in Japan in 1690 (Kaempfer, 1712). A specimen was subsequently planted in Utrecht, Holland. Unfortunately, Kaempfer's book has never been translated into English, and remaining manuscripts in Latin are quite rare.

Subsequently, the trees spread throughout Europe and the United States, including one in west Philadelphia in 1784. It has become extremely popular as a street tree due to its unique resistance to insect pests, plant diseases, and pollution. As Li stated (1956, p. 7), "It is ironical that the oldest living species of trees is better suited to the most modern man-made habitat than almost any other tree." As a final testament, it is reported that the first green growth to appear in the spring of 1946 near the epicenter of the atomic explosion in Hiroshima were sprouts of ginkgo that grew into a normal tree (Schulz, Hänsel, and Tyler, 1998).

Early Chinese medicinals advised the leaves for afflictions of the heart and lungs. A leaf decoction was inhaled to treat cough and asthma (Huh and Staba, 1990).

It has only been in the past three decades that Western research, primarily spearheaded by the Dr. Willmar Schwabe GmbH & Co. in Germany, has developed the ginkgo extracts and their modern indications. Ginkgo was used for cardiovascular treatment in 1972 (Huh and Staba, 1990), and its employment for intermittent claudication, memory problems of aging, and other uses has followed.

Preparation of Extracts

See Phytochemistry.

Studies in Normals

A French study (Warot et al., 1991) examined single 600 mg doses of two *Ginkgo biloba* extracts versus placebo in a double-blinded fashion with twelve normal adult females. Various tests of vigilance, reaction time, memory, and self-ratings were employed to assess the extracts' effects. No changes were seen in tests of vigilance, supporting a lack of significant sedation, even at this high dose (ten times the normal single dose). Memory scores were maintained after 1 h with EGb 761 ginkgo extract but were diminished with Ginkgo brand and placebo.

An important finding reported in 1992 (Kleijnen and Knipschild, 1992a) pertained to pharmacokinetics of *Ginkgo biloba* components. The authors reported that, after oral use of EGb 761 80 mg, ginkgo flavone glycosides had a bioavailability of greater than 60 percent and elimination half-life of 2 to 4 h. Similarly, ginkgolides A and B were greater than 98 percent bioavailable, with elimination half-life of 4 to 6 h. Finally, bilobalide was 70 percent bioavailable, with a 3 h half-life. Altogether, these findings support the advisability of frequent dosing with ginkgo preparations but may not truly reflect their cognitive or other cerebral effects.

A study focusing on electroencephalographic effects of three gingko extracts was published in 1995 (Itil and Martorano, 1995). Twelve normal volunteers were studied by computerized EEG brain-mapping techniques. After 1 h, all subjects receiving EGb 761 showed increased alpha activity (the pattern of normal quiet wakefulness). This was compared to other nootropic agents (used to enhance learning) employed in dementia treatment that similarly increase alpha activity, while decreasing slow waves in the EEG associated with drowsiness or areas of abnormal brain function. Agents that affect the EEG in this manner are termed cognitive activators.

Similar findings and results were documented for EGb 761 in a French study (Luthringer, d'Arbigny, and Macher, 1995). In subacute treatment over 6 h, an increase in alpha power persisted in normal volunteers and was accompanied by a decrease in theta power, correlating with patterns of drowsiness. The authors believed this supported an enhancement of vigilance and improvement of cognitive skills by gingko.

The American group extended its observations (Itil et al., 1996) and was able to demonstrate computerized EEG changes lasting up to 7 h with single doses of EGb 761. Up to 240 mg, there was a dose-related increase in alpha power and cognitive activation.

Studies in Clinical Disease

EGb 761 was employed in a placebo-controlled, double-blind crossover study of ninety patients with "cerebrovascular insufficiency" for forty-five days (Arrigo, 1986). Improvement was measured in terms of subjective symptoms, by patients, and eight psychometric tests. The ginkgo group showed measurable improvements in memory plus reductions in complaints of headache, dizziness, and anxiety.

A group of researchers in France compared the roles of EGb 761, 160 mg per day, and memory-training exercises for three months in the function of eighty otherwise healthy, ambulatory elderly people with memory complaints (Israel et al., 1987). The group was able to demonstrate significant improvements with EGb 761 alone, a greater improvement with memory-training exercises without medication, and yet a better effect with the two modalities combined. Results were significant ($p < 0.01$ to 0.001). Sustained effects, however, were not evident in the study.

In England, fifty-eight elderly patients with cognitive impairments were enrolled in a double-blind, randomized placebo-controlled study employing 40 mg of EGb 761 three times a day for twelve weeks (Wesnes et al., 1987). (Interestingly, three patients soon dropped out of the trial due to perceived side effects of medication. Subsequently, all proved to have been on placebo!) The Crichton Geriatric Rating Scale plus a battery of computerized and pencil-and-paper tests were employed to evaluate results. By the end of the study period, improvements seen in the drug treatment group were complemented by an increase in the interest patients displayed in their daily activities. The authors offered this as evidence of the utility of EGb 761 in the early stages of dementia.

A German study (Halama, 1990) examined twenty middle-aged to elderly patients with depression refractory to drug treatment in a double-blind, randomized pilot study with EGb 761, 80 mg tid. Zung self-rated depression scales (SDS), psychometric tests, and P 300 electroencephalographic testing were combined to assess efficacy. The treatment group showed improvements in psychometrics by week eight, along with a reduction in depression and in the latency of P 300 values in the right hemisphere (assumed to represent improvement in memory processing).

Another British study examined EGb 761, 40 mg tid, in a six-month double-blind, placebo-controlled parallel group of thirty-one patients over age fifty with mild to moderate memory impairment. Drug treatment improved response on digit-copying tests and response speeds on a computerized classification task compared to placebo.

A German study of EGb 761 in seventy-two outpatients with cerebral insufficiency in a double-blind randomized placebo-controlled protocol of twenty-four weeks (Grassel, 1992) demonstrated statistically improved short-term memory in the treatment group by six weeks and in learning rate after twenty-four weeks. The author emphasized the implication that longer treatment times are warranted in treating cognitive impairment with ginkgo.

In 1992, Kleijnen and Knipschild (1992b) reviewed the existing studies employing ginkgo to treat cerebral insufficiency. They found forty such studies, nearly all of which had reported positive results. Only eight, however, passed their rigorous criteria to be labeled "well performed." They suggested treatment trials of at least four to six weeks. As a final nod to the results, these critics acknowledged that if faced with this disorder themselves, they both would choose to take ginkgo.

A French study examined the role of single doses of EGb 761 (320 or 600 mg) in eighteen elderly patients with "slight age-related memory impairment" (Allain et al., 1993, p. 549), using a dual-coding test measuring the speed of information processing. The study showed an improvement in the speed 1 h after treatment. They stated, "The values obtained after treatment with the ginkgo extract were closer to the values observed in young healthy subjects" (Allain et al., 1993, p. 556).

The LI 1370 ginkgo extract was employed in a 1994 study of ninety outpatients with cerebral insufficiency over twelve weeks in a double-blind protocol (Vesper and Hänsgen, 1994). Improvements were noted in the treatment groups with respect to numerous parameters: attention to tasks, visual memory, and subjective perceptions of patients' own performance. Analysis of measures after six and twelve weeks of total rating, long-term and short-term memory, concentration power, maximum stress, mental flexibility, family problems, and satisfaction revealed no overlap whatsoever between control and drug treatment groups. Controls showed stable or deteriorating values, while treated patients only demonstrated improvement, with greater improvement resulting from the longer treatment interval.

Another German study (Kanowski et al., 1996) examined 216 outpatients with SDAT or MID, using a higher dose of daily EGb 761, equivalent to 240 mg per day, divided twice a day (bid) for twenty-four weeks. Various cognitive tests were combined with the Clinical Global Impressions (CGI) scale. Therapy responders strongly favored EGb (p < 0.005). Pharmaco-EEG analysis also revealed positive changes in the treatment group.

It was not until 1997 that the first significant clinical trial of ginkgo was published in the United States (Le Bars et al., 1997). This had a significant impact when combined with the tremendous interest of the lay press in herbal treatments. This placebo-controlled double-blind study employed EGb 761, 40 mg tid, in a full-year study of 309 patients with dementia secondary to SDAT or vascular effects. A variety of cognitive function measures and caretaker evaluations were combined to measure changes. On the Alzheimer's Disease Assessment Scale—Cognitive subscale (ADAS-Cog), the EGb group was not significantly changed, whereas the control group demonstrated a significant deterioration (p = 0.006). In some disease processes, maintaining without exacerbation represents a significant victory.

On the Geriatric Evaluation by Relative's Rating Instrument (GERRI), mild improvement occurred in the EGb group, while placebo again declined (p = 0.02). Results were similar and still significant when the SDAT group was separately analyzed. A high safety profile was observed in the treatment group. One stroke and one subdural hematoma occurred in study patients, both in placebo groups.

Although this study has been criticized in some quarters (*Medical Letter,* 1998) for the fact that treatment benefits were not evident by a test called the Clinician's Global Impression of Change (CGIC), objective measures and caretakers' assessments were both positive. Perhaps that is more valid: the people responsible for care of the demented (often family members) should see benefit from the drug treatment.

Overall, the authors demonstrated cognitive changes in ginkgo-treated patients equivalent to a six-month delay in progression of the dementia. They concluded, "EGb appears to stabilize and, in an additional 20 percent of cases (vs. placebo), improve the patient's functioning for periods of 6 months to 1 year" (Le Bars et al., 1997, p. 1332). Current standard pharmaceuticals are no more impressive in treating this difficult disorder.

Finally, a 1998 study specifically targeted the issue of ginkgo efficacy with respect to Alzheimer's disease (Oken, Storzbach, and Kaye, 1998) through a retrospective review of all available clinical studies in any language. Using rigorous inclusion criteria, fifty studies were culled down to just four (Hofferberth, 1994; Kanowski et al., 1996; Le Bars et al., 1997; Wesnes et al., 1987). These contained 212 patients each in ginkgo and control groups. Pooling the data allowed a significant effect size ($p < 0.001$) that provides strong evidence of treatment benefit.

Recent reports (Emerit, Arutyunan, et al., 1995; Emerit, Oganesian, et al., 1995) have demonstrated a protective effect of EGb 761 on radiation-induced clastogenic factors in workers exposed to radiation in Chernobyl. This finding raises the possibility that ginkgo would demonstrate protective effects and cognitive sparing in instances of cranial irradiation. Clinical trials of this hypothesis seem warranted.

An additional topic of interest for this book pertains to the prospects of *Ginkgo biloba* as a treatment for sexual dysfunction. Past reports hint at the benefits of ginkgo for impotence in male patients. A recent report discusses a rare complaint associated with SSRI antidepressant treatment, genital anesthesia (Ellison and DeLuca, 1998). A female patient suffered this side effect on high-dose fluoxetine (Prozac), and failed ameliorative attempts with the drugs cyproheptadine and yohimbine. She began taking EGb, 180 to 240 mg a day, with the fluoxetine and, within two weeks, "improved her level of desire, reestablished arousal with lubrication, and reversed the delay of her orgasms while restoring her previous level of vaginal, vulvar, and clitoral sensation" (Ellison and DeLuca, 1998, p. 199). The authors hypothesized any number of mechanisms, both circulatory and neurohumoral, that might account for this improvement.

In a subsequent open trial of ginkgo for sexual dysfunction in sixty-three patients (Cohen and Bartlik, 1998) taking SSRI antidepressants, the authors noted a 91 percent improvement in women, 76 percent in men, and 84 percent in composite. They observed,

"*Ginkgo biloba* generally had a positive effect on all 4 phases of the sexual response cycle: desire, excitement (erection and lubrication), orgasm, and resolution (afterglow)" (Cohen and Bartlik, 1998, p. 139). Inasmuch as complaints of sexual dysfunction are common on SSRIs and other pharmaceutical antidepressants, these results appear compelling. Sexual dysfunctions not attributable to anti-depressant medication are also possible and deserve scrutiny. This area is likely to generate further public excitement for *Ginkgo biloba* as the information becomes more widely available.

In summary (Squires, 1995, p. 13), "*Ginkgo biloba* has the wisdom of time locked in each leaf of this primordial tree and plays an important role, both in the prevention and treatment of many diseases."

Toxicity and Side Effects

As previously mentioned, ginkgo leaves and other plant parts contain ginkgotoxin, $4'$-O-methylpyridoxine, which has a neurotoxic, antivitamin B_6 action (Arenz et al., 1996). This is believed to be the source of a peculiar poisoning syndrome called Ginnan-sito-toxism. This has occurred sporadically in the Far East under conditions of famine when people ingested large quantities of ginkgo nuts. Convulsive seizures and even death have resulted.

It bears emphasis that small amounts of ginkgotoxin occur in leaves, but the heating of the industrial extraction process largely inactivates it. Its possible presence as a contaminant remains a compelling reason for the consumer to seek out standardized extracts corresponding to EGb 761 or LI 1370.

In recent times, a handful of reports on bleeding complications attributed to ginkgo have appeared in the literature (Matthews, 1998; Rosenblatt and Mindel, 1997; Rowin and Lewis, 1996; Vale, 1998). These occurred, variously, in a sixty-one-year-old man who had a subarachnoid hemorrhage while taking ginkgo, a seventy-year-old man on aspirin and ginkgo who developed bleeding from the iris, and a seventy-eight-year-old woman with dementia, gait problems, and heart disease on warfarin anticoagulation who developed an intracerebral hemorrhage. Although these reports received a lot of notice in medical circles and were mentioned in the *Medical Letter*'s (1998) review of ginkgo, many European scientists have downplayed any etiological association, since none was clearly proven. (In the case of subdural hematomas, increased bleeding time with ginkgo was documented [Rowin and Lewis, 1996].) However, the preparation employed was not specified beyond its dosage. No previous such reports appeared in Europe in the decades since the introduction of EGb. Such bleeding disorders do occur spontaneously in the aged, particularly in those on anticoagulation or antiplatelet therapy. One writer commented, "With the usual dose of *Ginkgo biloba,* no inhibitory effect on platelet aggregating factor can be shown. . . . I believe that there is hardly any suspicion at all that the ordinary extracts of *Ginkgo biloba* cause any form of hae-morrhage, and I am not aware of any reliable reports on increased bleeding tendency caused by them" (Skogh, 1998, pp. 1145-1146).

The question remains and deserves further study. The author would ask whether ginkgo could actually replace aspirin as a more effective and safer agent for CVA (cerebrovascular accident) and myocardial infarction prophylaxis. This would be a very worth-while investigation.

In the meantime, medical and legal constraints make it advisable for any practitioner to warn patients taking aspirin or anticoagulation drugs to exercise caution and good judgment in concomitant usage of ginkgo.

In normal usage, other side effects of ginkgo are minimal and may include gastrointestinal complaints, transient headache, or diz-ziness. The incidence in most studies has been 1 to 2 percent, considerably less than placebo.

No specific drug-herb interactions have been convincingly re-ported with *Ginkgo biloba.*

Costs/Comparison to Existing Pharmaceuticals

Studies directly comparing *Ginkgo biloba* to other nootropic agents have been few in the literature. In 1990, ginkgo was tested against dihydroergotoxine (Gerhardt, Rogalla, and Jaeger, 1990). According to one interpretation (Kleijnen and Knipschild, 1992a), in a study of middle-aged to elderly people with the symptoms of cerebral insufficiency, both medication groups demonstrated simi-lar degrees of improvement after six weeks of treatment.

Murray (1995) noted that improvements in memory have been attributed to the nutraceutical agent phosphatidylserine, but that he rarely recommended it in comparison to ginkgo, due to a cost of $75 per month for the former supplement. EGb 761 in the United States would average $25 to $50 per month for 120 to 240 mg per day.

Recently, a group compared ginkgo to tacrine (Cognex, tetra-hydroaminoacridine), the first modern drug approved in the United States for treatment of dementia (Itil et al., 1998). That agent increases levels of acetylcholine in the brain but is hampered by gastrointestinal and other side effects that have limited its use. Clinical results have been meager and short-lived in the hands of most neurologists. This study examined the use of single doses in demented patients on the quantitative pharmaco-electroencephalo-gram (QPEEG). Both drugs produced nootropic responses, but 240 mg of EGb produced a more pronounced cognitive activation.

In 1997, the estimated cost of tacrine (Cognex) plus its required blood monitoring was approximately $5,000 per patient for the six-month trial suggested to test its utility (the drug cost itself accounts for $900 of that). In the United States, paying the highest retail price for EGb 761, at 240 mg per day, without any monitoring, the equivalent cost would be about $456 (or perhaps considerably lower). This is not very comparable. Even as a mainstream neurologist prescribing pharmaceuticals, this author found that his clientele would not choose to initiate treatment with tacrine once informed of this difference.

Subsequently, a newer, more tolerable agent, donepezil (Aricept), has been approved in the United States. Although no head-to-head studies comparing it to ginkgo have yet been published, Oken, Storzbach, and Kaye (1998) extrapolated data that suggested the clinical effect of ginkgo and donepezil would be comparable. The cost of donepezil is $131 per month. If comparative studies show equivalent efficacy, ginkgo may represent significant savings for dementia patients and their families.

In the area of sexual dysfunction, few drugs have had the splash of publicity upon their release enjoyed by Viagra (sildenafil). This has occurred despite the reports of some deaths concomitant with its use. Its cost is high, irrespective of fatalities. Assuming, for the sake of argument, a usage of three doses per week by a given individual with erectile impotence, an annual cost of about $1,200 would be projected. Costs of EGb 761, 120 to 240 mg per day, for a year in the United States would be $275 to $550. Once again, the natural method deserves a closer look.

Panel and Regulatory Information

In 1994, the German Commission E stated that the following effects of ginkgo were experimentally established (Blumenthal et al., 1998, p. 137):

- Improvement of hypoxic tolerance, particularly in the cerebral tissue
- Inhibition of the development of traumatically or toxically induced cerebral edema, and acceleration of its regression
- Reduction of retinal edema and of cellular lesions in the retina
- Inhibition in age-related reduction of muscarinergic cholino-ceptors and 2-adrenoreceptor, as well as stimulation of choline uptake in the hippocampus
- Increased memory performance and learning capacity
- Improvement in the compensation of disturbed equilibrium
- Improvement of blood flow, particularly in the region of microcirculation
- Improvement of the rheological properties of the blood
- Inactivation of toxic oxygen radicals (flavonoids)
- Antagonism of the platelet-activating factor (PAF) (ginkgolides)
- Neuroprotective effect (ginkgolides A and B, bilobalide)

Commission E approved ginkgo for use in the treatment of symptoms of dementia, whether primary degenerative (SDAT), vascular, or mixed; treatment of intermittent claudication; and vertigo and tinnitus in elderly patients.

Additional national statements with regard to *Ginkgo biloba* are likely forthcoming. See Table 6.1 for a summary of ginkgo information.

TABLE 6.1. Ginkgo Summary

What it is:

A 50:1 standardized leaf extract taken 120 to 240 mg per day divided bid/tid, useful in treatment of dementia, memory problems, intermittent claudication, vertigo and tinnitus in elderly patients, and, quite possibly, as a treatment of sexual dysfunction of multiple etiologies and traumatic and vascular brain injuries.

What it does:

Improves cerebral and peripheral blood flow, reduces damage of oxygen-free radicals, protects cerebral membrane integrity, improves alertness and memory, reduces age-related decline in muscarinic function, etc.

What it does not do:

Reverse all negative effects of aging.

What to look for:

Only standardized extracts corresponding to EGb 761 or LI 1370 are recommended. Consumers should seek preparations that will provide 120 to 240 mg of *Ginkgo biloba* extract per day, with 24 percent ginkgo flavone glycosides and 6 percent terpenoids.

Cautions:

All unnecessary exposure to ginkgotoxin should be avoided. Ginkgo should be used with caution in people on chronic aspirin or anticoagulation treatment.

Recommendations:

More extensive use of standardized preparations of *Ginkgo biloba* extract may benefit many patients in our society.

GOTU KOLA:
Centella asiatica (L.) Urban Apiaceae

Synonyms

- *Hydrocotyle asiatica*
- *Gotu kola* (Sinhalese)
- *Brahmi* (Sanskrit)
- *Mandukaparni* (Sanskrit)
- Indian pennywort (English)
- *Indischer Wassernabel* (German)

- *Tsubo-kusa* (Japanese)
- *Luei gong gen* (Chinese)
- *Tungchian* (Chinese)

Botany

Centella asiatica is a tender creeping perennial herb of South and Southeast Asia. It is also found in Madagascar and the southeastern United States. It is particularly suited to marshy sites, growing as a weed in areas up to an elevation of 600 m (Diwan and Karwande, 1991; Kartnig, 1988). It may be utilized as a cover crop.

Phytochemistry

Gotu kola contains a variety of organic acids, triterpenes, and flavonoids: asiatic acid, madacassic acid, asiaticoside, madecasso-side, brahmoside, brahminoside, terpene acetate, camphor, cineole, kaempherol, and quercetin (Anonymous, 1996a; Duke, 1985; Medical Economics Company, 1998). It also contains an essential oil with an unidentified terpene acetate (36 percent), trans-beta-farne-sine, germacrene D, beta-caryophyllene, *p*-cymol, alpha-pinene, methanol, and allyl mustard oil (Kartnig, 1988).

History of Use

Centella asiatica is truly of ancient usage. The Ayurvedic text *Sushruta Samhita,* dated 600 to 400 B.C.E., prescribes a daily regimen of prayer and expressed juice of *Manduka-parni* for three months (*Sushruta Samhita,* Volume 2, 1991, p. 524), "This would ensure a long life of a hundred years in the full vigour of retentive memory and intellectual faculties, and would impart a god-like effulgence to the complexion."

Centella asiatica is employed in many other cultures of Asia. Folk beliefs continue to the present day, particularly employment in wound healing. These nonpsychotropic uses of *Centella asiatica* have been extensively reviewed by Kartnig (1988).

This herb was a component of the herb mixture *Fo Ti Tieng,* one of the "miracle elixirs of life" leading to a purported 256-year lifespan for Li Ching Yun (Duke, 1985, p. 109).

Centella asiatica is ingested raw, cooked, or in tea in many cultures and has a reputation as a restorative for rejuvenation purposes. One preparation or another is alleged to "improve the colour of the body, youth, memory and give long life" (Nadkarni and Nadkarni, 1954, p. 664). The Konkan of India maintain that a leaf or two each morning will cure stuttering (Duke, 1985). The Lahu tribe of Thailand, Burma, and Yunnan Province of China allege (Anderson, 1993, p. 170), "if you eat *Centella asiatica* at every meal of every day for three years, then you become invulnerable. You cannot be shot, cut, or hurt in any other way." Duke (1985) does indicate that *Centella asiatica* is a rich source of potassium and B vitamins.

As with any good thing, perhaps it can be abused. Grieve (1971, p. 425) maintains, "In small doses, it acts as a stimulant, in large doses as a narcotic, causing stupor and headache and with some people vertigo and coma."

Deservedly or not, the herb has taken on a reputation in the West as a "psychic energizer." These claims are certainly not supported by a great deal of documented research.

Finally, as frequently occurs in the herbal realm, confusion has arisen with respect to common names. The "kola" part of Gotu kola has suggested synonymy with *Cola* spp., caffeine-bearing nuts of West Africa. Siegel (1976, p. 474) placed kola nut and gotu kola together as a "Smoke, tea, or capsules as stimulant." He also reported a case of a man afflicted by chronic nervousness and insomnia attributed to intake of gotu kola capsules, identified as containing powdered *Cola* spp. True gotu kola is exclusively derived from *Centella asiatica* and contains no caffeine.

Preparation of Extracts

The leaves are used fresh or sun dried. Some companies provide gotu kola in capsule form. A standardized extract reportedly contains 40 percent asiaticoside, 29 to 30 percent asiatic acid, 29 to 30 percent madecassic acid, and 1 to 2 percent madecassoside (Anonymous, 1996a), with a recommended dose of 60 to 120 mg a day.

Basic Science and Animal Studies

Ramaswamy and colleagues examined the effects of *Centella asiatica* glycosides in rodents. Intraperitoneal injections in rats reduced exploration behavior without incoordination for 12 to 18 h (Ramaswamy, Periyasamy, and Basu, 1970). In mice, at high doses, there was some antagonism of amphetamine stimulation. Hexabarbitone (hexabarbital) sleeping time was also increased. The authors postulated sedative actions via cholinergic mechanisms.

Diwan and Karwande (1991) examined the effect of an aqueous extract of *Centella asiatica* in doses up to 50 mg·kg^{-1} ip, as compared to diazepam 4 mg·kg^{-1} ip, in mice. Results indicated that the herb had a comparable effect in reducing height and frequency of spontaneous motor activity. Its antianxiety effect was said to equal that of diazepam. Its prolongation of pentabarbital (pentabarbitone) sleep time by 120 minutes, on average, was believed to support a hypnotic effect ($p < 0.001$). In the immobility swimming test of behavioral despair, *Centella asiatica*, similar to diazepam, had no effect.

Cott employed a NovaScreen to demonstrate high affinity of the crude *Centella asiatica* extract to glycine and CCK_A (cholecystokinin) receptors (Cott, 1995).

Studies in Normals

None were discovered.

Studies in Clinical Disease

Two studies from India were identified. In the first, researchers examined the effects of *Centella asiatica* in double-blind fashion on thirty institutionalized mentally retarded children without known complicating neurological or biochemical syndromes (Appa Rao, Srinivasan, and Koteswara, 1977). At the end of one year, a difference in intelligence quotient (IQ) was noted between the supplemented and placebo groups ($p < 0.05$). A similar improvement was noted in "overall general adjustment" in treated patients. After withdrawal, some loosely defined benefits were observed for several months.

Results of the second study were strikingly different. Sharma and colleagues (1985) also studied *Centella asiatica*, as a crude powder, in twelve "educable mentally retarded children" in India. After being given 100 mg/kg body weight of the powder in two divided doses per day for six months, eight of twelve children improved, and markedly so. Malin's Intelligence Scale for Indian Children scores jumped some thirty points per category, representing gains of two standard deviations ($p < 0.001$ to 0.005). Bender-Gestalt Tests improved as well ($p < 0.005$), as did Raven's Colour Progressive Matrices $p < 0.05$). If true, these results would be unprecedented in psychopharmacological history. Unfortunately, the total lack of subsequent replication studies in the intervening years make the benefits highly suspect.

Toxicity and Side Effects

Occasionally, *Centella asiatica* is implicated in cases of contact dermatitis. No other significant risks are identified (Medical Economics Company, 1998).

Benefits

Given the dearth of available information, it must be stated that benefits of this herb are quite unclear at present. Further research is recommended.

Cost

The herb is inexpensive. One brand is $7 for 100 435 mg capsules. It is easily grown in suitable locales.

Panel and Regulatory Information

None is available.

HUPERZINE:
Huperzia serrata (Thunb.) Trev.
Lycopodiaceae

Synonym

- *Lycopodium serratum* Thunb.
- *Shuangyiping* (China)

Summary

Huperzia serrata is a club moss found in China, known as *qian ceng ta,* that has been used since ancient times as an anti-inflammatory and febrifuge. Although the latter indications have not been substantiated by modern assays, the plant yields an alkaloid, huperzine A, with very marked anticholinesterase activity (Skolnick, 1997). In fact, it may be more potent and specific in its action than tacrine (Cognex), and donepezil (Aricept), which are marketed for this effect in treatment of Alzheimer's disease. Neuroprotective effects have also been claimed. One source (Tang, 1996) refers to traditional usage of *Huperzia serrata* in treatment of schizophrenia.

Most of the literature on huperzine *(Shuangyiping)* is from China, where animal studies have been performed (Zhang et al., 1994; Zhu, 1991). Subsequent study has demonstrated not only increases in acetylcholine levels in rat cortices but in levels of norepinephrine and dopamine as well (Zhu and Giacobini, 1995). Good recent reviews of huperzine are available (Patocka, 1998; Tang, 1996).

At least one clinical study in humans has been reported (Zhang et al., 1991). In the latter, fifty-six patients with multi-infarct or senile dementia were studied in double-blind fashion. Wechsler memory quotients were significantly improved after treatment with huperzine (p < 0.01). Slight dizziness was reported as a side effect in some patients.

Although huperzine is commercially available in China, it has not been found in European or American markets until recently. At least one commercial manufacturer offers huperzine in a dose of 50 µg as an additive to a *Ginkgo biloba* preparation.

Approval as a pharmaceutical is possible in the future. Home experimenters are cautioned that there is no scientific information from TCM or other data to support usage of the *Huperzia serrata* club moss itself to treat dementia, myasthenia gravis, or other diseases.

Chapter 7

Anxiety

Anxiety is, at least, an occasional emotional pitfall in all people and serves a necessary function to focus attention on an area of concern. This is reflected in the number of its synonyms: disquietude, care, trouble, apprehension, misgiving, and so forth. Unlike many of the conditions in this book, acute anxiety displays clinical signs that anyone may recognize. They are part of our fight-or-flight reaction mediated by epinephrine release ("the adrenaline was running"), producing racing heart, sweaty palms, and tremors. The theatrical portrayal of someone else's anxiety is always good for a laugh. Many comedians have made a living describing their battles with it. The accumulated angst of Woody Allen has launched a score of movies.

Anxiety as an occasional affliction is something of which we are happy to be rid, but as a chronic disorder, it may paralyze an individual. When fear and dread become focused on a specific object or thought, this is called a phobia. For example, generalized anxiety severe enough to prevent the afflicted individual from leaving the home is termed *agoraphobia* (from the Greek terms for "fear of the marketplace"). Finally, anxiety may manifest itself in discrete, incapacitating panic attacks, with attendant rapid pulse, heart palpitations, chest pressure, shortness of breath, shakiness, and other symptoms, frequently encountered in hospital emergency rooms.

Pharmacological management of chronic and acute anxiety has always been essentially synonymous with sedation. Even the alcohol that a man may drink before he finds the nerve to approach a woman will have a sedative "downside" when the "liquid courage" has taken its course.

Although antidepressants may be extremely effective in treating anxiety, the latter does not always obviously overlap with depression, and physicians frequently attempt to treat anxiety in isolation. Until recently, this has usually meant the prescription of addictive sedatives, whether barbiturates or a successive string of benzodiaz-epines, for example, Valium (diazepam). All may be effective, espe-cially on initial usage, but most display tachyphylaxis, or loss of effect, over time. More ominously, all are difficult to discontinue, reinforced by the fact that their withdrawal symptoms parallel those of anxiety itself. The vicious circle is set, and the result is that many patients end up taking these medicines chronically.

A relatively nonsedating, nonaddictive pharmaceutical agent has recently appeared on the scene, buspirone (BuSpar). Unfortunately, its benefits are too subtle in many patients, and it has no protective value in panic disorder.

Apparently, the field of treatment for anxiety is wide open. An herbal candidate that may meet many of the prerequisites of an ideal antianxiety agent is emerging on the scene in the form of kava, *Piper methysticum.*

KAVA-KAVA:
Piper methysticum Forest. f. Piperaceae

Synonyms

- *Kava* (Polynesian)
- Kava-kava
- *áva* (Hawaiian, Tahitian)
- *Awa* (Hawaiian, Tahitian)
- *Yangona* (Fijian)
- *Yanqona* (Fijian)
- *Piperis methystici rhizoma* (Latin)

Botany

Kava, or kava-kava, is a South Seas derivative of the rhizomes and rootstocks of *Piper methysticum,* or mystical pepper, from the black pepper genus, with over 2,000 species (Griffiths, 1994). Kava prefers a deep, well-drained soil, rich in humus, with a pH of 5.5 to

6.5, and it has a heavy water requirement (greater than 2,000 milli-meters [mm] annually). It prefers temperatures of 20 to 35°C and relative humidity above 70 percent (Lebot, Merlin, and Lindstrom, 1997). It grows best at altitudes of 150 to 300 m (Singh and Blumenthal, 1997) and, thus, may be absent from coral atolls.

The shrub, with its large leaves shaped similar to valentine hearts, may attain a height of 4 m, but it grows slowly and is often harvested after three to five years at a height of 2 to 2.5 m (Singh and Blumenthal, 1997; Singh, 1992). The shrub, however, may increase in mass and flavor after that time. A three-year-old plant can yield 10 kg of fresh rootstock (Lebot, Merlin, and Lindstrom, 1997).

Kava plants have a life span estimated up to fifteen to thirty years, depending on the strain (Lebot, Merlin, and Lindstrom, 1997). They are vegetatively propagated by stem nodes, sometimes in the hollowed trunk of a tree fern or in pits of decaying material. Lebot and colleagues have provided extensive coverage on the cultivation of this "pacific elixir" (Lebot, Merlin, and Lindstrom, 1997).

According to painstaking research (Lebot, 1991; Lebot, Merlin, and Lindstrom, 1997), it has been conclusively established that kava, *Piper methysticum,* represents a sterile cultivar (cultivated variety) of the species *Piper wichmannii,* which similarly prefers a shady, wet location and also contains kavalactones. The normal chromosome complement in the *Piper* genus is thirteen, whereas both *Piper methysticum* and *P. wichmannii* are decaploid, with 130 chromosomes (Lebot, Merlin, and Lindstrom, 1997).

Furthermore, oral traditions in Vanuatu indicate that *Piper wichmannii* was employed to produce the kava root beverage by island forefathers (Lebot, 1991). Although some have suspected kava originated in New Guinea, very few strains are found there, being confined largely to coastal areas (Lebot, 1991).

Although kava displays a dioecious character, with sexes on separate plants, the rare cases of successful pollination by hand led to premature flower drop. No seed production has ever been documented (Lebot, 1991).

Kava is thus reproduced from cloned plants, selected primarily due to their clinical effects, which correlate closely with kavalactone composition. Lebot (1991, p. 189) stated, "Evolutionary changes in plants involve morphological or chemical changes according to the selection pressures applied." Simply stated, kava plants whose roots produce appreciated effects are propagated, while those lacking desirable features are left to rot. The best clones are shared with family and neighbors.

Different strains may be distinguished on the basis of external appearance (morphotypes), enzyme representation (zymotypes), or chemical composition of kavapyrones (chemotypes). The latter will be considered under Phytochemistry.

Extensive research by Lebot and colleagues (Lebot and Cabalion, 1986; Lebot and Lévesque, 1989) has allowed an extremely interesting portrait of kava's natural history to emerge. Lebot identified 122 kava clones from 29 Pacific islands and were able to conclude that the northern part of Vanuatu was the origin of its dissemination. That archipelago represented 80 out of 118 known cultivars at one stage in the reckoning, and 247 kava cultivars in 82 morphotypes overall (Lebot, Merlin, and Lindstrom, 1997).

Other conclusions reached by Lebot and colleagues are summarized as follows (Lebot, 1991; Lebot, Merlin, and Lindstrom, 1997):

1. *Piper methysticum* is restricted to Pacific islands and represents a sterile cultivar of the wild form, *Piper wichmannii.* These are the sole representatives of the genus known to contain major psychoactive kavalactones.
2. Chromosome studies and enzyme homology do not support taxonomic division of *Piper methysticum* from *Piper wichmannii.* By the rules of taxonomic precedence, both could be consolidated under *Piper methysticum.*
3. Kava's genetic diversity is a direct result of human manipulation, primarily for biochemical characteristics.
4. Vanuatu is the center of kava distribution to other Pacific islands and back to New Guinea, the likely source of wild-type *Piper wichmannii.*
5. Kava may be up to 3,000 years old as a "human creation."

History of Use

As noted earlier, kava seems to have originated in the northern portion of Vanuatu, previously known as the New Hebrides, and has been in continuous use for some 3,000 years based on biochemical, linguistic, and possible archeological evidence (Lebot, 1991; Lebot, Merlin, and Lindstrom, 1997). Seafaring Polynesians progressively disseminated the shrub throughout the Pacific islands, and it is used today in Micronesian and Melanesian cultures. The etymology of kava probably relates to the Polynesian word, *ava,* denoting bitter or inebriating drink (Lebot, 1991). Origin myths relating to kava frequently contain elements of death and rebirth, or the observation of a rat or pig eating its roots, leading to the human discovery of its ability to allay unhappiness.

As pointed out by Singh and Blumenthal (1997), Oceania, besides North America, was one of the few places in the world not to have a tradition of exposure to alcoholic beverages before the era of European exploration. Unfortunately, even modern articles may falsely portray kava as a fermented product with presumptive alcohol content.

Traditionally, kava is prepared by collecting fresh rhizomes and chewing or grinding them. Dried rhizomes are also employed. The rhizome pith contains starch cells, and the chewing or grinding releases the active lipid soluble kavalactones (or kavapyrones). Many cultures specify that the chewing be performed by healthy virgin women or young men with strong teeth.

In 1616, while sailing the South Pacific in the Horne Islands (currently known as Wallis and Fortuna), Dutch explorers Jacob LeMaire and William Schouten were the first Europeans to view and document the ceremonial preparation of kava. This was captured in an etching displaying the islanders chewing the roots and spitting into a common bowl (Schouten, 1771). Schouten (1771, p. 45) wrote, "They presented also their desirable drink to our people, as a thing rare and delicate, but the sight of their brewing had quenched their thirst."

The voyages of Captain Cook led to the first scientific description of kava in Tahiti by Parkinson (Parkinson, 1773). On a second voyage on the ship *Resolution,* a father and son team of German botanists, J.R. Forster and Johann Georg Adam Forster, accompanied Cook. The latter provided the first botanical description of kava and dubbed it *Piper methysticum,* or intoxicating pepper. Cook was possibly the first Westerner to actually partake of kava, on Tonga, and he recorded his observations as follows (Cook, 1955):

> The manner of Brewing or preparing the liquor is as Simple as it is disgusting to a European and is thus; several people take of the root or stem adjoining to the root and chew it into a kind of Pulp when they spit it out into a platter or other Vessel, every one into the same Vessel, when a sufficient quantity is done they mix it with a certain proportion of Water and then strean the liquor through some fiberous stuff like fine shaving and it is then fit for drinking which is always done immediately; it has a pepperish taste rather flat and insipid and intoxicating. (Volume 2, p. 236)

> . . . [they] presented to each of us a Cup of the liquor, but I was the only one who tasted of it, the manner of brewing had quenished the thirst of every one else. (Volume 2, p. 247)

The ship's surgeon on Cook's third voyage, David Samwell, offered an early medical opinion (Cook, 1955), writing that kava "has a strong bitter sickly taste peculiar to itself, it exhilerates the Spirits [and] is perfectly intoxicating tho' it partakes more of the Effects of Opium than of Spiritous Liquors, causing Drowsiness and Stupidity" (Volume 3, Part 2, p. 1035).

Use of kava has fluctuated historically among indigenous populations according to supply and the relative prohibition or license of their colonial overseers. Frequently, missionary zeal has militated against its use (especially preparation by mastication), which has resulted in its virtual disappearance from Tahiti and Hawaii. Lewin stated that, in 1924, "The missionaries did all they could to suppress the use of kava, probably not to the benefit of the natives. . . . There is no doubt whatever, that the physical and moral state of the natives has been, and is, far more damaged by the use of alcohol than by the consumption of kava" (Lewin, 1998, p. 182).

Kava has been subject to many use taboos. In the early history of Hawaii, employment of *awa* was confined to the highest social echelons, but, typically, when abundant, kava use has been democratically widespread in indigenous populations. All have used it as a convivial beverage of social relaxation, but its use has taken on ceremonial importance in matters of commerce, exchange, and celebration, as well as in the search for inspiration and medicinal benefits, particularly by the *kahunas,* or priests, of traditional Hawaiian culture, as it was their charge to maintain communication with the gods.

Lebot (1997, p. 155) noted an effect on the creative processes of Vanuatu's songwriters: "they often retire to a place in the forest that they know ancestors frequent and there cook a fowl, drink kava, and settle back to await inspiration. They hope to overhear, while drunk on kava, some ancestor singing fragments of a song they can learn and subsequently share with others."

Some societies restrict female use, often to postmenopausal women or those who have attained a certain political station.

As mentioned, the preparation of kava by mastication of the rhizome has been socially condemned by Westerners. Only certain pockets of traditional usage remain in central and southern Vanuatu and isolated parts of New Guinea (Lebot, Merlin, and Lindstrom, 1997). Pharmacologically, something may be missing. Lewin (1998) stated, "It is even said that in infusion of scraped kava in water and masticated kava are as dissimilar in their effects as currant wine and champagne."

On the island of Pentecost in Vanuatu, a lichen species of the genus *Usnea,* with its lactonic acids, may be added to kava to produce a synergy that boosts its potency (Lebot, Merlin, and Lindstrom, 1997).

Lebot (1991) has provided an excellent contemporary account of kava's effects:

> When the beverage is not too concentrated drinkers attain a state of happy unconcern, well-being and contentment. They feel relaxed and free of any physical or psychological excitement.
> . . . Drinkers remain masters of their conscience and reason.
> . . . The beverage soothes temperaments and drinkers never become angry, unpleasant, noisy or quarrelsome. Kava is considered as a means of easing moral discomfort and killing anxiety.

In many cases, it helps thought processes and solves the problems of everyday life as drinkers can talk to each other without any nervous tension. The following day, drinkers awaken in excellent shape. (pp. 182-183)

The initial result of kava drinking is a local anesthetic effect in the mucous membranes, which is followed by reductions in troubling anxiety and fatigue, which are replaced by pleasant, social feelings. One account is as follows (Lemert, 1967, p. 333):

The head is affected pleasantly; you feel friendly, not beer sentimental; you cannot hate with kava in you. Kava quiets the mind; the world gains no new color or rose tint; it fits in its place and in one easily understandable whole.

Celebrities who have taken part in traditional kava ceremonies include Queen Elizabeth, Pope John Paul II, Hillary Rodham Clinton, and Lady Bird and Lyndon Johnson. I have personally heard, however, that President Johnson merely feigned participation by touching the bowl to his lips without drinking.

The ceremonial and social use of kava is on the rise throughout Oceania. Forgotten pockets of renowned kava cultivars, such as Ko'uko'u on Kauai, Hena on Oahu, Lanakila on Maui, and Puna on Hawaii (Singh, 1992), may yet be revived. Reportedly, Lebot has recently discovered cultivars on the Big Island of Hawaii that are among the most potent extant (Richard Liebmann, personal communication).

Kava is becoming increasingly important to island economies. On Vanuatu, Lebot and colleagues noted a kava plant density of 100 plants per hectare (ha) (about 2.5 acres), with a yield of 10 kg of fresh root per plant, at $1 per kg. This would lead to a net profit of $7,000 per ha, and kava matures more rapidly than tree crops. Thirty tons are purchased from Vanuatu annually by the French pharmaceutical industry alone (Lebot, Merlin, and Lindstrom, 1997).

The *nakamals,* or kava bars, of Vanuatu, where men go to drink before the evening meal, represent an alternative to alcohol-based establishments that may serve as an example to other islanders in Oceania, and, perhaps, eventually the world at large.

Kava has been used as a sedative and antihypertensive in Europe since 1920. It appeared for a time in the *British Pharmacopeia* and the *United States Dispensatory* as a treatment for chronic urinary tract complaints secondary to gonorrhea (Lebot, Merlin, and Lindstrom, 1997). Kava was included as a recognized drug in the *National Formulary* from 1916 to 1936 (Varro E. Tyler, personal communication, 1999).

In a final aside, Siegel (1976) listed kava as having a suggested use as a smoke or tea, as a marijuana substitute, and reported mild hallucinogenic effects. There is no substantiation whatsoever for such usage or effects.

Phytochemistry and Basic Science Studies

The phytochemistry of kava is certainly as complex as that of other botanical psychotherapeutic agents but is almost unique, in that the identity of the molecular components, if not their mechanisms, is well known. Although alkaloids are often the point of departure in the search for active medicinal phytochemicals, none were found in kava until 1979. Pipermethystine is found in the leaves but has no role in the traditional or phytopharmacological application of kava.

Fresh kava is 80 percent water, while dried kava roots contain 43 percent starch, 20 percent fiber, 12 percent water, 3.2 percent sugars, 3.6 percent protein, 3.2 percent minerals, and 3 to 20 percent kavalactones (Lebot, Merlin, and Lindstrom, 1997).

The active components of kava root are termed kavapyrones or kavalactones. Research in this area began in the 1860s with Gobley and Cuzent, followed by Lewin in the 1890s (who did the first pharmacological experiments on kava activity and demonstrated that active components were lipid soluble), and Borsche and colleagues from 1914 to 1933. Hänsel undertook an extensive review in 1968 (Hänsel, 1968). The older literature is replete with errors, accusations, and name changes for various chemicals and is not germane in this arena.

Acceptable kava rhizomes contain 5.5 to 8.3 percent kavalactones, primarily kawain (or kavain), dihydrokawain (or dihydrokavain), and methysticin (Bone, 1993-1994). The rootstock color varies from white to dark yellow, according to the content of kavalactone-containing resin (Lebot, Merlin, and Lindstrom, 1997). A total of fifteen such chemicals have been positively identified, but six are of key interest and account for 96 percent of the content (Lebot, 1991): demethoxyyangonin (DMY = 1), dihydrokawain (DHK = 2), yangonin (Y = 3), kawain (K = 4), dihydromethysticin (DHM = 5), and methysticin (M = 6). A unique synergism of these components is observed. Clinical experimentation in the field and laboratory has allowed this statement (Lebot, 1991, p. 187): "In fact, each element is so dependent on the presence of the others that the extract used without the slightest alteration gives much better results than any single one of these substances isolated."

Kawain and methysticin, taken as synthetic drugs, are said to lack the effects of the raw extract (Lebot, Merlin, and Lindstrom, 1997).

Hänsel (1968) pointed out that alpha-pyrones (kavalactones) contain no nitrogen but behave similarly to alkaloids in some biochemical tests. In another twist on phytochemistry, he asserted, "*Kawa* pyrones appear to be precursors of flavonoids with one less acetate unit" (p. 296). Hence, we have a couple of chemical explanations for the baffling and pharmacologically unique aspects of these agents.

Physiological effects of kavalactones include potentiation of barbiturate sleep time, analgesic effects (twice as potent as acetylsalicylic acid, and one fortieth the potency of morphine [Hänsel, 1968]), local anesthetic effects (comparable to cocaine [Hänsel, 1968]), muscle relaxant effects, and antifungal activity.

Studies of Lebot and Lévesque (1989) have established the chemotypes of kava and demonstrated desirable and undesirable component ratios. These ratios are genetically determined and are generally resistant to environmental influences, although poor growth of a given clone may lead to a limited yield or crop failure.

The chemical composition analyses nicely parallel the ethnobotanical reports of kava effects. Lebot (1991) provided several examples. For instance, the 521634 cultivar is avoided by indigenous users because the most abundant chemicals, DHM and DHK, produce nausea. Interestingly, these components predominate in the wild-type *Piper wichmannii.* Similarly, the 256431 cultivar is known in the Bislama pidgin of Vanuatu as *tudei* ("two day") for its long duration of activity.

Kawain and dihydrokawain are the kavalactones that reportedly cross the blood brain barrier most easily (Lebot, Merlin, and Lindstrom, 1997).

The more desirable kava clones have low DHM content and a high percentage of kawain. The most desirable chemotypes for kava beverage are said to be 426 (kawain, yangonin, methysticin) or 642 (methysticin, kawain, yangonin), both strongly represented among the clones employed by traditional kava drinkers throughout Polynesia.

Kava produces a muscle relaxant effect, which was investigated in 1983 (Singh, 1983) in frog preparations. An extract of dried stems produced a depression of end-plate and miniature end-plate potentials, while greatly prolonging duration of both. This effect was likened to that of local anesthetics, such as cocaine. The muscle relaxant properties were believed to be due to a direct action on contractility via a reduction in postjunctional sensitivity rather than any interference with neuromuscular transmission. A protective effect against ventricular fibrillation was hypothesized.

Jamieson and colleagues (1989) compared the effects of aqueous and lipid extracts of kava and concluded that the pharmacological activity resides in the lipids. An aqueous extract containing no kavalactones given by injection did reduce spontaneous activity in mice and produced mild analgesia, but it did not have an effect on muscle tone, produce the convulsive effects of strychnine, or affect sleep tendency. Most important, the aqueous extract was essentially inactive orally. In contrast, the lipid-soluble fraction was effective orally and produced a decrease in movement, reduced motor control, and induced sleep.

It had frequently been observed that the muscle relaxant, anti-anxiety, and anticonvulsant effects of kava mirrored those of benzodiazepines. Many postulated a common mechanism of action. This hypothesis was tested by Davies and colleagues (1992) and was found wanting. Inasmuch as benzodiazepines produce effects by potentiation of gamma-aminobutyric acid (GABA), a major CNS inhibitory neurotransmitter, particular attention was directed toward kava activity on those mechanisms in rat and mouse brain tissues.

Three sets of experiments were undertaken: in vitro with synaptosomal membrane preparations, ex vivo with brain homogenates from mice pretreated with kava administration, and in vivo examinations of mice brains after kava.

The scientists confirmed that selected kavapyrones accumulated in brain tissue. $GABA_A$ receptors in the forebrain were the only sites affected at all by kava components, and only slightly. $GABA_B$ binding was unaffected. Yangonin and methysticin were most active in displacement of benzodiazepine binding in vitro, but in ex vivo experiments after injection of kavapyrones or resin, no subsequent benzodiazepine binding was observed.

Similarly, in vivo trials showed no displacement of benzodiazepine receptor ligands after administration of appropriate doses of kava resin.

One important positive feature of this study was its confirmation that "facilitated entry of pyrones in to brain occurs when administered together, (as in the crude resin) rather than individually" (Davies et al., 1992, p. 124). As to having similar mechanisms or interactions with benzodiazepines, the authors concluded that the pharmacological actions of kava components were not due to a direct effect on GABA receptors (Davies et al., 1992).

Kava has proven remarkably nontoxic. Citing a German study, Bone (1993-1994, p. 149) noted, "The LD-50 of kavalactones given by ip injection to various test animals ranged from 300-400 mg/kg. In the average human, this would range up to 28 grams of pure kavalactones."

Seitz and colleagues studied the effect of the individual kavapyrones kawain and methysticin on monoamine uptake in rat synaptosomes (Seitz, Schüle, and Gleitz, 1997). Whereas the authors cited kawain as demonstrating some ability to inhibit uptake of tritiated noradrenaline (norepinephrine), the effect was 10,000-fold less than that of the reference compound, desipramine (a tricyclic antidepressant). Thus, the likelihood of a significant clinical effect via this mechanism is remote. Similarly, neither natural kavalactone inhibited serotonin uptake to a significant degree.

Hänsel (1997-1998) has attributed to kavapyrones the action of sodium channel blockade and implicates this as a mechanism responsible for their local anesthesia and neuroprotective effects.

Schirrmacher and colleagues (1999) have recently demonstrated that the kawain component of *Piper methysticum* reduces current through voltage-activated sodium and calcium channels in rat spinal ganglia cells. The authors felt that effects on sodium channels supported anticonvulsant effects of kava, and perhaps its psychotropic actions. Similarly, kava's calcium antagonism would provide explanation of its activity in both epilepsy and anxiety.

Preparation of Extracts

Many islanders prefer fresh rhizomes as more potent than dried. Mastication produces an emulsification of kavalactone-containing resin that aids absorption. This process may be reproduced in modern times by grinding the root and employing lecithin or coconut milk as emulsifiers in preference to saliva (Lebot, Merlin, and Lindstrom, 1997).

Fresh rhizomes may be prepared for export by washing, slicing, and quickly sun drying the stump to a moisture content under 12 percent (Lebot, Merlin, and Lindstrom, 1997). Dried material may also be ground to produce an instant product, with addition of water and subsequent filtration.

Pharmaceutical extracts are produced from dried rhizomes (or inferior-quality lateral roots) concentrated 12 to 20:1 in ethanol and water to produce 30 percent kavapyrones, or in acetone and water for a 70 percent kavapyrone yield (Schulz, Hänsel, and Tyler, 1998).

Studies in Normals

Shulgin (1973) examined the effects of alpha-pyrones, individually and in combination, in human volunteers. Absorption after oral intake was very rapid for kawain and dihydrokawain and slower for methysticin and dihydromethysticin. He classified dihydromethysticin, kawain, and methysticin as major components; 5,6-dehydromethysticin, demethoxyyangonin, dihydromethysticin, flavokawin A, and yangonin as minor components; and flavokawin B, 11-methoxynoryangonin, and 11-methoxyyangonin as trace elements. Bone (1993-1994, p. 149) summarized research findings by stating, "bioavailability of lactones, as measured by peak plasma concentrations, is up to three to five times higher for the extract than when given as single substances." This synergism of kava components is a common theme in source literature.

Herberg examined the effect of a standardized extract of kava, WS 1490, 100 mg tid over eight days, in twenty adults in a placebo-controlled double-blind study to assess the effects of safety-related performance (driving and operating machinery) after administration of ethanol. This was designed to attain blood alcohol levels of 0.05 percent (below legal levels of intoxication in the United States). Ultimately, no negative effects were demonstrated in various test batteries. In fact, in a test of concentration, the WS 1490 group showed a significant advantage over the placebo group receiving only alcohol ($p < 0.01$). Thus, kava lacked deleterious effects in conjunction with low-level alcohol ingestion and may even improve attention in that condition.

Münte and colleagues (1993) compared kava extract WS 1490, 200 mg tid, to oxazepam (Serax) in a double-blind crossover study of twelve normal adults in event-related potentials (ERPs) in a word recognition task. ERPs are an elaborated electroencephalographic (EEG) technique employed, in this instance, to assess cognitive processes. In behavioral measures of reaction times, oxazepam produced slowing, while results in the kava group were not significantly different from those in the placebo group. The difference between responses in the oxazepam and kava groups was highly significant ($p < 0.001$). In the word recognition paradigm, tested electrophysiologically, reaction times and correct responses were notably reduced for oxazepam, while the actual number of correct responses in the kava-treated group actually increased. The authors stated (Münte et al., 1993, p. 52), "Thus, the behavioral indices in the word recognition paradigm suggest enhanced memory performance under kava medication and a greatly impaired performance in the oxazepam condition."

Lebot and colleagues estimate that half a coconut shell, or an estimated volume of 100 to 150 ml, of some kava varieties contains 1 to 1.5 g of resin and is sufficient to produce deep sleep in 30 min (Lebot, Merlin, and Lindstrom, 1997).

Studies in Clinical Disease

Warnecke (1991) examined kava's effects on symptoms of the female climacteric (menopause) in a randomized, placebo-controlled double-blind study of twenty patients. A standardized extract, WS 1490, 100 mg tid, was employed in the kava group. Assessment of anxiety scores (HAMA), depressive mood (DSI), severity of disease (CGI), and specific scales of menopausal symptoms and subjective assessment via diaries demonstrated a high degree of efficacy in the treatment group in the eight-week trial. Specifically, HAMA scores fell from 30 to 8 in the kava group versus from 30 to 21 in the placebo group ($p < 0.01$).

Kinzler and colleagues used the WS 1490 standardized extract in a similarly controlled trial to assess twenty-nine patients with anxiety symptoms (Kinzler, Krömer, and Lehmann, 1991). Once again, HAMA scores diverged after one week in the treated group as compared to placebo, with the difference becoming more pronounced over the four-week study. No kava side effects were noted.

An important article in German by Woelk and colleagues (1993) has been nicely summarized by Schulz, Hänsel, and Tyler (1998). In this study, 210 mg per day of kavapyrones in the form of WS 1490 were administered to patients and compared to the effects of oxazepam, 15 mg a day, and bromazepam, 9 mg a day, in a double-blind trial. After 164 trials over six weeks, symptom relief was virtually identical in the three groups, with HAMA scores falling about 10 points.

Volz (1996) examined 100 outpatients with anxiety in a randomized, placebo-controlled double-blind study over six months, employing WS 1490, 100 mg tid, corresponding to 210 mg of kavalactones per day. Patients were screened and included those with diagnoses of generalized anxiety, social phobia, or agoraphobia by DSM-III-R criteria. A HAMA score of 18 or greater was a prerequisite to entry. After twenty-four weeks of treatment, HAMA scores demonstrated a clear superiority of the kava group over the placebo group ($p < 0.0015$). Scores indicative of compulsivity and depression were also significantly benefited by kava. Volz (1996, p. 186) concluded, "This indicates that kava special extract WS 1490 can be a basic therapy for patients with anxiety disorders, and one especially useful for outpatient general medical and psychiatric practices."

Lehmann and colleagues examined an additional fifty-eight patients with anxiety in a one-month trial of standardized 70 mg tid of kavalactones versus placebo. Statistically significant differences were noted in HAMA scores, Adjectives Check List, and CGI without any adverse reactions (Lehmann, Kinzler, and Friedemann, 1996).

In an unpublished study, Singh and colleagues (1997) examined the effects of Kavatrol, a U.S. commercial preparation, in a randomized, double-blind placebo-controlled study of four weeks' duration in sixty adults. The authors stated, "Current research suggests that kava can be used in a safe and effective manner at therapeutic doses of up to 400 mg of kava-lactones per day" (p. 2). In this study, kava group patients took two capsules bid, equivalent to a daily dose of 240 mg kavalactones. Remarkable differences were noted after treatment in favor of Kavatrol, in measures of Interpersonal Problems, Personal Competency, Cognitive Stressors, Environmental Hassles, Varied Stressors, Weekly Stress Index, and State Anxiety (all $p < 0.0001$). Trait Anxiety, a parameter said to be a "fairly fixed attribute and . . . not amenable to dramatic change" (p. 9), was not significantly different in the Kavatrol and placebo groups. No one in the treatment group experienced increases in twenty-seven side effects.

Although these results may increase public acceptance of this particular product, they are scientifically difficult to assess because Kavatrol is a combination product that contains, in addition to kavalactones, a "base" of hops as well as passion flower, chamomile, and schisandra. The concentration of these other components was not specified in the article, nor is it on the packaging. The question as to whether these other components are pharmacologically relevant remains.

Lebot (1991) listed a large variety of conditions in the islands for which kava is administered as a traditional medicine. These include gonorrhea, cystitis, other urinary complaints, menstrual cramps, migraines, sleeping problems, asthma, tuberculosis, intestinal problems, and a variety of local applications for skin conditions. A great opportunity for clinical experimentation is thus available for this versatile botanical.

Readers interested in a simple review of clinical kava use may refer to Constance Grauds' *Kava and Anxiety* (1999).

Toxicity and Side Effects

Bone (1993-1994, p. 151) has stated, "Long-term use of a dose equivalent to 400 mg or more of kava lactones per day is likely to cause a scaly skin rash in some patients." This effect has been examined in detail in a superb article by Norton and Ruze (1994), which is also laden with historical treasures. Apparently, Forster, on Cook's voyage, observed this effect: "the skin dries up and exfoliates in little scales." Medically this affliction is termed *reversible ichthyosiform eruption, kava dermopathy.* According to a Tongan myth (Norton and Ruze, 1994, p. 90), "those that drink much kava become scaly like a leper just as the kava grew from the body of a leperous woman."

Kava-related skin changes are readily cured by a short period of abstinence in every report. Early observations documented that kava dermopathy leaves a smooth clear skin after the scales drop off, and some indigenous skin diseases have been successfully treated in this manner. No modern study of this effect has been undertaken (Norton and Ruze, 1994), but certainly the benefits of exfoliatives, such as tretinoin, in the treatment of acne and other dermatological afflictions suggest a promising role for kava derivatives.

The underlying pathogenesis of kava dermopathy remains obscure. Ruze (1990) hypothesized a niacin deficiency and supplemented afflicted Tongans with nicotinamide in a placebo-controlled double-blind experiment. No benefits were observed. A possible effect on cholesterol metabolism was hypothesized.

Kava skin lesions are called *kani kani* in Fiji (Lebot, 1991) and are said to be "very uncommon." To elaborate further, Singh and Blumenthal (1997) specified that its appearance was a result of daily use of kava over many months.

Mark Blumenthal, executive director of the American Botanical Council and editor of *HerbalGram* stated of "kawaism," "It occurs only when kava is consumed as a beverage; there is no evidence to date that it is associated with ingestion of alcoholic extracts of kava root, currently the most popular form sold in the United States" (1997, p. 15).

Recently, two case reports revealed allergic reactions with lymphocytic infiltration of dermis and sebaceous glands in patients taking commercial preparations of kava (Jappe et al., 1998). One had a positive lymphocyte transformation test with kava extract, and the other a positive patch test, both supporting a true allergy to kava. This study was well documented, but such reactions are notably rare.

Four cases of extrapyramidal movement disorders attributed to kava preparations have also been reported (Schelosky et al., 1995). However, two had a previous history of such reactions, one being parkinsonian and predisposed to their development by virtue of concomitant eight-year use of levodopa (L-dopa). Two of the patients had spontaneous dyskinetic movements after kava and denied use of other medications. The authors postulated that "the sedative effects of kava might result from dopamine antagonistic properties of the extracts from the *Piper methysticum* plant" (Schelosky et al., 1995, p. 640). Evidence of the latter is not apparent in the previous literature review.

On New Year's Eve 1996, some concertgoers in Los Angeles took a distributed drug called "fx." It was alleged to contain kava as a primary ingredient. Fifty people complained of dizziness, nausea, shortness of breath, and so on. Many were hospitalized. Samples were assessed by the American Botanical Council (Anonymous, 1997) and were found to contain caffeine, plus a toxic compound, 1,4-butanediol, which is catabolized in humans to gamma-hydroxybutyrate (GHB), a sedative drug. No kava whatsoever was detected. Unfortunately, this latter fact was not widely reported by the media.

A letter to the editor titled "Coma from the Health Food Store: Interaction between Kava and Alprazolam" was published by *Annals of Internal Medicine* (Almeida and Grimsley, 1996) and serves as an example of hyperbole and poor science for the sake of vindictive sensationalism. In essence, a fifty-four-year-old man was admitted in a "lethargic and disoriented state" (p. 940), (not comatose), with stable vital signs and normal laboratory parameters. Chronic medications included alprazolam (benzodiazepine), cimetidine (H_2 antagonist antihistamine), and terazosin (antihypertensive also employed to reduce bladder outlet obstruction). Apparently he had been taking store-bought kava for three days and denied taking any medication above recommended dosages. Drug screening confirmed the presence of benzodiazepines, but no effort was made to quantify levels. The patient apparently "became more alert after several hours."

The authors cited the study of Davies and colleagues (1992) as supporting that "kava might have additive effects with benzodiazepines" and that this "signals the potential for dangerous interactions between kava and prescription drugs. The growing popularity of kava increases the danger" (Almeida and Grimsley, 1996, p. 940). It requires repetition that Davies and colleagues (1992, p. 124) stated "the results [of assays] indicate that the pharmacological activity of the active components of kava are not due to direct interaction of the kava pyrones with benzodiazepine or GABA receptors." In short, the study does not support their contention of similar mechanisms for kava.

Webb has addressed the issues of this letter (Webb, 1997). She quoted Dr. Werner Busse, who observed:

> In general I gained the impression from recent publications in conventional and medical journals in the U.S. that they seem to be eagerly accepting *poorly substantiated and documented reports* about possible side effects of botanicals, whereas the same journals have been rather reluctant in the past to accept reports on the efficacy of botanicals due to "methodological drawbacks" in the study design as detected by statisticians. (p. 2)

To expound on other explanations for the observed effects, terazosin has sedative actions in its own right, and encephalopathic effects are sufficiently common with cimetidine (Tagamet) that it was almost barred from release as an over-the-counter (OTC) medicine in the United States.

Cimetidine and alprazolam compete for the cytochrome P450 metabolic pathway in the liver, and the former has been notorious for its action to potentiate alprazolam activity, including sedation. Thus, it seems eminently more likely that the chronically administered conventional drugs produced the patient's sedation, as opposed to kava usage for three days.

Unfortunately, poor science is often perpetuated. The Almeida and Grimsley report was cited in a recent review article (Heiligenstein and Guenther, 1998) as a "possible interaction." Certainly, caution is advisable, but perhaps the pendulum should swing in a manner that makes the public more suspicious of benzodiazepines and their dangers, while more inclined toward kava as an herbal alternative that is equally effective and safer.

A recent review (Winslow and Kroll, 1998) has claimed kava to be hallucinogenic, but there is no historical or chemical basis for the allegation. Once again, truth and scholarship are casualties of the conflict that conventional medical journalism has chosen to wage on rational phytotherapy.

Costs/Comparison to Existing Pharmaceuticals

Contrasts of kava with benzodiazepines have been discussed previously, and include a lower incidence of side effects, sedation, and virtual lack of known addiction potential. A head-to-head study of kava versus buspirone (BuSpar) would be interesting. The author's bias would suggest greater efficacy for kava.

Costs for benzodiazepines are about $36 per month for generic brands of alprazolam, $116 for brand-name Xanax (*Medical Letter,* 1999a), and $21 for generic diazepam (Valium). Buspirone (BuSpar), a nonbenzodiazepine agent for anxiety, costs about $109 per month (*Medical Letter,* 1999a).

Kava also compares quite favorably to alcohol as a convivial beverage of social interaction. Kava presents a much lower risk of abuse, associated accident rate, and toxicity. To quote a Hawaiian proverb (Titcomb, 1948, p. 124), "The man who drinks *áwa* is still a man, but the man who drinks liquors becomes a beast."

Panel and Regulatory Information

The German Commission E approved kava-kava in 1990 (Blumenthal et al., 1998) for conditions of nervous anxiety, stress, and restlessness. Contraindications were noted for pregnancy, nursing, and endogenous depression. Side effects were "none known," aside from those of chronic kavism. The Commission stated, "Potentiation of effectiveness is possible for substances acting on the central nervous system, such as alcohol, barbiturates and psychopharmacological agents" (Blumenthal et al., 1998, pp. 156-157). The Commission recommended duration of administration of not more than three months without medical advice.

The American Herbal Products Association (AHPA) has recommended that total consumption of kavalactones should be limited to 300 mg per day. Other suggestions included avoidance under age eighteen, when driving or operating heavy equipment, or in combination with alcohol (Anonymous, 1999). See Table 7.1 for a kava information summary.

TABLE 7.1. Kava Summary

What it is:

The rhizomes or extract from *Piper methysticum,* the "mystical pepper" of the Pacific, employed as a safe, nonaddictive antianxiety agent.

What it does:

Safely treats acute and chronic anxiety states, including social phobia, and, perhaps, panic states, without significant sedation in normal doses.

What it does not do:

Eliminate life's troubles in totality.

What to look for:

Standardized alcohol extracts, such as WS 1490, have the best record of clinical investigation and validation. Typical daily doses are 70 mg of kavalactones tid. Tincture preparations (1:2) may be taken at dosages of 3 to 6 ml per day (Bone 1993-1994). Dried roots are also available from some sources in doses up to 3 g per day but may be subject to quality control issues. Powdered extracts and tinctures present some danger of adulteration.

Cautions:

Allergic hypersensitivity reactions are possible, but rare. Although "kavism" has been observed to date only in excessive usage of kava rhizome itself, consumers should be cautious with chronic usage of any kava product, monitoring for cutaneous changes. Withdrawal from any antianxiety agent should be gradual and judicious. Usage of kava products with any other sedative substance risks additive effects.

Recommendations:

Kava is a psychotropic herb that deserves greater attention by medical providers and consumers as a safe, effective antianxiety agent.

Chapter 8

Adaptogens

The drive to feel better and boost performance is a very strong one in modern Western society. How can people enhance their status, "sharpen their edge," or "get a leg up"? The modern lexicon is filling with such phrases as more people are asking the questions.

The concept of adaptogens was popularized in the former Soviet Union after World War II, especially through the work of Lazarev and Brekhman. An adaptogen is defined, to paraphrase Foster (Foster, 1996e), as follows:

1. An adaptogen is an agent that is benign in its effects and does not impair basic functions.
2. An adaptogen displays nonspecific actions but serves to reduce stress and enhance performance in a wide array of clinical contexts.
3. An adaptogen normalizes function in either direction; that is, it will provide energy to the fatigued or calm the overanxious.

Many will recognize these properties as those of the panacea, the tonic cure-all. Traditionally, most examples have been hyperbolic, leading to eventualities such as the "snake oil" scandal of the prior century. Is there any substance to modern claims? As we shall see, positive evidence for adaptogens is modest, particularly with respect to allegations of cognitive benefits. These agents are included herein mainly for completeness, and due to their apparent popularity, rather than for their obvious scientific merit.

CHINESE GINSENG:
Panax ginseng C.A. Meyer Araliaceae

Synonyms

- Chinese ginseng
- Asian ginseng
- Korean ginseng
- *Ginseng radix* (Latin)
- *Ginsengwurzel* (German)

Botany

One of five to seven perennial herbs in the genus, *Panax ginseng* is rare in the wild. It is grown for its branching, carrot-shaped, occasionally anthropomorphic, aromatic, and mucilaginous root, with a bittersweet taste. The plant reaches 60 cm in height and has five-lobed leaves, three to five in number on a single stem, and drupaceous fruits (berries), which are red when ripe (Griffiths, 1994). It is native to eastern China. The aerial portion dies back annually. Plants flower after three to four years.

Panax derives from Greek terms for "cure-all" and, our familiar term, "panacea." The term *sêng* refers to a group of Chinese herbs with fleshy roots and tonic effects. *Ginseng* is, then, "the essence of the earth in the form of a man" (Foster, 1996b; Hu, 1976).

Hu (1977) has written an important document outlining the exacting cultural requirements of this unique tonic plant of Asia. All species of the genus prefer a cool temperate climate and dense shade of hardwood forests on north or northeast slopes with rich, damp soil. *Tilia* (linden) is an "indicator" species, whose presence in the environment supports the prospect of successful ginseng cultivation. The ginseng plant is propagated exclusively from fresh seed, preferably collected from four- to five-year-old plants. Potential growers may consult the previous reference for additional particulars on soil preparation and fertilization regimens.

Harvested plants are allowed to grow three to six years, and are then picked from August to October. A plantation may last twenty years, but then it must be left fallow for an additional ten years (Hu, 1977).

National production of ginseng in China in 1985 was 1,560.9 tons (Liu and Xiao, 1992). One author cited ginseng as being responsible for 15 to 20 percent of the $1.5 billion botanical herb market in the United States (Gillis, 1997). One million pounds were imported into the United States in 1994.

Phytochemistry

Ginseng is unusual because, although its phytochemistry is decidedly complex and represents a mixture of active ingredients, at least the identity of those agents is known. These are the ginsenosides, triterpene saponins, or glycosides of the dammaran series, representing two to three percent of the root content. The most important are Rg_1, Rc, Rd, Rb_1, Rb_2, and Rb_0 (Bisset and Wichtl, 1994). The ginsenosides (or panaxosides, in the Russian literature) are named according to their migration patterns on TLC (thin-layer chromatography). Liu and Xiao (1992) noted a total of twenty-eight ginsenosides, whose yield is often highest after four to five years of plant growth. They resemble steroids in structure.

Ginseng also contains an essential oil, 0.05 percent, with limonene, terpineol, citral, and polyacetylenes, as well as sugars, starches, and ginsenoynes (Bisset and Wichtl, 1994). Flavonoids include kaempferol, trifolin, and panaxasenoide (Liu and Xiao, 1992).

Panax ginseng root cultures provide the same ginsenosides as the native root (Ma et al., 1996). Ginsenosides Rb_1, Rc, Rg_1, Rb_2, Re, and Rd predominate.

History of Use

Ginseng, along with cannabis, is possibly the agent of most ancient vintage in this text. Both plants' use is documented in the *Pen-ts'ao-ching* of Shên-nung (the divine plowman), a Chinese emperor who, according to legend, introduced the people to 365 herbs around 2800 B.C.E. This book is perhaps the world's oldest materia medica, written in the late Han Dynasty, in the first century (Hu, 1977, p. 7). Hu's translation represents the complete citation on ginseng:

Ginseng is also called *Jen-hsien* (man gag), or *Kuei-kai* (demon's umbrella). It tastes sweetish, and its property is slightly cooling. It grows in the gorges of the mountains. It is used for repairing the five viscera, *quieting the spirit, curbing the emotion, stopping agitation, removing noxious influence, brightening the eye, enlightening the mind, and increasing the wisdom* [italics added]. Continuous use leads one to longevity with light weight.

The anthropomorphic shape of the ginseng root was very symbolic to the ancient Chinese and remains a classic example of the Doctrine of Signatures, a pan-cultural tenet of medical herbalism which purports that a plant's appearance may dictate its usage.

The plant was already rare in the wild about the time that formal cultivation became widespread 2,000 years ago. In the T'ang Dynasty of the seventh to tenth centuries, ginseng sold for its weight in silver (Hu, 1977). Then, as now, the roots of the plant were used bleached, boiled, steamed (red ginseng), or cured in sugar. The author included various prescriptions of the root as a sole agent or essential component of various compound herbal prescriptions.

The first Western account of ginseng was by Père Jartoux, a Jesuit priest, who wrote to a superior from his posting in Beijing in 1711, describing his experiences two years earlier near Korea. We will examine excerpts of this long account:

> The most eminent Physicians in *China* have writ whole Volumes upon the Virtues and Qualities of this plant. . . . They affirm, that it is a Sovereign Remedy for all Weaknesses occasion'd by excessive Fatigues either of the Body or Mind; that it dissolves Pituitous Humours; . . . that it is good against Dizziness of the Head and Dimness of Sight, and that it prolongs Life in old Age.
>
> No Body can imagine that the *Chinese* and *Tartars* would set so high a Value upon this Root, if it did not constantly produce a good Effect. Those that are in Health often make use of it to render themselves more vigorous and strong. (Jartoux, 1714, p. 238)

Simultaneously, Jartoux advanced the argument of ginseng efficacy (a variant of the current-day "One billion Chinese people cannot be wrong!") and understanding of the concept of its use as a tonic preparation.

Unlike many skittish contemporaries, Jartoux pursued a series of personal bioassays. He noted (Jartoux, 1714, pp. 238-239):

> I observed the rate of my Pulse, and then took half of the Root, raw as it was and unprepar'd: In an Hour after I found my Pulse much fuller and quicker; I had an Appetite, and found my self much more vigorous, and could bear Labour much better and easier than before. . . . But four days after, finding myself so fatigued and weary that I could scarce set on Horse back, . . . I took half of it immediately, and an Hour after I was not the least sensible of any weariness. I have often made use of it since, and always with the same success.

Hu (1976) described in detail the various preparations of ginseng: *Yuan-sêng* (cultivated ginseng), *Hung-sêng* (red ginseng), *Shêng-sai-sêng* (raw sun-dried ginseng), *T'ang-sêng* (sugared ginseng), *T'ao-p'i-sêng* (loose rind ginseng), and *Yeh-shan-sêng* (wild ginseng). In China today, ginseng is often sold in thin slices.

Indications for ginseng use remain legion: as a tonic to regain strength, improve appetite and sexual performance, alleviate nervous agitation and forgetfulness, and "quiet the spirit and give wisdom" (Hu, 1976, p. 22).

Western medicine engaged in ginseng bashing shortly after its "discovery" (Anonymous, 1898). The *Journal of the American Medical Association* noted a Western-trained Chinese physician to observe that "in his experience he has failed to observe any definite results obtained by the use of ginseng. Its use among the Chinese is entirely empiric, and its efficacy depends upon the imagination of the patient" (Anonymous, 1898, p. 1492).

Since the 1960s, ginseng has been subjected to more scientific scrutiny. The present review will focus almost exclusively on cognitive and neurochemical effects.

Preparation of Extracts

Ginseng is available in innumerable forms, including chewable lozenges, and remains popular as a root infusion. Quality control has been a critical issue: *no herb in this book is more subject to adulteration and misrepresentation than ginseng.* Ginsenoside content in many brands on the U.S. market is low to negligible (Anonymous, 1995).

High-quality standardized preparations often contain 4 to 7 percent ginsenosides. One, named G 115, is the most frequently studied. The German Commission E suggests that the root should contain at least 1.5 percent ginsenosides, calculated as Rg_1 (Blumenthal et al., 1998). Our literature review will emphasize standardized preparations as the only reasonable method of scrutinizing content of ginseng, the most complex and controversial of the phytomedicinals.

Basic Science and Animal Studies

Bulgarian researcher Petkov has made many important contributions to the ginseng literature. In a 1978 study, Petkov examined the effect of a standardized dry extract in an oral dose of 20 to 100 mg/kg for three days on learning and memory retention in rats. As compared to controls, the treated rats at the lower dosage improved in five of seven learning measures. Interestingly, performance deteriorated at the highest dose. Obviously, this implies that dosing parameters are critical to possible clinical success with this agent.

In parallel experiments, Petkov (1978) demonstrated that ip dosing of the extract at 30 mg/kg for five days produced increased levels of dopamine and norepinephrine in the brainstem, while slightly increasing serotonin content in the cerebral cortex. Transport of phenylalanine, a catecholamine precursor, across the blood brain barrier was also significantly increased.

Petkov (1978) noted an inhibitory or sedative effect on cognitive parameters of ginsenoside Rb_1, while ginsenoside Rg_1 had stimulatory actions on learning and stamina.

Nikaido and colleagues (1984) demonstrated an inhibitory effect of ginseng saponins on cyclic adenosine monophosphate (AMP) phosphodiesterase.

Tsang and colleagues (1985) posited an influence of ginsenosides on central neurotransmission, given their demonstrated effects on protein synthesis and incorporation of glucose into lipids in the CNS. An *n*-butanol extract reduced uptake of neurotransmitters in rat brain synaptosomes as follows: GABA > glutamate ≥ dopamine > norepinephrine = serotonin. Another fraction, with 80 percent ginsenoside Rd reduced neurotransmitter uptake: GABA = norepinephrine > dopamine > glutamate > serotonin. The authors offered these observations as explanations for the central effects of ginseng.

Liu and Xiao (1992) cited Rg_1 and Rb_1 as the principle nootropic agents of ginseng, able to improve memory and learning, especially in the cognitively impaired. The claimed effects included stimulation of synthesis of acetylcholine, decrease in brain serotonin, promotion of protein and nucleotide metabolism, and decreases in oxygen free radicals.

Gillis (1997) reviewed the role of ginseng in antioxidant effects linked to nitric oxide synthesis. An effect of ginseng to relax the corpus cavernosum was believed to be an explanation for purported aphrodisiacal effects.

Studies in Normals

D'Angelo and colleagues (1986) examined the effect of the standardized extract G 115, 100 mg bid, for twelve weeks in sixteen young healthy volunteers in a double-blind placebo-controlled study. A variety of psychomotor assessments were employed to assess performance effects. No side effects were reported, and a large number of screening laboratory tests remained normal during the trial. While cancellation, digit symbol substitution, tapping, and simple reaction time tests were unaffected. Choice reaction time did decrease significantly in the G 115 group ($p < 0.05$), while logical deduction similarly improved. The former, a test of attention, was the most significantly altered as compared to the control values. These results would support a very modest boost to specific mental functions in the normal population.

A variety of modern studies have supported an improvement in arterial and venous oxygen saturation of hemoglobin under the influence of G 115. Von Ardenne and Klemm (1987) demonstrated a 29 percent increase, suggestive of benefit to athletes and elderly people.

Wiklund and colleagues studied the effects of a dietary supplement containing ginseng extract G 115 versus placebo in a double-blind study of almost 400 adult volunteers over twelve weeks (Wiklund, Karlberg, and Lund, 1994). General well-being on the Psychological General Well-Being (PGWB) index test improved in both groups. Sleep was slightly improved in both as well. The ginseng group improved significantly versus placebo in alertness (p = 0.05), relaxation (p = 0.02), and overall score (p = 0.03). It was also observed that changes were most pronounced in those with the lowest baseline scores.

Bahrke and Morgan (1994) have extensively reviewed the past research of ginseng effects on athletic performance, noting many contradictory or equivocal results, frequently due to methodological and quality control issues. Some better-documented cognitive benefits of G 115 included decreases in reaction times in middle-aged adults, along with subjective improvements in vitality, concentration, sleep, and mood. They also reported on a Swedish paper in which benefits were observed in a double-blind study on spiral trace and letter cancellation tests. Their overall impression was guarded: "Although the psychotropic effect of the ginseng root has been frequently reported, there is an absence of compelling experimental evidence supporting these anecdotal observations" (Bahrke and Morgan, 1994, p. 238). Better research designs including double-blind placebo controls were suggested.

Sørensen and Sonne (1996) studied a "pure ginseng preparation" versus placebo in 112 healthy subjects over forty in a double-blind randomized trial over two months. A variety of cognitive tests were administered, but only two parameters showed significant differences. The most rapid auditory reaction times (tenth percentile) were improved over placebo (p = 0.04), while total errors on the Wisconsin Card Sorting Test (of abstractions) were reduced in the ginseng group (p = 0.02). The authors once more asserted that ginseng effects are expected to be most prominent in the ill or elderly.

The prominent and respected herbalist Amanda McQuade Crawford has stated (Collura, 1997, p. 96), "I never recommend Panax ginseng to young people. It's like giving Geritol to a toddler. But for those who are 45 and older, it can help people age more gracefully."

Studies in Clinical Disease

Unfortunately, little unequivocal information can be presented in this section. Caso Marasco and colleagues (1996), in Mexico, assessed 525 adult volunteers characterized as "known to be subject to increased physical and mental stress and/or to present fatigue symptoms" (p. 326). A vitamin-mineral complex was studied versus the same preparation including ginseng extract G 115, taken once a day. In a profound oversight, the dose of G 115 was not specified. Starting at two months, and continuing to the four-month visit, successive improvements were seen in eleven quality-of-life indices in the ginseng group ($p < 0.0001$). The authors recommended the ginseng-vitamin-mineral mixture as an effective treatment for patients experiencing physical and mental stress.

Toxicity and Side Effects

The greatest danger from ginseng preparations arises due to adulteration or misrepresented products.

The LD50 of ginseng in mice was estimated to be 10 to 30 g/kg of whole root and was attributed to gastrointestinal distention rather than pharmacological toxicity (Bahrke and Morgan, 1994). Chronic feeding of G 115 in dogs was without important deleterious observations (Hess et al., 1983).

Solely because it is so often cited in the literature, we will include mention of the "ginseng abuse syndrome" (Siegel, 1979). A variety of subjective reports of persistent heterogeneous symptoms, including hypertension, anxiety, insomnia, diarrhea, and dermatological reactions, were allegedly related to ginseng use. Subsequent authors have denounced these reports (Gillis, 1997) because huge doses of the preparation (up to 15 g per day) were employed, no placebo control was used, and, most important, the source and quality of the ginseng was not specified.

A letter to the editor in the *Journal of the American Medical Association* reported on a supposed association of ginseng with resistance to diuretic therapy in a man with renal failure (Becker et al., 1996), which the authors surmised was due to its germanium content. The preparation in question, taken in high doses, was called "Uncle Hsu's Korean Ginseng." However, once again, it seems that medical journalistic jingoism is more important than solid scholarship or good science: the alleged ginseng preparation was not assayed for ginsenosides or germanium content.

In a brief account, actually better documented than any others, Janetzky and Morreale (1997) reported on a case in which a patient on warfarin anticoagulation showed a 50 percent drop in the International Normalized Ratio (INR) while taking an extract of G 115 ginseng, at a dose 1.5 times that recommended. The laboratory abnormality abated once the patient discontinued the supplement, and no thrombosis or other adverse clinical signs supervened. Pharmaton, the manufacturers of the ginseng product, indicated no history of previous similar reports.

Rare side effects of ginseng consist of insomnia, nervousness, diarrhea, or menopausal bleeding, but only in instances of high dosage or prolonged use (Bisset and Wichtl, 1994).

The German Commission E (Blumenthal et al., 1998) indicates no contraindications, no known side effects or drug interactions, but suggests employment of ginseng for no more than ninety days continuously.

Benefits

The author has gone through many cycles of ginseng skepticism and ginseng belief. At best, it can be said that ginseng has modest, but demonstrable benefits for some cognitive and athletic measures. It is worthy of consideration for use in the aged or infirm, those wishing to aid recovery after chronic illness, or elite athletes.

Cost

Ginseng from a reliable source is expensive. Prepared supplements with specified ginsenoside content frequently cost $16 to $30 monthly in the United States.

Panel and Regulatory Information

Ginseng is not on the GRAS list in the United States (Bahrke and Morgan, 1994). That notwithstanding, the International Olympic Committee has failed to list ginseng as a banned substance for its athletes (Bahrke and Morgan, 1994).

The German Commission E published its monograph on *Panax ginseng* in 1991 and approved its use, as 1 to 2 g of root or equivalent per day, for up to three months, with repeat courses possible (Blumenthal et al., 1998). Its use is "[a]s tonic for invigoration and fortification in times of fatigue and debility, for declining capacity for work and concentration, also during convalescence" (Blumenthal et al., 1998, p. 138). See Table 8.1 for a summary of ginseng information.

TABLE 8.1. Ginseng Summary

What it is:
The prepared root or standardized extract of *Panax ginseng.*

What it does:
Modestly aids recovery and cognition in chronic illness or stress.

What it does not do:
Act as a true panacea.

What to look for:
Genuine *Panax ginseng* root, or a standardized preparation of 4 to 7 percent ginsenosides, such as extract G 115, 100 mg bid.

Cautions:
Genuine root or, better, standardized extracts should be used, not exceeding dosage guidelines, and preferably for a limit of three months at one time.

Recommendations:
The very sick or very competitive may wish to try ginseng on a trial basis.

AMERICAN GINSENG:
Panax quinquefolius L. Araliaceae

Synonyms

- Canadian ginseng
- Sang (American colloquial)

Botany

American ginseng is a hardy perennial herb of eastern North America, reaching 60 cm in height, bearing bright red fruits in summer (Griffiths, 1994). Its name means five-leaved cure-all. After five to seven years of growth, its root may be harvested. The plant is rare in its range outside of the Cumberland Gap region (Foster, 1996a) and is listed in Convention on International Trade in Endangered Species (CITES) II as endangered. It is cultivated in various areas. In the neighborhood of 1,200 metric tonnes are exported from North America to Asia annually (Li and Harries, 1996). Foster (1996a) cited the market value in 1995 as $44 million of cultivated root and $31 million of wild American ginseng. Its popularity in Asia may be attributable to its relatively sweeter taste, making it more "yin" as compared to the "yang" of Asian ginseng. It is reportedly used pharmaceutically, but also in soups and salads (Li and Harries, 1996).

The age of wild *Panax quinquefolius* can be estimated by counting leaf scars (Anderson et al., 1993).

Commercially, demand is highest for wrinkled, coarse roots of *Panax quinquefolius* that are brown on the surface yet creamy-golden internally (Reynolds, 1998b).

Phytochemistry

Similar to its Asian cousin, *Panax quinqefolius* contains ginsenosides, particularly Rb_1, Rb_2, Rb_3, Rc, Rd, Re, Rg_1, Rg_2, Ro, and F_2 (Foster, 1996a). Ginsenoside yields are reportedly higher in wild as opposed to cultivated specimens, and maximal about the fifth year of growth.

Awang (1998) indicates that Rf and Rg_2 are totally absent in American ginseng, while Rb_1, Rc, Rd, and Re predominate. Ma and colleagues (1996) found Rb_1 and Re content of up to 2 to 3 percent of dry root.

L. Bruce Reynolds (1998a, b) has recently examined the effects of drying conditions and harvest time on physical and phytochemical characteristics of *Panax quinquefolius*. Drying at 44°C lowered ginsenoside content and produced an undesirable darkening of the root. Conversely, drying at 32°C increased the ginsenoside content significantly, but only for ginsenoside Ro. Drying at 38°C seemed to yield the optimal chemical and physical results (Reynolds, 1998a).

Ginsenoside content was observed to rise from 3 percent in the first year to nearly 8 percent in the fourth (Reynolds, 1998b). Harvest in Canada in mid-August to mid-September produced roots with darker internal color but avoided the 14 percent loss in total ginsenoside content associated with November harvests.

History of Use

Native Americans apparently employed this agent extensively (Moerman, 1998). The Cherokee used it for headache, convulsions, weakness, and nervous conditions. Many saw it as a panacea, and the Iroquois smoked it. The Menominee cited it as a "strengthener of mental powers." The Meskwaki, Pawnee, and Seminole tribes employed American ginseng as love medicine. The latter tribe gave it to children to alleviate dreams of raccoons and opossums.

In a bit of botanical prescience, Père Jartoux (1714), while in China, predicted the discovery of ginseng in North America. He wrote, "if it is to be found in any other Country in the World, it may be particularly in *Canada*, where the Forests and Mountains, according to the relation of those that have lived there, very much resemble these here" (p. 376).

Another Jesuit missionary followed his lead and found American ginseng near Montreal in 1716, after a three-month search (Foster, 1996a). Samples of the roots of the plant went through a chain of command; they were sent to Jartoux, met Chinese approval, and the exportation of American ginseng began, becoming a major industry of the nineteenth century (Gibbons, 1966). However, it was never a popular medicinal agent in its own land except as a bitter stomachic. *Panax quinquefolius* was in the USP from 1842 to 1882 (Foster, 1996a).

Preparation of Extracts

Preparation is similar to that of *Panax ginseng.*

Basic Science and Animal Studies

In general, authors attribute to American ginseng properties similar to those of Asian ginseng.

Awang refers to claims in books on ginseng that support the ability of Rb_1 to increase stress resistance through enhancement of respiration via adenosine triphosphate (ATP) (Awang, 1998). Rb_1, which predominates in American ginseng, was said to suppress aggressive activity in mice and rats and, possibly, increase rates of learning.

Studies in Normals

None were identified.

Studies in Clinical Disease

None were identified.

Toxicity and Side Effects

These are assumed to be similar to those of Asian ginseng.

Benefits

American ginseng seems to be a possibly promising herbal commodity, but one that requires additional investigation in placebo-controlled double-blind trials in humans.

Cost

A couple of prominent American herbal companies sell fifty *Panax quinquefolius* capsules for $16.

Panel and Regulatory Information

None is available.

ELEUTHERO:
Eleutherococcus senticosus
Ruprecht et Maximowicz Araliaceae

Synonyms

- Siberian ginseng
- Devil's shrub
- Eleutherococ
- Wild pepper
- *Acanthopanax senticosus*
- *Hedera senticosa*
- *Eleutherococci radix* (Latin)
- *Eleutherococcus-senticosus-Wurzel* (German)
- *Ci-wu-jia* (Chinese)

Botany

Eleuthero, as most herbal cognoscenti prefer to call it, is a 1 to 3 m dioecious shrub of the mixed mountain forests of the Asian Far East, especially Siberia, Manchuria, Northern China, and Japan. Although also a member of the Araliaceae, it is not a ginseng. Furthermore, its medicinal root is woody, not fleshy, and, as such, it is not considered a *sêng* in traditional Chinese medicine (TCM) (Anonymous, 1996b; Foster, 1996e; Medical Economics Company, 1998).

Phytochemistry

A series of eleutherosides labeled A through M have been isolated from the roots of *Eleutherococcus senticosus*. Although this system intentionally resembles the nomenclature of ginsenosides, the eleutherosides are chemically heterogeneous. They include triterpene saponins, steroid glycosides, a phenylacrylic acid derivative, and lignans (epimeric diglucosides of syringaresinols) (Medical Economics Company, 1998). Also present in the roots of eleuthero are eleutheranes A through G, polysaccharides with reported immunomodulating effects.

According to the *Lawrence Review of Natural Products* (Anonymous, 1996b), eleuthero root activity decreases in July and is maximal in specimens harvested in October.

The American Botanical Council is currently employing HPLC assays to assess components of eleuthero, as is also occurring with true ginsengs.

History of Use

Eleuthero is mentioned in the *Pên-tsao Ching* of Shên-nung, much as Asian ginseng (Foster, 1996e), making its term of use at least 2,000, and perhaps up to 5,000, years. It is cited as *cu-wu-jia,* an herb of the first class. Its use in TCM is related to its supposed benefit on *qi* (vital energy, or *chi*) and its ability to alleviate "yang" deficiencies and normalize bodily functions (Foster, 1996e).

This agent was popularized in the former Soviet Union after World War II, primarily as an adaptogen. The supportive literature is in Russian but has been nicely interpreted for nonspeakers (Robbers and Tyler, 1999). Some 2,000 healthy patients were studied with respect to stressful adaptations, work capacity, and athletic performance, employing oral doses of 33 percent alcohol extracts of eleuthero for up to two months. Another 2,000 patients with chronic disease states were similarly studied. A wide variety of claims were made regarding blood sugar stabilization, immunomodulation, and response to ergogenic stress. However, such benefits have not been totally substantiated under subsequent scrutiny. In addition, the studies were not double-blinded. These possible deficiencies notwithstanding, eleuthero is reportedly still popular throughout Russia today (Foster, 1996e).

Preparation of Extracts

The root may be ground for tea, or aqueous alcohol extracts may be employed. Apparently, standardization for this agent has not occurred to any degree (Foster and Tyler, 1999).

Basic Science and Animal Studies

These are equivocal and will not be intensively reviewed. One study in mice showed increased sleep latency and duration. Another, in rats, failed to improve endurance in swimming tests or to boost longevity, but it did increase aggressive behavior (Anonymous, 1996b).

Studies in Normals

The most comprehensive studies are those just discussed, but these are methodologically suboptimal. Injections in human volunteers reportedly boosted immune function parameters (Anonymous, 1996b).

Studies in Clinical Disease

Little in the way of well-documented modern research has been performed since those studies previously discussed.

Toxicity and Side Effects

Rare cases of fatigue or drowsiness after dosing, perhaps due to a hypoglycemic effect, have been reported (Anonymous, 1996b). Many cases of supposed toxicity attributed to this agent have proven to be secondary to misidentification.

The German Commission E notes no known side effects or drug interactions but limits suggested use to three months (Blumenthal et al., 1998). The Commission does note a contraindication for patients with hypertension, based on a few case reports.

Benefits

The author believes this agent is possibly promising but requires further study. The evidence of cognitive effects is paltry.

Cost

Siberian ginseng frequently appears in combination with other ginsengs. Eleuthero may be available for under $10 for 100 capsules.

Panel and Regulatory Information

The German Commission E approved eleuthero in 1991 (Blumenthal et al., 1998, p. 124), "[a]s a tonic for invigoration and fortification in times of fatigue and debility or declining capacity for work and concentration, also during convalescence."

Chapter 9

Miscellaneous Herbal
Psychotropic Agents

DAMIANA:
Turnera diffusa Willdenow
Turneraceae

Synonyms

- *Turnerae diffusae folium* (Latin)
- *Damianablätter* (German)
- *Hierba de la pastora* (Mexican/Spanish)

Botany

Damiana is a shrub of Mexico and the arid southwestern United States, reaching a height of 0.6 to 2 m. Leaves are harvested during flowering (Lowry, 1984; Medical Economics Company, 1998).

Phytochemistry

Damiana contains triacontane, beta-sitosterol, hexacosanol-1, and 5-hydroxy-7,3′,4′-trimethoxy-flavone; an essential oil with alpha-pinene, *p*-cymene, beta-pinene, and 1,8-cineol (Domínguez and Hinojosa, 1976); tannins, resins, arbutin, and barterin (Medical Economics Company, 1998).

History of Use

Damiana may be the only herbal entry in this volume for which a therapeutic indication was merely fabricated. Although Moerman refers to other agents in the Native American pharmacopoeia as aphrodisiacs (Moerman, 1998), no entry appears for *Turnera diffusa*. Lowry (1984) submitted an extensive two-page review of the herb's history, alleging documentation of ancient use in Mexico, but close inspection reveals that the oldest documents cited were actually all of modern vintage.

Tyler indicates that damiana was introduced as an aphrodisiacal elixir in the United States by a Washington, DC, druggist in 1874 (Foster and Tyler, 1999) and was soon exposed as a fraud. If so, it is one that has been widely perpetuated. Most often, the herb appears as one part of a greater potion with alleged benefits on the lovelorn or impotent, without ever having the backing of scientific proof. Tyler quoted the famous pharmacist John Uri Lloyd, who wrote, in 1904, "Damiana is a homely, domestic remedy, innocent of the attributes under which, in American medicine, it has, for a quarter of a century, been forced to masquerade" (Foster and Tyler, 1999, p. 136).

Lloyd would probably be appalled to discover that the masquerade has continued through another century. The aphrodisiacal power of damiana remains such a common citation in herbal texts that it prompted one doctor to assert (Lowry, 1984, p. 267), "Herbal books constitute a literature somewhere halfway between witchcraft and science." He described additional "proof " of its efficacy, including one herbalist who attributed an increased "lust level" to five days' usage. Another testimonial referred to a sixty-nine-year-old male who, by virtue of two cups of damiana tea a day, attained "three orgasms a night with a young lover" (p. 267). No data were provided as to whether the damiana made this gentleman unusually fortunate as well as merely potent.

Finally, Lowry (1984, p. 268) indicated that the herb is an ingredient in a Mexican liqueur whose bottle was previously "shaped like a woman's torso, possibly for those with reading disabilities."

Siegel (1976, p. 474) reported on herbal smoking agents: "Damiana *(Turnera diffusa)* is advertised as producing a marihuana-like euphoria lasting 60 to 90 minutes, but such effects are little more than anecdotal at this time." He also listed it as a "mild stimulant."

Preparation of Extracts

No data were discovered.

Basic Science and Animal Studies

None were discovered.

Studies in Normals

None were discovered.

Studies in Clinical Disease

None were discovered.

Toxicity and Side Effects

One source noted no known side effects or hazards (Medical Economics Company, 1998). This author considers that to be wishful thinking. Past damiana admixtures have included strychnine and a variety of other toxic components. The drive to attain a perfect sexual prowess drives people (read: men) to exercise poor judgment in their choices of medicine.

Comparison to Existing Pharmaceuticals

No comparisons exist. Those seeking improvement in sexual function through herbs would be well advised to consider use of ginkgo and ginseng as safer, surer, and possibly even effective in the case of the former.

Benefits

None are proven.

Panel and Regulatory Information

The German Commission E evaluated *Turnera diffusa* in 1989 and concluded, "Since the effectiveness of Damiana preparations for the claimed applications is not documented, a therapeutic administration cannot be recommended" (Blumenthal et al., 1998, pp. 325-326).

AROMATHERAPY AND ESSENTIAL OILS

Essential oils have been mentioned frequently throughout this volume in relation to various plant components. They represent a volatile, usually highly fragrant, and often pharmacologically important fraction of medicinal herbs. Essential oils are derived from the leaf, fruit, flower, twig, bark, wood, or root, usually through distillation, but also by maceration, carbon dioxide extraction, or "phytonic process." They may also be found in the literature as ethereal oils or essences and are the *huiles essentielles* of the French.

Aromatherapy as a healing discipline was developed in France in the twentieth century, especially by Gattefossé (1993) and Valnet (Valnet and Tisserand, 1990), whose works were largely ignored in the United States until their recent translations into English. They wielded essential oils as agents for internal use and local applications as medicines. Tisserand and others have further developed this branch of healing science (Tisserand, 1977, 1988), which, in the United Kingdom and the United States, now emphasizes external use through aromatherapy massage and vaporization of essential oils.

However, even through massage, cutaneous absorption of essential oils has been demonstrated in humans and in test animals (Bronaugh et al., 1990), as has pulmonary absorption of aerosols (Buchbauer et al., 1993). Aromatherapy needs to be distinguished from *aromachology,* a term employed in the fragrance (perfume) industry, which espouses a belief that synthetically derived chemical fragrances are equally therapeutic. This is anathema to the natural preferences of aromatherapists, and, hence, the two disciplines remain at odds.

It is certain that odors have strong psychological effects. This is difficult for the author to admit, since he is prone to say, "Nothing is psychological; everything that occurs in the brain is ultimately biochemical."

Odors arise from volatile chemicals that interact with olfactory cells in the nose. They follow a straight path from the olfactory lobes into the heart of the limbic system, the seat of emotions, without previous processing through higher cognitive or rational centers. In her popular book *A Natural History of the Senses,* Diane Ackerman (1990) chose to address smell first. A few quotations should prove illustrative of the issues: "Smell is the mute sense, the one without words. . . . Smells are our dearest kin, but we cannot remember their names" (p. 6). "A smell can be overwhelmingly nostalgic because it triggers powerful images and emotions before we have time to edit them" (p. 7). In passionate prose, Ackerman explains the fecund sexuality of a flower: "We inhale its ardent aroma and, no matter what our ages, we feel young and nubile in a world aflame with desire" (p. 13). Powerful medicine, indeed, this sense that Helen Keller once termed "a fallen angel" (p. 37).

The lay literature on aromatherapy from the past decade is extensive and ranges from lively, lovely, lofty prose to an amalgamation of fatuous New Age gobbledygook. The author does not need to level additional criticism, for it has been ably done elsewhere. King (1994, pp. 411-413) has reviewed the scientific status of the field: "aromatherapy is permeated too by a certain religious feeling. Its writings are inspired by sentiments of love, peace, and gentleness. . . . Aromatherapy has the strength and attractiveness of the green movement, flower power, and religion rolled into one. . . . Aromatherapy is a shadowy world of romantic illusion, its magic easily dispelled by the harsh light of science."

However, is it really as bad as all that? The author thinks not, and he sees a great deal of promise and research opportunities for essential oils. Although it is true that unsubstantiated claims abound in some current aromatherapy literature, and that a few "studies" betray poor technique and equally poor results, as for some of the "worthless weeds" previously discussed, pharmacological verification does exist for essential oils and deserves discussion.

The following are general reviews and recent applications of aromatherapy in nursing: Cawthorn, 1995; Price, 1998; Tisserand, 1995; Tobin, 1995; Trevelyan, 1993; Trevelyan and Booth, 1994; Welsh, 1997.

Three critical reviews with a great deal of supportive scientific analysis include an article by Martin (1996), another article (Vickers, 1997), and a book (Vickers, Van Toller, and Stevensen, 1996). The latter also examines therapeutic claims of massage, which is a key component of aromatherapy in the United Kingdom and the United States, but it will not be addressed here as it is outside the scope of this book's subject. Schnaubelt's (1998) book has a more scientific focus, while Tisserand and Balacs' *Essential Oil Safety* (Tisserand and Balacs, 1995) is a treasure trove of necessary information on essential oil components, their toxicity, and proper handling. It is mandatory reading for all pursuing this modern therapeutic art.

This review will focus on the more scientific research on essential oils as psychotropics. This area of treatment, that of anxiety, insomnia, and depression, is certainly important in aromatherapy practice and is addressed at length in most current popular offerings.

As a brief survey of therapeutic claims in this area, Table 9.1 was compiled by consulting two classic sources (Gattefossé, 1993; Valnet and Tisserand, 1990), and several modern manuals of aromatherapy practice (Keville, 1996; Lawless, 1995; Tisserand, 1985). Assignation is based on frequency of citation, and particular emphasis on a given oil by an author is illustrated by italic type.

The following examination of essential oils will first address lavender, the aromatherapy superstar, and then will turn to a concise discussion of the scientific literature on other agents.

Lavender: **Lavandula angustifolia *Mill. Lamiaceae***

Synonyms

- *Lavandula vera* DC.
- *Lavandula officinalis* Chaix
- English lavender
- French lavender
- True lavender
- *Lavandulae flos* (Latin)
- *Lavande* (French)
- *Lavendelblüten* (German)

TABLE 9.1. Essential Oils for Psychotropic Usage

Anxiety	Depression	Insomnia
Highest Echelon	**Highest Echelon**	**Highest Echelon**
Cypress Lavender Marjoram	*Lavender*	Neroli
High Echelon	**High Echelon**	**High Echelon**
Bergamot Rose	*Neroli* Sandalwood Ylang-Ylang	*Chamomile, German* *Lavender* Marjoram Melissa Valerian Violet Rose
Middle Echelon	**Middle Echelon**	**Middle Echelon**
Basil *Benzoin* *Cedarwood, Atlas* *Cedarwood, Texas* Cedarwood, Virginia *Chamomile, German* *Chamomile, Roman* Cinnamon, Leaf Geranium Jasmine *Melissa* Neroli Orange, Bitter Orange, Sweet Sandalwood Thyme Violet Ylang-Ylang	Basil Borneol Chamomile, German Chamomile, Roman Geranium Grapefruit Melissa Patchouli Petitgrain *Peppermint* *Rose* *Rosemary* Sage, Clary Spruce, Hemlock Thyme	*Chamomile, Roman* *Hops* *Nutmeg* Petitgrain Sandalwood Yarrow Ylang-Ylang
Lower Echelon	**Lower Echelon**	**Lower Echelon**
Ambrette Angelica Asafetida Balsam, Canadian (?) Balsam, Copaiba Balsam, Peru Borneol	Ambrette Angelica Asafetida Balsam, Canadian (?) Cassie Cinnamon, Leaf Citronella	Asafetida Basil Bergamot Calamint Cinnamon Cloves (?) Elemi

TABLE 9.1 *(continued)*

Lower Echelon	Lower Echelon	Lower Echelon
Calamint	Coriander	Frankincense
Cananga	Cumin	Galbanum
Cardamom	Cypress	Lemon
Cassie	Elemi	*Linden*
Elemi	Eucalyptus, Blue	Mandarin
Frankincense	Eucalyptus, Peppermint	Myrrh
Galbanum	Frankincense	Orange
Helichrysum	Ginger	Perilla (?)
Hops	Helichrysum	Rosewood
Hyacinth	Hyacinth	Sage, Clary
Juniper	Lavandin	Thyme
Lemongrass	Lavender, Spike	Vanilla
Linaloe	Lemon	Vetiver
Linden	Lemongrass	
Mandarin	Marjoram	
Mimosa	Nutmeg	
Myrrh	Orange	
Opopanax	Palmarosa	
Palmarosa	Pine, Scotch	
Patchouli	Spearmint	
Peach	Tangerine	
Peppermint	Vetiver	
Petitgrain	Violet	
Pine, Scotch		
Rosemary		
Rosewood		
Sage, Clary		
Spearmint		
Spruce, Hemlock		
Storax, Levant		
Valerian		
Vetiver		

Sources: Based on information in Gattefossé, 1993; Valnet and Tisserand, 1990; Keville, 1996; Lawless, 1995; Tisserand, 1995.

Notes: Italic type indicates that a particular oil was given special emphasis by an author; question marks indicate that placement is questionable.

Botany

Lavender is a member of the mint family, from a genus of some thirty species (Griffiths, 1994). It grows as an herb to 60 cm, or as a shrub to about 2 m. Lavender is native to the Mediterranean region but has been naturalized around the world. The flowers represent the prime herbal product, and harvest occurs, optimally, as they are just opening. The species name means "narrow-leafed lavender," while the genus name, *Lavandula,* probably refers to ancient use of the herb as a bathing substitute.

Lavandula angustifolia should be distinguished from other useful species in the genus, such as *Lavandula latifolia* Medik. (or *Lavandula spica* DC.), the spike lavender, and *Lavandula intermedia,* a hybrid.

Phytochemistry

The primary components of interest derive from the essential oil, with a yield of 1 to 3 percent. This consists of linalool, linaloyl acetate, ocimene, caryophyllene, cineole, camphor, and so on, in varying proportions (Bisset and Wichtl, 1994; Medical Economics Company, 1998).

History of Use

The genus is of ancient use, but spike lavender was probably the choice of the ancient Greeks (Theophrastus, 1948). Passionate debate continues to this day as to whose national crop (French, English, or other) is superior.

Hildegard, in the twelfth century, noted lavender to be unpalatable, but of strong odor, useful as an insecticide to kill lice, stating, "It curbs very many evil things and, because of it, malign spirits are terrified" (Hildegard, 1998, p. 25).

Gerard (1931) observed its utility in treating migraine and epilepsy, with various admonitions. He continued:

> The floures of Lavander picked from the knaps, I meane the blew part and not the husk, mixed with Cinnamon, Nutmegs, [and] Cloves, made into pouder, and given to drinke in the distilled water thereof, doth helpe the panting and passion of the heart, prevaileth against giddinesse, turning, or swimming of the braine, and members subject to the palsie. (p. 147)

Culpeper's (1994, p. 210) views were similar as to its employment: "Two spoonfuls of the distilled water of the flowers help them that have lost their voice, the tremblings and passions of the heart, and fainting and swoonings."

Grieve (1974, p. 471) supported various indications of lavender essential oil: "admirably restorative and tonic against faintness of a nervous sort, weak giddiness, spasms and colic. It . . . provokes appetite, raises the spirits and dispels flatulence."

Lavender remains a fixture and workhorse of modern aromatherapy practice. Its uses are legion, making it the ginseng of essential oils. Tisserand and Lawless have both suggested its application to patients with variable moods, even bipolar illness (manic depression) (Lawless, 1994; Tisserand, 1977).

Preparation of Extracts

The flowers, once dried, are processed for herbal use or distilled to obtain the essential oil. Lavender is a component of many proprietary herbal offerings in Europe.

Basic Science and Animal Studies

In an early study, Macht and Ting (1921) examined the effect of inhaled lavender on rat maze running and observed a mild depressant effect.

Atanassova-Shopova and Roussinov (1970b) examined the effect of lavender oil in rodents. The ratios of components in essential oils are key to observed results. Theirs contained 23.4 percent linalool and 15.2 percent terpinenol. Solutions were made with the oils, saline, and Tween-80, a detergent, and these were administered ip. Anticonvulsant effects were noted. In addition, at a dose of 50 mg/kg, linalool did not alter spontaneous motor activity, while 100 mg/kg cut it in half. Amphetamine stimulation was also curtailed. Similar measures with caffeine showed minimal differences with linalool and terpinenol. The former, at a dose of 100 mg/kg, doubled hexobarbital sleep time. Both components doubled narcotic effects of alcohol. Overall, linalool and terpinenol responses paralleled those of lavender itself. The authors believed these were the active components.

In two similar studies from a team in France (Delaveau et al., 1989; Guillemain, Rousseau, and Delaveau, 1989), the authors cited the 1890 work of Cadeac and Meunier that demonstrated sedative effects of intravenous essential oil of lavender in dogs. In their own studies in rodents with oral doses, similar antianxiety and sedative effects were observed. Lavender reduced sleep latency ($p < 0.03$) and prolonged sleep duration ($p < 0.05$). The potentiation of pentobarbital sleep time by lavender abated after five days of consecutive administration. The authors believed that lavender could be characterized as "neurodepressive," and that linalool and terpinene-1-ol-4 components were primarily active.

Jirovetz and colleagues (1990) examined blood levels of lavender components in mice after inhalation. Linalool and linalyl acetate components were noted in concentrations of 1 to 12 ng/ml. The authors concluded that "the observed sedation of the test animals was a direct pharmacological effect and not only a reflectoric one" (p. 922).

Additional evidence of sedative effects of lavender were subsequently reported after experiments with inhalation in mice (Buchbauer et al., 1991). Correlation was found to linalyl acetate and linalool content; sedative effects were observed even at these single-digit ng/ml concentrations. Inhalation of these components also countered induced hyperactivity secondary to ip injection of caffeine. The research group posited a synergism of lavender essential oil components. They also commented on stimulatory effects of lavender oil that have occasionally been claimed, attributing them to a 1,8-cineole component in some lavender chemovars.

In the most comprehensive article of its type yet performed, Buchbauer and colleagues (1993) examined the sedative or stimulatory effects of forty-two essential oils and compounds in mice. Interestingly, oils were applied by vaporization, so as to mimic aromatherapy practices. Motility was assessed after 1 h of vapor exposure. Decreases in motility were observed for lavender (-78.4 percent) and its components, linalool (-73 percent) and linalyl acetate (-69.1 percent), exceeding all other compounds tested. The three also diminished caffeine overstimulation in the mice: lavender (-91.67 percent), linalool (-56.67 percent), and linalyl acetate (-46.67 percent).

The researchers also examined serum levels of essential oil compounds in the mice after exposure by GC-MS and other techniques and were able to show significant results: linalool (4.22 ng/ml) and linalyl acetate (3.43 ng/ml).

Studies in Normals

Studies of lavender in humans have been few. Ludvigson and Rottman (1989) examined the effect of vapor of lavender and cloves on various parameters in college students. As the authors stated, "the prevailing wisdom has held—and still holds in many sectors—that olfaction is primarily a curious vestige of our dim evolutionary past, a source of ephemeral pleasure or annoyance at best, and certainly of no great consequence for all that we cherish as distinctly human" (p. 525). Nevertheless, statistically relevant results emerged from their studies. Cognitive responses, especially arithmetic, were depressed in subjects first exposed to lavender (and less so to cloves), but not on a second encounter. Neither essential oil vapor had major effects on mood. Subject appreciation of the experiment was enhanced on first exposure to lavender but was diminished in those whose first session was placebo with no odorant. The authors surmised that effects were very subjective and state related, resisting simple categorization. That notwithstanding, they stated, "Lavender is relaxing, since conceivably greater relaxation could be detrimental to cognitive functioning while at the same time engendering a favorable affective reaction" (p. 534).

Lorig and Roberts (1990) examined the contingent negative variation (CNV) (an EEG measure of alertness, vigilance and expectation) of normal volunteers exposed to odors of lavender, jasmine, galbanum, and a mixture of the three oils. Results were mixed and subject to expectation factors, but they suggested that the lavender odor was arousing and distracting. Jasmine was also found to be stimulatory.

Torii and colleagues (1991) examined the effects of inhaled lavender oil in seven normal subjects on their CNV. Lavender produced relaxation and sedation, but without the reductions in reaction time or heart rate observed with benzodiazepines.

Karamat and colleagues (1992) published an abstract of experiments on ten normal subjects' reaction times. Lavender increased reaction time (sedative effect), while jasmine reduced it (stimulatory effect). No statistics were cited.

Knasko (1992) tested normal subjects and their responses to lavender and lemon essential oils, and to dimethyl sulfide, a synthetic chemical with an unpleasant odor. Tests of mood revealed an elevation in the lavender group (p = 0.02), while subjects exposed to lemon reported fewer health symptoms as compared to unscented tests (p = 0.02). No effects of any substance were observed on tests of creativity, but lavender exposure promoted fluency and originality (p < 0.01). Malodor lowered mood ratings, and intermittent exposures seemed to accentuate observed effects.

Studies in Clinical Disease

Hardy (1991) performed one of the few clinical studies of lavender effects on elderly, demented nursing home residents with sleep disorders. Four subjects received their normal medication for two weeks' observation, then no medication for two weeks, and finally were exposed to lavender vapor in the subsequent two weeks. Although no statistical analysis was performed, very significant improvements were noted in sleep duration with lavender as compared to control, and these paralleled duration with previous sedative medication. A cost savings compared to medication was also realized in the experiment.

In 1995, Flanagan reported on successful use of aromatherapy with lavender and other oils in the treatment of thirteen patients on an Alzheimer's disease ward. Unfortunately, only qualitative narrative data were presented in support of improvement.

Lindsay and colleagues (1997) compared four therapy approaches in four people with severe developmental disabilities. Their aromatherapy trial involved rubbing patients' hands with essential oils of orange flower, lemongrass, and lavender. No benefits were noted. However, the pharmacological doses of the applied oils were likely negligible and should not be taken as proof positive that more compelling application of aromatherapy techniques in the same population might not prove effective.

That same year, another group assessed the effects of lavender inhalation, massage, and nontreatment on behavior of four severely demented patients (Brooker et al., 1997). The treatments increased agitation in two patients. Only one patient showed significant improvement ($p < 0.05$), and the addition of massage (with a tiny concentration of lavender essential oil) did not offer further benefit. Few basic conclusions should be drawn from a small study of this type.

Toxicity and Side Effects

A detailed examination of the toxicology of linalool was published in 1985 (Powers and Beasley, 1985). An LD_{50} in rats was 2,790 mg/kg orally (this would be the equivalent of 195 g in a human). Toxic signs included ataxia, immobility, and respiratory depression. This essential oil component is nonsensitizing to the skin and has no mutagenic effects.

The German Commission E lists lavender as having no contraindications, side effects, or drug interactions (Blumenthal et al., 1998).

Comparison to Existing Pharmaceuticals

Lavender may have the potential to reduce reliance on sedative drugs with addictive potential, such as the benzodiazepines.

Cost

All essential oils are expensive on a per ml basis, lavender less so ($6 to $12 per 15 ml), and amounts required are very small. Lavender has proven to be very economical in most clinical applications.

Panel and Regulatory Information

Lavender attained GRAS (generally recognized as safe) status in the United States in 1965.

The German Commission E (Blumenthal et al., 1998, pp. 159-160) first ruled on lavender in 1984 and revised the findings in 1990. Its use was approved for mood disturbances, such as restlessness or insomnia, and functional abdominal complaints. Use was suggested as a tea of 1 to 2 teaspoons of herb per cup, 1 to 4 drops of essential oil (20 to 80 mg) on a sugar cube, or 20 to 100 g of herb as a bath additive. See Table 9.2 for a summary overview of lavender.

TABLE 9.2. Lavender Summary

What it is:

An essential oil employed as a vaporant, massage, or oral ingredient, or an herbal tea.

What it does:

Produces mild sedation or sleep promotion.

What it does not do:

Significantly impair motor or learning responses at low doses.

What to look for:

Dried herb or quality essential oil from a reliable source.

Cautions:

All essential oils must be handled with care, kept cool, and stored away from light and children.

Recommendations:

Lavender is an agent that deserves greater consideration as a safe sedative and sleep aid, especially in institutional settings.

Other Essential Oil Research

Animal Studies

In 1921, Macht and Ting tested maze-running effects of inhaled vapors of several substances. Results were reported qualitatively. Distinct depression was observed with valerian, and even stronger effects with asafetida (*Ferula assa-foetida* L. Apiaceae). Violet (*Viola odorata* L. Violaceae) odor produced a mixed effect, either stimulation or depression, while rose had distinct sedative effects.

Valnet and Tisserand (1990) reviewed the remaining early history of experiments with essential oils in animal nervous systems. Results relied to a large degree on autonomic responses, such as heart rate changes, and are difficult to interpret in terms of current issues. More modern studies have relied on a variety of techniques.

Atanassova-Shopova and Roussinov (1970a) examined effects in mice of clary sage (*Salvia sclarea* L. Lamiaceae) injected ip. Linalyl acetate was the primary component (55.5 percent). Large doses depressed motor responses and increased sleep times of soporific drugs.

Their oil also contained 2.4 percent thujone, a rather high amount for this component, with unusual narcotic properties. It was the main ingredient in absinthe, the banned drink of wormwood (*Artemisia absinthum* L. Asteraceae). It had been suggested that thujone might have effects on cannabinoid systems in the brain, but that has been recently disproved (Greenberg, Mellors, and McGowan, 1978; Meschler and Howlett, 1999).

The analgesic and sedative effects of frankincense, *Boswellia serrata* Roxb. Burseraceae, have been examined (Menon and Kar, 1971) by ip injection in rats. Higher doses, 300 mg/kg, produced sedation comparable to 7.5 mg/kg of chlorpromazine hydrochloride (Thorazine). Sedative effects of boswellia were partially blocked by nalorphine (an opiate antagonist), while analgesic effects were not. Secobarbitone (barbiturate) sleep times were increased by boswellia in moderate doses ($p < 0.01$) and high doses ($p < 0.001$). These results may serve to support the touted benefits of frankincense as an aid to meditation.

Binet and colleagues (1972) studied the effect of mice treated with injected essential oil components. Citronellol, farnesol, feranil, linalool, nerol, nerolidol, and rhodinol demonstrated sedative effects on motility, most pronounced with farnesol. The latter is a sesquiterpene alcohol found as a minor component of various essential oils: citronella [*Cymbopogon nardus* (L.) Rendle Poaceae], linden [*Tilia* spp.], and lemongrass [*Cymbopogon citratus* (DC. ex Nees) Stapf. Poaceae], neroli (*Citrus aurantium* L. Rutaceae), rose and petitgrain (*Citrus aurantium* var. *amara* Rutaceae) (Tisserand and Balacs, 1995).

Ludvigson and Rottman's (1989) finding that odor failed to stimulate contextual clues of memory is puzzling, perhaps undermining the wisdom of Shakespeare's Hamlet (Act IV, Verse 174): "There's rosemary, that's for remembrance . . . and there is pansies, that's for thoughts." However, rosemary (*Rosmarinus officinalis* L. Lamiaceae) was tested and found to have pharmacological stimulatory effects (Kovar et al., 1987). These authors examined the effect of rosemary oil in mice. Increases in locomotor responses were seen when rosemary essential oil was administered by vaporization or orally, and both techniques produced significant serum levels of the component 1,8-cineole.

Sedative effects have been demonstrated for the essential oil of *Calamintha sylvatica* Bromf. ssp. *ascendens* P.W. Ball (Lamiaceae) by ip injection in mice (Ortiz de Urbina et al., 1989). Doses of 0.4 to 0.6 ml/kg produced significant inhibition of locomotion, said to be comparable to the effects of chlorpromazine. Data supported that pulegone, menthone, and eucalyptol components were responsible for the sedative effect.

Jäger and colleagues (1992) studied the essential oil of neroli (bitter orange blossom, *Citrus aurantium* L. ssp. *aurantium* Rutaceae) and its components. Mice were exposed to vaporized oil, and their motility assessed: neroli reduced activity by about two-thirds, while citronellal and phenylethyl acetate components cut it in half. The effect lasted 30 min, until evaporation of the oils. Significant serum concentrations were noted for the three test substances. Citronellal is a strong component of citronella [*Cymbopogon nardus* (L.) Rendle Poaceae], *Eucalyptus citriodora* Hook. Myrtaceae, and *Melissa officinalis* essential oils (Tisserand and Balacs, 1995).

Returning to the work of Buchbauer and colleagues (1993), a large variety of essential oils and components were assessed for effects on mice after vaporization, with measurement of blood levels. Noteworthy decreases in activity were noted for the following: lavender (-78.4 percent), neroli (-65.3 percent), linalool (-73 percent), linalyl acetate (-69.1 percent), citronellal (-49.8 percent), benzaldehyde (-43.7 percent), 2-phenylethyl acetate (-45 percent), alpha-terpineol (-45 percent), and sandalwood oil (*Santalum album* L. Santalaceae) (-40 percent). Increased activity was seen for orange terpenes (+35.3 percent), thymol (+33 percent), isoborneol (+46.9 percent), and isoeugenol (+30.1 percent). Lavender, isoeugenol, linalool, maltol, carvone, and linalyl acetate reduced agitation of caffeine administration in the mice, whereas this effect was potentiated by anthranilic acid methyl ester, farnesol, linden oil, and nerol.

Interestingly, the folk use of rose oil as a sedative was not confirmed. Marguerite Maury (1989, p. 87) wrote, "But the rose procures us one thing above all: a feeling of well being, even of happiness, and the individual under its influence will develop an amiable tolerance."

Maury (1989, p. 96) also observed, "We shall see the anxiety dispelled, thanks to the benzoic. This essence creates a kind of euphoria; it interposes a padded zone between us and events." Her contention is certainly supported by the calming effects of the components of benzoin (*Styrax benzoin* Dryand Styracaceae), noted previously, on both activity and overstimulation by caffeine.

The importance of the study by Buchbauer and colleagues (1993) is threefold:

1. Confirmation of stimulatory and inhibitory effects of essential oils and components by inhalation
2. Demonstration of appropriate serum levels of essential oil components
3. Their claim of "a direct pharmacological interaction of fragrance molecules with bodily tissues and disproving the assumption of reflective interaction caused by a pleasant feeling" (p. 663)

Studies in Normals

Smith and colleagues (1971) attempted to map human cerebral responses to olfactory stimulants through EEG techniques, but this effort to produce an "olfactory evoked response" was unsuccessful. They established that certain noxious stimuli produced brain potentials, but through stimulation of the trigeminal, not olfactory, nerves.

Numerous studies have been attempted to examine the role of odorants on human memory. Results have been difficult to evaluate and indicate that set, setting, mood, and conditioning all play important roles (Ehrlichman and Halpern, 1988; Kirk-Smith, Van Toller, and Dodd, 1983; Knasko, 1993).

Steele (1984) used standard EEGs to assess the effect of essential oils. Findings included an increase in beta activity, probably denoting activation, with basil (*Ocimum basilicum* L. Lamiaceae), rosemary, black pepper, and cardamom [*Elettaria cardamomum* (L.) Maton. Zingiberaceae]. Antidepressant euphorics that promoted slower EEG rhythms included orange flower (neroli), jasmine (*Jasminum officinale* L. Oleaceae), and rose.

Warm and colleagues tested normal volunteers with respect to performance on a visual task involving sustained attention (Warm, Dember, and Parasuraman, 1990). Barely statistically significant improvements (p < 0.05) were obtained in some measures with fragrances of peppermint (*Mentha* × *piperita* L. Lamiaceae) and *muguet* (french for lily of the valley).

Warrenburg and Schwartz (1990) published an abstract examining the effects of three odorants, apple spice (synthetic), neroli, and galbanum *(Ferula galbaniflua* Boiss. & Bushe or *G. gumosa* Boiss. Apiaceae), in twenty-eight normal volunteers. Subjects that appreciated the scent of neroli were said to be more relaxed and attentive during its application.

Miyake, Nakagawa, and Asakura (1991) examined sleep latency in normals with EEG techniques. Spike lavender, sweet fennel, linden, valerian, bitter orange, and marjoram essential oils were vaporized for the tests. Only bitter orange was said to promote sleep significantly.

Nagai and colleagues (1991) assessed the effects of sweet fennel oil *(Foeniculum vulgare* Mill. Apiaceae) on mental stress and fatigue in twelve normal subjects. Vaporization reduced respiratory sinus arrhythmia component (p < 0.05) and decreased the ratio of pupillary constriction (p < 0.01). The authors felt that sweet fennel reduced parasympathetic stimulation due to stress.

As discussed previously under lavender, Lorig and Roberts (1990) examined CNV in humans with different essential oils. CNV amplitude was decreased with lavender but increased with jasmine, supporting its stimulatory effect. Similarly, Karamat and colleagues (1992), as previously discussed, examined actions of essential oils in humans. While lavender had depressant effects, jasmine decreased human reaction time and stimulated animal activity. Jasmine *(Jasminum officinale* L. Oleaceae) is widely used in aromatherapy as an antidepressant and aphrodisiac (Lawless, 1994). It is one of the most complex essential oils, with over 100 components (Lawless, 1995).

Also discussed earlier, Knasko (1992) examined effects of lemon [*Citrus limon* (L.) Burm. Rutaceae] essential oil, with positive effects on feelings of health and cleanliness.

A study of essential oils in demented patients was attempted by Mitchell (1993), using disparate methods of application of lavender and melissa oils versus control. Mild subjective improvements in behavior and communication were claimed for the oil treatments, but these would not meet modern standards of scientific investigation.

Rose and Behm (1994) reported a very different aromatherapy application, that of inhalation of vapor from essential oil of black pepper (*Piper nigrum* L. Piperaceae) to reduce cravings in smokers deprived of their cigarettes. Results compared to placebo and a mint/menthol mixture were very significant ($p < 0.01$) but were thought to relate to an irritating effect of the black pepper oil on the subjects' bronchial tree as a substitute for burning tobacco. They did not address the psychopharmacological effects of black pepper, which are prized in modern aromatherapy. Lawless (1994, p. 196) observed "The warm, penetrating odour has an intellectually stimulating effect that increases alertness, and concentration."

The beneficial uses of a variety of essential oils used to improve atmosphere and behavior in institutionalized Alzheimer's patients were reported by Flanagan (1995), without statistical analysis.

In contrast, a very compelling article from Japan in the same year documented fairly striking objective results of clinical use of lemon oil spiked with other citrus components (Komori et al., 1995). Depressed inpatients, by DSM-III-R criteria, were exposed to the citrus fragrance on a daily basis for a period of four to eleven weeks. By trial end, nine of twelve patients so exposed no longer required supplemental antidepressant medication. Hamilton Rating Scale for Depression showed no significant differences between the aromatherapy group and patients merely remaining on regular doses of standard antidepressants. Levels of urinary cortisol and dopamine were lowered by citrus fragrance, and measures of cytological immunity were also improved. The authors posited that such treatment could substitute for antidepressant administration in some patients, with few or no side effects and additional immunological benefit.

Sano and colleagues (1998) demonstrated that an essence of cedar produced sedative effects in rats and shortened the time needed to achieve deeper stages of sleep in napping humans.

Mehta and colleagues commented on the use of essential oils in anesthesia induction in children (Mehta, Stone, and Whitehead, 1998).

An Aside

Large doses of nutmeg (*Myristica fragrans* Houtt. Myristica-ceae), or its spice sister, mace, have long been known to be hallucinogenic (psychedelic/entheogenic) when ingested. Earlier studies revealed sedative and MAOI effects in rodents (Seto and Keup, 1969; Sherry and Burnett, 1978). The topic of nutmeg psychoactivity has been reviewed at length (Ott, 1996; Tisserand and Balacs, 1995). The authors of the latter book engaged in some self-experimentation with nutmeg and its essential oils. They found no support for minor component myristicin and elemicin alone producing such effects. Some additional component apart from the essential oil may be operative, and the latter certainly seems to be safe in routine clinical usage (Tisserand and Balacs, 1995).

However, the story does not end there. Ten different essential oil components merely need be aminated to produce amphetamines, those chemicals with a variety of stimulant and hallucinogenic effects. The brilliant biochemist of psychotropics Alexander Shulgin has reviewed the situation at length in his *PIHKAL: A Chemical Love Story* (Shulgin and Shulgin, 1991). Agents of the TMA (3,4,5-trimethoxyamphetamine), MDA (3,4-methylenedioxyamphetamine), and DOM (2,5,-dimethoxy-4-methylamphetamine) ("STP") series may all be synthesized from essential oil precursors (Ott, 1996). Many have speculated whether similar reactions occur in our brain de novo when we employ essential oils. Given the incredible diversity of oils and their ingredients, research opportunities abound.

Conclusions

The author hopes that the previous review will serve as some measure of scientific validation for a branch of herbal medicine that has suffered the dual difficulties of public unfamiliarity and technical underinvestigation. This area seems ripe for further development on a clinical basis. The Japanese and Europeans seem to understand this, but the field of essential oil research has been poorly funded in the United States. More studies with good methodology should assist in bringing this therapeutic modality more into the main-stream of clinical practices.

CANNABIS: A BREED APART

Cannabis sativa L. and *Cannabis indica* Lam. are most recog-nized in our society as the recreational drug called marijuana. This agent has been employed medicinally throughout much of the world for a large variety of maladies. Although the herb remains a political pariah, the trend toward "medical marijuana" has recently revealed some important secrets about our internal chemistry. One key active component of cannabis is THC, tetrahydrocannabinol, which was synthesized in the laboratory by Raphael Mechoulam in the 1960s (Mechoulam and Burstein, 1973). The question remained regarding how this unusual chemical affected the mind of man. It was not until 1993 that Devane and colleagues (1992) discovered anandamide, an endogenous cannabinoid, which revealed that mari-juana works by mimicry of our own natural chemical machinery. Though the herb has been demonized, the investigation of the can-nabinoid neuromodulatory system has resulted in monthly revela-tions about normal neurochemistry and its perturbations. Therapeu-tic breakthroughs in the treatment of nausea and weight loss in AIDS and chemotherapy patients, new knowledge about the im-mune system, control of pain, prevention of brain damage from stroke and trauma, and many other benefits are imminent as a result of these discoveries.

Anandamide activity is highest in the hippocampus, parahippo-campal cortex, thalamus, striatum, and cerebellum, suggesting, among other activities, that cannabis may modulate motor, memory, and cognitive functions (Consroe, 1998).

It has also been shown that endogenous cannabinoids and their inactive metabolites combine to enhance biochemical activities' responses (the "entourage effect") (Mechoulam and Ben-Shabat, 1999). Considering the possible contributions of other cannabis components, such as flavonoids and essential oils, to therapeutic effects on mood (reviewed in McPartland and Pruitt, 1999), one must readily assent to the following observation (Mechoulam and Ben-Shabat, 1999, p. 136):

> This type of synergism may play a role in the widely held (but not experimentally based) view that in some cases plants are better drugs than the natural products isolated from them.

The fact is that we owe these advances in basic psychopharmacology to a plant, without which the understanding of a major biochemical system that is crucial to our well-being would have eluded our grasp for a much longer period of time.

Although cannabis represents a departure from the format of examination of commercially available therapeutic psychotropic herbs, the author feels that a reexamination of its potential benefits is warranted. Furthermore, a liberalization of legislation on medical cannabis use is occurring in many countries, if most slowly in the United States. Although this discussion will necessarily be truncated, the interested reader is referred to upcoming analyses in the *Journal of Cannabis Therapeutics* (Russo, 2000). Those concerned with the dangers of cannabis usage may be reassured by the book *Marijuana Myths, Marijuana Facts* (Zimmer and Morgan, 1997) and the Institute of Medicine Report (Joy, Watson, and Benson, 1999), as well as a recent article examining cognitive function in long-term cannabis smokers (Lyketsos et al., 1999).

Let us examine the history of this most controversial agent. The first records of medicinal use of cannabis may occur in the *Pên-tsao Ching,* the Chinese herbal based on the oral traditions passed down from Emperor Shên-nung in the third millennium B.C.E., written down in the first or second centuries. It was noted that the plant fruits "if taken in excess will produce hallucinations (literally 'seeing devils')" (Li, 1974, p. 446).

The *Atharva Veda* (passage 11, 6, 15), dated to between 2000 to 1400 B.C.E., provides the first mention of cannabis as a psychotropic herb under the name *bhanga,* according to G. A. Grierson (Indian Hemp Drugs Commission, 1893-1894, Appendix 3, p. 246):

> We tell of the five kingdoms of herbs headed by Soma; may it and *kuca* grass, and *bhanga* and barley, and the herb *saha* release us from anxiety.

Use of cannabis in ancient Assyria has been claimed in numerous sources. Most notably, Campbell Thompson (Thompson, 1924, 1949) documented twenty-nine citations of cannabis in ancient Assyrian medical texts of Sumerian and Akkadian vintage (early second millennium B.C.E.), as well as psychogenic effects by various methods, including fumigation. Thompson stated (1924, p. 101):

> The evidence thus indicates a plant prescribed in AM [Assyrian manuscripts] in very small doses, used in spinning and rope-making, and at the same time a drug used to dispel depression of spirits. Obviously, it is none other than hemp, *Cannabis sativa*, L.

Campbell asserted cannabis to be "an intoxicant and drug for mental exhilaration."

Herodotus, the Greek historian (circa 450 B.C.E.), documented a funeral rite of the Scythian people. They erected tents, heated stones, and placed cannabis seeds or the flowering tops upon them to produce smoke (Herodotus, 1954, p. 95):

> for when they have parties and sit round a fire, they throw some of it into the flames, and as it burns it smokes like incense, and the smell of it makes them drunk just as wine does us; and they get more and more intoxicated as more fruit is thrown on, until they jump up and start dancing and singing.

This passage lends credence to cannabis's reputation as an "assuager of grief."

Jābir ibn Hayyān in the *Kitab al-Sumum* in the eighth century also cited the psychoactive effects of cannabis (Lewis et al., 1971).

Cannabis also figured in the medical writings of Avicenna (ibn Sīnā) in the tenth century, wherein the inebriating effects of the plant leaves were noted (Ainslie, 1826), as they were, too, in the works of Maimonides (Moses ben Maimon) in the twelfth century (Meyerhof, 1940).

Leclerc documented various Arab authors' experiences with cannabis, for example, he quoted Ed-Dimachky (Leclerc, 1881, p. 118), who stated that cannabis "purifies the brain if one injects its decoction in the nose" (translation E. B. R.).

Cannabis was not without controversy in the early Islamic world and has been vilified by many contemporary authors, some even claiming that it actually provoked melancholy (Lozano Camara and Instituto de Cooperación con el Mundo Arabe, 1990).

Europeans were reminded of the psychoactivity of cannabis by Garcia da Orta (1913), a Spanish Jew who explored India in the sixteenth century. The author documented sedative and appetite-stimulating properties in his 1563 book.

In Indonesia, then known as the Dutch East Indies, Georg Everard Rumpf studied the flora, writing (Rumpf and Beekman, 1981, p. 194):

> The Indians [loose term for peoples of the East] deem this Fool's-Herb to be their *Nepenthes* which serves to drive away sorrow and bring them jollity.

Robert Burton (1907) did not neglect the therapeutic benefits of cannabis ("bange") in his encyclopedic *Anatomy of Melancholy* of 1621: "Bange is like in its effects to opium, causing a kind of ecstasy, an inclination gently to laugh" (p. 593).

In 1712, Engelbert Kaempfer published his *Amoenitatum Exoticarum Politico-Physico-Medicarum,* in which he described the psychotropic nature of cannabis as utilized in Persia and India (Dolan, 1971; Kaempfer, 1996).

In 1839, the medical use of cannabis, or Indian hemp, was re-introduced to the West from India (O'Shaughnessy, 1838-1840). He examined the effects of cannabis extract in treatment of a variety of desperate medical cases. Recoveries were documented in cases of delirium tremens (alcohol withdrawal) and tetanus. Even in rabies, which remains virtually universally fatal to this day, patients were able to attain rest, comfort, and, in terminal events, an easier passage.

In England, Clendinning (1843) used a tincture of Indian hemp to advantage in a variety of illnesses, even in cases of morphine withdrawal symptoms:

> I have no hesitation in affirming that in my hand its exhibition has usually, and with remarkably few substantial exceptions, been followed by manifest effects as a soporific or hypnotic in conciliating sleep; as an anodyne in lulling irritation; as an

antispasmodic in checking cough and cramp; and as a nervine stimulant in removing languor and anxiety, and raising the pulse and spirits; and that these effects have been observed in both acute and chronic affections, in young and old, male and female. (p. 209)

The French physician Jacques-Joseph Moreau de Tours was the first to systematically examine the role of cannabis in psychiatric practice in his 1845 book *Du Hachisch et de l'Alientation Mentale: Études Psychologiques.* Moreau (1973) mused about its applications:

One of the effects of hashish that struck me most forcefully and which generally gets the most attention is that manic excitement always accompanied by a feeling of gaiety and joy inconceivable to those who have never experienced it. I saw in it a mean of effectively combatting the fixed ideas of depressives, disrupting the chain of their ideas, of unfocusing their attention on such and such a subject. (p. 211)

He went on to report that initial trials had mixed results.

Subsequently, some years later, Moreau (1857) reported in detail the case study of a young man with intractable lypemania, a sort of obsessive melancholia, and its remarkable cure with cannabis. Could the same result have occurred spontaneously? Perhaps, but subsequent evidence supports a rational basis for its efficacy.

Many judged Moreau's efforts to be an ultimate failure, but not all. In 1926, Professor E. Perrot of the *Faculté de Pharmacie de Paris* stated:

The Indian hemp, to take but one example, quite cheated the hopes of Moreau de Tours, but it would be imprudent to affirm that it will not be better utilized by the psychiatry of tomorrow! (Rouhier, 1975, p. IX) (translation E. B. R.)

In 1853, François Allemand, a French physician, wrote a utopian treatise, *Le hachych,* which was published in Paris. In it, a fictional Dr. Lebon speaks of hashish's psychotropic effects, when asked about its benefits:

What pleasure? Without hashish, I should have died of melancholy a hundred times. . . .

The most constant and remarkable property of hashish is to exalt the dominant ideas of the person who has taken it, to make him see in the clearest way his most complicated plan come to fruition without difficulty, his dearest project realized without obstacle, to furnish him with the precise intuition he seeks. Finally, it lets him taste in thought the absolute possession of everything according to his wishes, and habitual passions, and according to the direction of his thoughts at the moment the hashish acts on him. (Kimmens, 1977, pp. 117-118)

A physician in Ohio reported a notable therapeutic success with cannabis in the treatment of "hysterical insanity," a case that we would currently recognize as bipolar disease (manic depression) (McMeens, 1860). Concluding an extensive review of cannabis therapeutics, the author stated:

In those mixed and indefinable paroxysms of an hysterical nature, I have found no remedy to control or curtail them with equal promptness and permanency. . . . In sleeplessness, where opium is contraindicated, it is an excellent substitute. . . . As a calmative and hypnotic, in all forms of nervous inquietude and cerebral excitement, it will be found an invaluable agent, as it produces none of those functional derangement or sequences that render many of the more customary remedies objectionable. (McMeens, 1860, p. 95)

John Russell Reynolds, who was to become personal physician to Queen Victoria, initially reported on various successes with an extract of cannabis in depression, lassitude, and senile restlessness (Reynolds, 1868).

In 1870, a Professor Polli of Milan documented at length another fascinating case of a young widow with an advanced melancholia with obsessional features and anxiety. She was successfully treated over ten days with *dawamesk,* an Egyptian confection composed of hashish (Polli, 1870, p. 99):

with a steady and progressive amelioration of all the phenomena; the nights became tranquil, the intelligence just, the affec-

tions natural. There only remained for a few days a little lo-
quacity, some inclination to laugh unnecessarily, and a slight
muscular feebleness.

Some months afterwards this lady was perfectly well, lively,
and in flourishing health. The cure was permanent.

Indian hemp proved to be a useful agent in treatment of delirium
tremens (alcohol withdrawal) and for treating opiate addiction. One
author, citing his experience and that of his colleagues, stated, "the
effect was marvellous" (Tyrell, 1867, p. 244).

Referring to *Cannabis indica,* it was said (Strange, 1883, p. 14):

> in cases of melancholia, and, indeed, in all cases of mental
> depression with sleeplessness, I have found a valuable and
> almost certain ally in this drug.

By 1890, Reynolds had employed cannabis medicinally for almost forty years. As a treatment for senile insomnia, he wrote, "in
this class of cases, I have found nothing comparable in utility to a
moderate dose of hemp" (Reynolds, 1890, pp. 637-638). He related
its effectiveness over long periods of time without resort to escalat-
ing dosages.

The same year, the treatment of delirium tremens was described
(Aulde, 1890, p. 526):

> In all probability the first dose will be sufficient to arrest the
> vomiting, and, if the drug is pushed, the patient will gradually
> fall in to a natural-like sleep, and awake several hours after
> greatly refreshed and entirely free from the threatening symp-
> toms presented a few hours previously.

Suckling reported successes with Indian hemp in the treatment of
mania and melancholia, in quaint prose that would raise eyebrows
nowadays for its misogyny:

> almost a specific in that form of insanity peculiar to women,
> caused by mental worry or moral shock. (1891, p. 12)

Mattison (1891) reviewed cannabis therapy in detail. One indication he advocated was treatment of addiction to cocaine, chloral

hydrate, and opiates. He stated, "In these, often, it has proved an efficient substitute for the poppy." He concluded with a flourish:

> Indian hemp is not here lauded as a specific. It will, at times, fail. So do other drugs. But the many cases in which it acts well, entitle it to a large and lasting confidence.
>
> My experience warrants this statement: cannabis indica is, often, a safe and successful anodyne and hypnotic. (p. 271)

At the turn of the twentieth century, a British pharmacologist touted smoking cannabis (Dixon, 1899, p. 1356):

> In cases where an immediate effect is desired the drug should be smoked, the fumes being drawn through water. In fits of depression, mental fatigue, nervous headache, and exhaustion a few inhalations produce an almost immediate effect, the sense of depression, headache, feeling of fatigue disappear and the subject is enabled to continue his work, feeling refreshed and soothed.

An interesting description of cannabis intoxication provided by Lewis in 1900 is telling in its potential for therapeutic effects:

> A feeling of joyful anticipation of some unknown yet great pleasure is experienced, and there seems to be an end of all trouble and care. Without taking cognizance of the fact, past events and details grow very unimportant and the most pressing obligations are forgotten. The mind seems wholly taken up with the thoughts of the moment. Very frequently a great inexplicable sense of relief is felt, the sensation many times being identical with that experienced by one who suddenly awakes from a horrible dream to the feeling of gratitude which is always felt at its unreality. (p. 247)

Although cannabis use was essentially outlawed in the United States in the late 1930s, it has remained an agent of ethnobotanical importance around the world. In a treatise titled *Indigenous Drugs of India,* Chopra and Chopra (1957, p. 91) stated, "cannabis is used in medicine to relieve pain, to encourage sleep, and to soothe restlessness."

In another book about medicinal plants of the subcontinent, the author asserted (Dastur, 1962, p. 67):

> Charas is the resinous exudation that collects on the leaves and flowering tops of plants [equivalent to the Arabic *hashish*]; it is the active principle of hemp; it is a valuable narcotic, especially in cases where opium cannot be administered; it is of great value in malarial and periodical headaches, migraine, acute mania, whooping cough, cough of phthisis, asthma, anaemia of brain, nervous vomiting, tetanus, convulsion, insanity, delirium, dysuria, and nervous exhaustion.

Similarly, cannabis retains many uses in the folk medicine of Southeast Asia, including smoking and ingestion as a tonic for chronic illness, after childbirth, as a soporific, and as a relaxant (Martin, 1975). In Vietnam, a use of cannabis seed was observed: "The preparation *(sac thuoc)* is used to combat loss of memory and mental confusion" (Martin, 1975, p. 172).

Despite cannabis prohibition in most countries, investigation has continued in modern times to some degree. In 1944, the LaGuardia Commission published an in-depth examination of marijuana and found its dangers vastly overstated. Therapeutic applications were even advanced (Mayor's Committee on Marihuana, 1944, p. 147): "the typical euphoria-producing action . . . might be applicable in the treatment of various types of mental depression."

As part of the study (Mayor's Committee on Marihuana, 1944), fifty-six inmates with morphine or heroin addiction were examined. A group treated with THC (tetrahydrocannabinol, the main psychoactive cannabinoid)

> had less severe withdrawal symptoms and left the hospital at the end of the treatment period in better condition than those who received no treatment or who were treated with Magendie's solution. The ones in the former group maintained their appetite and in some cases actually gained weight during the withdrawal period. (p. 147)

Efforts continue in a similar vein to treat withdrawal with cannabis and have been spearheaded by Tod Mikuriya, who has reported on a successful use of cannabis in the treatment of alcoholism (Mikuriya, 1970). Current governmental constraints in the United States have recently rendered formal clinical studies with cannabis an extreme rarity.

A clinical study in 1976 revealed statistically significant results (Regelson et al., 1976, p. 775):

> Delta-9-THC in cancer patients at acceptable dosage (0.1 mg/ kg tid, orally) had the effect of a tranquilizer and mild mood elevator, clearly without untoward effects on cognitive function- ing and apparently without untoward effect on personality or emotional stability—at least as can be measured by psychological tests.

Thousands of cancer survivors have anecdotally supported similar personal observations.

Cannabis use has often been cited as an implicated etiological or aggravating factor in the development of psychosis (schizophrenia). A recent study found otherwise (Warner et al., 1994). Among the findings, psychotic patients who used marijuana had lower hospital- ization rates than those who abused other substances, and they had lower rates of activation symptoms. Patients reported beneficial effects on depression, anxiety, insomnia, and pain.

Cannabis may improve night vision, according to reported ob- servations of night fishermen in Jamaica, as reported in the journal *Nature* (West, 1991). This proposition could be scientifically veri- fied by the use of ERG (electroretinography) testing in volunteers.

Any pharmacological discussion of cannabis is complicated by the fact that, as with any herb, it is subject to quality control issues. Cannabis is a mixture of myriad cannabinoids and essential oils that may contribute to its physiological effects. In addition, ratios of tetrahydrocannabinol (THC) and cannabidiol (CBD) are critical in observed medicinal activity. THC is primarily responsible for eu- phoric effects but may aggravate anxiety. CBD, in contrast, is less psychoactive, more sedative, and ameliorates anxiety. It also serves to modulate the "high" produced by THC. These relationships be- tween cannabis components have been extensively studied in Brazil by Zuardi and colleagues (Zuardi et al., 1981, 1982, 1993, 1995; Zuardi, Guimaraes, and Moreira, 1993; Zuardi and Karniol, 1983;

Zuardi, Rodrigues, and Cunha, 1991). Although these results are not easily summarized, and the interested reader is urged to examine the source material, a good review of CBD activity is available (Zuardi and Guimaraes, 1997).

CBD had a significant effect on anxiety in normal subjects in an experimental protocol, and without significant sedation (Zuardi, Guimaraes, and Moreira, 1993).

CBD also improved symptoms of psychosis in one patient, without induction of parkinsonian symptoms, as commonly occurs with standard antipsychotic agents. Improvement did not occur with addition of haloperidol to CBD (Zuardi et al., 1995).

Dr. Lester Grinspoon, a psychiatrist at Harvard University, has pioneered and spearheaded the medical use of marijuana. His writings have frequently included personal case studies of patients whose psychiatric illnesses have been successfully treated through cannabis use (Grinspoon and Bakalar, 1997). Although critics have derided testimonials of this type as anecdotal, many of the patients failed miserably on standard pharmaceuticals but successfully alleviated their symptomatology with cannabis. How much scientific verification do the patients themselves require?

Many of these accounts document the manner in which patients were relieved on cannabis, worse without it, and helped once more upon its resumption. This represents an "N-of-1 trial" (patient acts as own control and notes effects on and off the drug) that has been widely accepted as a valid research technique in pharmacological study of conditions that are extremely rare, or in which true double blinding is impossible, as is clearly the case for cannabis.

Dr. Grinspoon recently published another series of case studies of cannabis in the treatment of bipolar disease (manic depression) (Grinspoon and Bakalar, 1998). This author believes that these accounts are extremely compelling in supporting efficacy for cannabis in this most difficult clinical problem.

Consroe (1998) has nicely reviewed the topic of brain cannabinoids in neurological disease and points out that the effect of cannabis to impair short-term memory suggests the potential utility of cannabinoid *antagonists* in treatment of dementia. Interestingly, and contrary to logic, recent reports indicate that dronabinol (synthetic THC) actually decreased the severity of disturbed behavior in a dozen patients with Alzheimer's disease (Volicer et al., 1997). Cohen-Mansfield Agitation Inventory scores, expressed as a percentage of baseline, were diminished significantly (p = 0.05), while negative affect in the dronabinol group also decreased over placebo (p = 0.004). Dronabinol also produced weight gain in these previously anorexic subjects (p = 0.006). The results were sufficiently compelling to cause the drug's manufacturer to seek out a formal indication for its use in Alzheimer's disease from the FDA.

Finally, cannabis has been reported as effective in treatment of Tourette's syndrome (TS) (Hemming and Yellowlees, 1993; Moss et al., 1989; Müller-Vahl, Kolbe, and Dengler, 1997; Müller-Vahl et al., 1998, 1999; Sandyk and Awerbuch, 1988). This entity consists of a combination of involuntary movements, or tics, and pervasive features of obsessive-compulsive disorder (OCD). Cannabinoid receptors are heavily represented in the basal ganglia (Herkenham et al., 1990; Herkenham, 1993), and it has been hypothesized that this is the pathologically impaired site in TS patients.

Efficacy has been demonstrated anecdotally (Müller-Vahl et al., 1998) with cannabis in 82 percent of surveyed TS patients on both tics and OCD symptoms. The same was confirmed experimentally in one patient with dronabinol (Müller-Vahl et al., 1999). A few patients of this book's author report similar findings.

Such results have important implications. OCD represents one of the most recalcitrant disorders in psychiatry. Before 1980, no standard pharmaceuticals were significantly effective in its treatment. Nowadays, high, and sometimes massive, doses of clomipramine (a TCA) or SSRIs (Prozac and others) are required for its control.

Whereas a disorder of serotonin expression has been implicated as etiological in OCD, the necessity of these massive doses undermines that theory and, rather, supports the prospect that the current therapeutic drugs are producing secondary effects in another neurotransmitter system. What if OCD actually represents a disorder of the cannabinoid neurotransmitter system? After all, depression may be due to serotonin or norepinephrine deficiency, anxiety to GABA abnormalities, dementia to acetylcholine deficiency, and schizophrenia to dopamine excess. Conceivably, OCD and other illnesses (e.g., migraine and idiopathic bowel disease) may eventually be tied to a clinical cannabinoid deficiency state.

OCD is marked by an insurmountable preoccupation with fixed ideas (e.g., if I walk on the lawn, I will step on worms and something very bad will happen), no matter how preposterous, that withstand the patient's best efforts to submerge them through the application of logic. Cannabis, as no other substance yet discovered, allows a person to forget, and to laugh, even at one's own obsessions and compulsions. For OCD, it sounds like just what the doctor ordered.

PART III:
CLINICAL CASE STUDIES

Disclaimer

The information in this section is provided for illustrative purposes only.

The majority of the material in this book has emphasized a scientific analysis of herbs and use of standardized preparations along the lines of the German model of phytotherapy.

Practices in the United States, Canada, Australia, and other countries may be quite distinct. As such, *these case studies represent examples of how herbal treatment may be practiced rather than how it should be practiced.* Consumers have the prerogative to judge for themselves and apply all appropriate cautions.

Case Study 1

Episodic Use of Kava

The patient was a middle-aged professional. He reported a history of performance anxiety dating from childhood. This arose in relation to public speaking, musical performance, dangerous situations (rock climbing), and other similar situations. In his teen years, manifestations were often quite flagrant and included sweaty palms, manifest psychic distress, and tremor, often reaching the severity of "sewing machine knee."

Over time, he had overcome some degree of symptomatology through repetitive experience. However, he found that for certain public-speaking situations and court appearances that symptoms remained problematical. He was given metoprolol (Lopressor), a beta-blocker, in doses of 50 to 100 mg to employ for symptomatic relief. This was quite effective, allowing him to retain composure, even in the face of contentious testimony in the legal setting. No tachyphylaxis was observed.

He noted, however, that this approach had drawbacks. Although he enjoyed the relief that the beta-blocker afforded, it seemed to remove any positive emotion of relief after the lecture or trial appearance had been completed. In short, he felt cheated of his ability to celebrate once the event was over. Thus, he came to abandon this practice as undesirable and, eventually, unnecessary.

Some years later, he decided to experiment with kava. He took an extract of kava, 384 mg, standardized to 210 mg of kavalactones, for particularly stressful lectures and court appearances. He found this equally effective as the beta-blockers. As he put it, "On kava, it's hard to get too upset about anything." He reported no sedation, no deleterious effect on memory, and, most important, no decrement in his enjoyment of the relief related to completion of these tasks. He noted one other benefit: he had often experienced migraine headaches after such events due to the "release phenomenon," but these did not occur when kava was employed. Much as previously, over time, he found the necessity of kava treatment lessened as he became increasingly accustomed to "performing."

Editorial Comments

Although not a promoted indication for kava use, this case illustrates its efficacy for performance anxiety. Given this agent's safety in acute use (under three months), this type of application should be considered more widely.

Case of Dementia
Treated with *Ginkgo biloba*

This sixty-two-year-old male was first seen in 1996, referred for neurological evaluation of memory problems. Description of his condition included a short note from his doctor and additional information from the patient himself, who was a bit of a difficult historian due to his tendency toward rumination and slow responses.

The patient felt he had always had difficulty with memory, and that even though he became a veterinarian, he had to study harder and longer than his peers did. In school, he could remember things only until the examination was completed. In his clinical practice, he had been able to keep track of drug dosing, but with increasing difficulty. He occasionally left appliances or machines on but had not caused any accidents or mishaps. He had "wandering keys" syndrome but generally managed to find things he misplaced. He had difficulty orienting and problems driving in Seattle.

The patient's judgment was that he had a history of decreased focus and was easily distracted by background noise or other events. However, he claimed no evidence of significant work quality issues. He had always had difficulty taking notes, possibly due to inadequate spelling skills. The patient complained that he would continually recheck things and admitted to a degree of compulsivity in this. He also admitted to frequent rumination on certain issues. He experienced long-term depression and anxiety, especially in relation to minor events. He characterized himself as a loner, yet a person who was careful about what he said and who was sensitive to others. Interestingly, he had no previous drug treatment to speak of, although on one occasion he took Valium (diazepam). Subsequently, he was less anxious and able to perform better when playing golf.

The patient had previous mastoid surgery, by his description, but no history of diabetes, thyroid problems, seizures, meningitis, or encephalitis. He incurred minor injuries playing football but had no history of concussion. He had no current medications, nor allergies. He was primarily left-handed.*

Family history was noteworthy: one brother was compulsive and a workaholic, another brother was a paranoid schizophrenic, and his sister seemed to be very high functioning.

The patient was a veterinarian who expressed interest in retiring. He characterized himself as continually "on the move" in terms of his activity, often sleeping only 3 to 4 h a night. The patient had been on and off cigarettes, at that time smoking three to four a day. He drank alcohol lightly and had one to five cups of coffee a day.

Physical examination revealed a weight of 160 pounds (lb) and a blood pressure (BP) reading of 120/80. He was a generally pleasant, cooperative sixty-two-year-old male. His head was normocephalic without bruits. The ear, nose, and throat (ENT) exam was unremarkable. The neck was supple and carotids full without bruits. Heart sounds were normal.

On mental status testing, the patient seemingly gave no simple answers. He, with a lot of direction, was basically oriented, knew the presidents, and had normal right-left orientation and naming skills. However, he seemed hard of hearing and required an inordinate amount of redirection, repetition, or demonstration of commands, implying a significant dyspraxia (inability to carry out verbal instruction). He read a sixth-grade-level passage well, with partial recall, but required the examiner to draw out all the details. Serial 3s were quite slow initially, then better, but he tried to go through the 90s twice before correcting himself. He remembered two of three objects directly after 5 min, none with hints and the final one with a choice of three. He was very soft-spoken but tended to be circumlocutory ("talk around" a topic), anxious, subdued, distracted, and fidgety. He ruminated markedly upon his answers,

---

*Left-handedness may indicate brain injury in development or early life. Whether a person is right- or left-handed is a standard piece of information for neurologists.

which tended to wander, and there was a significant latency to responses.

Cranial nerves were unremarkable, except for being hard of hearing.

The patient experienced difficulty relaxing but ultimately seemed to have normal tone and strength, with no arm drift. Sensation was intact to fine touch, sharp/dull, vibration, position, and graphesthesia. Romberg was negative. The patient performed finger-to-nose quite slowly, with heel-to-shin normal. He had difficulty upon initiating pronation/supination on the right side. There was some mirroring on fine finger movements. Gait, including toe and heel, was normal, but tandem gait was slow and careful. Reflexes were 1+ and symmetric with down-going toes.

At the time, I did not see convincing evidence that this patient had a progressive dementia or degenerative disease. Rather, I thought that his problem resulted from a combination of obsessive-compulsive traits and considerable anxiety and depression. In addition, with his manifest dyscoordination, the patient showed some evidence of having attention-deficit hyperactivity disorder, residual form (ADHD-R). We discussed all of these implications at some length and the methods of assessment. The patient agreed to an audiogram and performance of some basic labs, but he decided to forgo other tests for treatable causes of dementia.

The patient acceded to trying sertraline (Zoloft), 50 mg po (by mouth) qd a.m. He was given written instructions to call in two weeks with plans to adjust upward, since I felt higher dosing might be necessary to produce significant improvement in obsessive-compulsive (OCD) symptoms.

After the conversation, the patient managed to leave his appointment card and prescription twice, in various areas of the clinic. During this interval he seemed particularly scattered and was unsure as to whether he was supposed to see his regular doctor. We planned to follow up subsequently.

On review of laboratory data, the patient had a normal chemistry panel, except for moderately elevated cholesterol and triglycerides, with no indication of liver or kidney disease. A complete blood count (CBC) revealed merely a mild increase in mean corpuscular hemoglobin (sometimes observed in vitamin B_{12} deficiency). Thyroid function tests (TFTs) were within normal limits.

A hearing test showed a significant high-frequency sensorineural loss bilaterally. This was symmetrical in the 250 to 300 Hz range, then dropped off to a mild loss on the right side around the 50 decibel (dB) range, with moderate loss to 70 dB on the left side. He was referred for hearing aid evaluation.

The patient was lost to follow-up for sixteen months. As he explained, "I dropped off the edge." When he returned, he admitted, "I need some help." The patient remained extremely tangential and digressive in providing history but imparted that he was having more memory and anxiety issues. He was not practicing veterinary medicine at that moment. He indicated, "I made some money," and apparently saved enough so that he was not in dire straits. He complained, "I need to get away from a number of little things," without being able to substantiate or explain this or other statements more explicitly.

On exam, the patient was alert and cooperative but remained very circumlocutory, fidgety, and eccentric in appearance, with marked latency. He thought that it was Monday, and was one day off, and really could not name the month. He was quite dyspraxic. He could name the president but remembered only one of three objects after 5 min, none with hints and the other two with choice of three. The remainder of the exam was unremarkable, except that he had a great deal of difficulty getting through the directions for finger-to-nose, his actions being quite disjointed, and his tandem walking was a little tentative.

The patient's situation remained undefined. I surmised that he certainly might have a primary dementia but could not rule out an extreme pseudodementia with features of anxiety, attention deficit, and OCD, much as before. The patient indicated having had an MRI (magnetic resonance imaging) scan that was reportedly negative. Subsequently, an EEG was performed during wakefulness. This was disorganized, with a moderately severe diffuse disturbance of brain function characterized by slowing of background activity, especially in frontotemporal areas.

Three days later, the patient's assistant called with her concerns. She needed to mark down his appointments because she knew he would forget. (He had arrived two hours early for his last appointment with me because he had forgotten where his sister lived along his route and was unable to visit beforehand.) She noted numerous problems. For example, he would forget the whereabouts of his own dog. One day he left it in the truck all day and had been calling all over to inquire its whereabouts of others. He had begun walking up to strangers on the street holding his pillbox, asking what day it was and whether he should take his Zoloft. One time, he was supposed to take home a year's worth of files, but they ended up in the dumpster instead. Frequently, he would arrive at the office flustered because he could not recall what he wanted to say or do. He had packed a bag before Thanksgiving in anticipation of his family coming to take him to Washington State. Every day for a week he would pace up and down waiting for his family and ask if they were coming, only to be told the date of the trip. Nevertheless, he would repeat the performance the next day.

Neuropsychological testing was performed utilizing the Wechsler Adult Intelligence Scale (WAIS-III), Wechsler Memory Scale (WMS-III), the Rivermead Behavioral Memory Test, the Mattis Dementia Rating Scale, Complex Ideation for the Boston Diagnostic Aphasia Examination, and select components of the Halstead-Reitan Neuropsychological Battery. These revealed a consistent picture of fairly severe dementia, mainly frontal lobe in location. It was felt that he would require medication and a supervised living situation.

Two months later, the patient had completed his testing with the neuropsychologist and had been referred back for consideration of medicines. I asked him about his testing results meeting, and he essentially was unable to remember anything substantial about the contents, merely circumlocuting around his deficit. A plan had been formulated in which the patient would continue living alone, but with close supervision by one of his employees and his brother. The patient had attempted the sale of his veterinary practice, but plans did not work out. Rather, he hoped to hire an associate. The patient remained on Zoloft but experienced periodic anxiety that seemed related to his memory problems.

The patient was alert and cooperative but remained very prone to hemming and hawing. He thought it was Thursday (one day off) and after a very long latency established the name of the facility. He knew the president's name. He remained quite dyspraxic. His finger-to-nose movement was disjointed, with a slight tremor, but the remainder of the exam was unremarkable.

Based on the testing, it was determined that the patient had a significant presenile dementia, Alzheimer's type. The situation was discussed with the patient and his guest. We discussed options, and it was agreed we would try donepezil (Aricept, a drug that increases levels of acetylcholine in the brain), 5 mg each evening, with supervision by his assistant. Alternatives such as *Ginkgo biloba* were discussed but tabled. We planned treatment for a month, before considering dose increases or additions.

He returned one month later. In the meantime, the patient had been taking donepezil, 5 mg a day; sertraline, 50 mg; and vitamin E, 400 IU (International Unit). The patient disclaimed any gastrointestinal symptomatology on the medicine. He felt improved, with less anxiety and greater organizational ability. He still had problems remembering names but was less upset by it. He had been doing lots of spring cleaning and brush burning.

The patient was obviously happier. He incorrectly thought it was a Saturday in December and could not name the year. He still had a long latency to responses, but a lot less hemming and hawing, and he appeared much more self-assured. He had difficulty registering the test words for memory but ultimately got two of three after 5 min, a third with choice of three. His praxis was fair. The remainder of the exam was normal, without tremor.

He was assessed as having modest but definite gains. He certainly seemed "less lost." We discussed the situation and decided to cautiously try him on donepezil, 10 mg a day.

In another month, the patient remained on sertraline, 50 mg a day; donepezil, 10 mg a day; and vitamin E, 400 IU. On the increased dose of donepezil, he complained that his stool was perhaps a little loose, but he had no discomfort, and no actual complaints.

The patient actually drove himself alone to the appointment that day, a distance of more than ninety miles, much to my consternation. Apparently he came via the airport rather than on the freeway, which was an obvious mistake in light of ongoing construction. He thought things were going well and that he was less anxious and more articulate. He still had problems with names but noted no new difficulties. He continued to work outside.

The patient was alert, much more fluent and articulate, but he was very hesitant, with long latency, in trying to figure out the date. He said initially it was March; with some prompting he said May. He could not name the date. He remained quite dyspraxic with some nonsequiturs in conversation. He remembered two of three objects after a long gap, failed with hint on the third, but got it with choice of three. The remainder was unchanged.

It was felt that the patient showed quite a bit of improvement in his adjustment, while dementia remained a significant problem. We discussed the situation, and it was agreed he would try *Ginkgo biloba* in the form of a standardized EGb 761 preparation, 60 mg PO bid. He was given the ordering information for a reliable supply. We planned to have someone in his office check that he ordered and administered the medicine.

Two months later, he arrived late to the appointment, with his brother, who had little corroboratory information. Apparently he had recently lost his billfold. He indicated that things had been going fairly well until recently. His two adult children had visited, and he claimed that things had been moved around his home, but whether this was true was unclear. He voiced some frustration. He was poorly cognizant of what his medicine was and whether he was really taking it consistently. As far as I knew, he was supposed to be on *Ginkgo biloba,* 60 mg bid; sertraline, 50; donepezil, 10 mg; and vitamin E, 400 IU a day.

The patient was alert but easily confused, with some word-finding difficulty and a great deal of circumlocution, leading to long yarns, the point of which were obscure to the examiner. He knew it was Tuesday but thought it was another month. He knew the president. With difficulty he remembered two of three objects after 5 min, the third with choice. His finger-to-nose movement was poorly carried out due to praxis difficulties. Reflexes were symmetric. Gait was normal.

I felt that the patient was probably at the point of maximal yield, if he was, in fact, taking the medicine. The case was briefly discussed with the examining neuropsychologist, who planned retesting with respect to safety issues. At the time, I was not satisfied that he was safe on his own in the home environment, without closer supervision. If he was not taking his medicines regularly, certainly he had to, and I emphasized this to him, as well as the idea that he should not get too hung up on details in his life that could best be avoided.

He was seen again, three months later, accompanied by his sister. Apparently, on his neuropsychological retesting, his memory was no better, but his anxiety was no worse. As best we could figure, he remained on gingko, 60 mg bid; sertraline, 50 mg; donepezil, 10 mg; and vitamin E, 400 IU. Someone was doing his cooking for him. The sale of his business was pending. It was apparent that he really did not want to take this step, but everyone in the family believed it was best, as did I. An interim driving evaluation that we had arranged had not been completed. In fact, although this was hard to conceive of, he had recently driven to Seattle and back, a round trip of some 1,000 miles.

The patient was alert and cooperative, displaying intermittent humor, but he was speaking in ironies and nonsequiturs to a fair degree. He was variably fidgety and quite dyspraxic. There was some latency to his responses and some circumlocution. He thought it was August 15, was confused by what I meant by the day of the week, thinking it was Thursday rather than Tuesday. He knew the president. With hesitation and some contradiction, he perhaps got two of three objects after 5 min, but he needed a choice of three for the third and still was not sure. His finger-to-nose movement was quite poorly done due to dyspraxia. Reflexes were 2+ and gaits were normal.

The patient seemed to be on optimal treatment. I indicated to him that it was my professional opinion that he should not be driving. I again encouraged him to sell the business because he was obviously preoccupied with it, and this would reduce his responsibilities. We planned to follow up in six months.

When he returned at that time, the situation had become increasingly desperate, but the patient refused to acknowledge the inadvisability of driving or remaining independent. He became very agitated in this discussion.

Editorial Comments

This case nicely illustrates the pitfalls in diagnosis of dementia. The patient initially presented with symptoms more suggestive of severe anxiety than of Alzheimer's disease. Such pseudodementia is important to recognize because it is one of the few treatable conditions presenting with memory loss, and because suitable pharmacotherapy with an antidepressant or antianxiety agent may quickly be effective.

The observed plateaus in functioning after optimal drug treatment, or even subsequent deterioration, are the rule in true dementia cases rather than the exception. This window of improvement may be critical, however, in the patient's family and business relationships before an inexorable deterioration erases memory, personality, and the possibility of meaningful communication. *Ginkgo biloba* did not prevent this deterioration, nor would it be likely that any future pharmaceutical could either.

Case Study 3

Head Injury
Treated with Ginkgo

This twelve-year-old female was referred by her pediatrician for neurological evaluation. The patient was well until a school bus accident of three weeks previously, when she was on the way to a science fair in a distant town. The vehicle overturned on an icy highway. The patient apparently hit her head and may have lost consciousness briefly, although the notes from the emergency room near the scene did not indicate this. In any event, she had complaints of headache, nausea, and dizziness when she arrived. A physical exam was negative aside from abrasions. Urinalysis was negative, as was a CT (computed tomography, "CAT scan") of the head without contrast. Apparently the patient returned to Missoula and performed as a dancer in *The Nutcracker Suite* that weekend despite continued headache, dizziness, nausea, and a bout of diarrhea. One week later, she had persistent headache in the left occiput and frontal areas. She noted some decreased recall of her math techniques and memorized musical pieces. There was some decrease in headache with Tylenol (acetaminophen). Another exam by her pediatrician was fairly normal, and it was recommended she take ibuprofen, 400 mg bid, with supplemental acetaminophen as needed.

The patient indicated no history of premorbid headache. By the time of the evaluation, she had no memory of getting out of the bus, as she had been observed to do. She continued to have headaches, usually every afternoon, but, with, perhaps, two- to three-day intervals without that complaint. They began in the left parietal area and were often initially sharp, with pounding if she were supine. Headaches had waves of intensity and might reach up to an 8/10 on a ten-point subjective pain scale. Nausea was occasional and she had a couple episodes of emesis. She denied visual blurring or photophobia. Pain lasted two hours or more and was most often present in the evening. She still complained of occasional dizziness. She has found the ibuprofen to be less effective than Tylenol and probably only got 500 mg just before bed. The patient had not danced since the one performance after the accident, but she continued with piano playing and other activities. She had performed reasonably well in school, making only one error that she thought was silly. She continued riding the bus to school and denied any emotional fallout from the event.

The patient was born after a normal pregnancy, labor, and delivery at a birth weight of 7 lb. She had had an appendectomy and suffered pneumonia earlier that year but otherwise had been quite healthy, with no other head trauma, seizures, meningitis, or encephalitis.

She was in the seventh grade, taking high school algebra, and usually received all As. She was right-handed.

Family history was negative for neurological conditions, including headache. She normally was quite active and slept about 10 h nightly.

A physical exam recorded a weight of 90 lb, height of 63 inches (in), and a BP of 110/70. There were no general abnormalities, except tenderness in the left parietal area.

Mental status: The patient was alert and oriented to the medical center. Initially she said it was November 18 (one month off), then corrected herself. She knew recent presidents, had normal right-left orientation, praxis, and naming skills. She read a sixth-grade-level passage well but missed one element and confabulated (filled in missing blanks with made-up material) slightly. She remembered three objects for 5 min. Serial 3s were well done. Her drawing of a cube and her cursive script were normal. She named thirteen animals in 30 seconds (sec), which is normal. Speech and affect were normal.

Cranial nerves: I—Intact. II—Acuity was measured as 20/20 OU (each eye). Fields and OKNs (optokinetic nystagmus) were normal. Fundi were benign. Pupils were equally reactive to light, and external ocular movements (EOMs) were full with no nystagmus. Remaining cranial nerves V and VII through XII were unremarkable.

Motor exam: Patient had normal tone and strength, with no drift. Sensation was intact to fine touch, sharp/dull, vibration, position, and graphesthesia. Romberg was negative. The patient performed finger-to-nose, heel-to-shin, and rapid alternating movement tests (RAMs) well. Gaits, including toe, heel, and tandem, were normal. Reflexes were 1+ and symmetric with down-going toes.

Assessment: This twelve-year-old female seemed to have a mild posttraumatic syndrome with headaches, and very mild cognitive effects. It was felt that this should be a self-limited affair, with possible resolution within three months of the event, but it was indicated to the patient and her mother that up to twelve months of healing are often required in situations of closed head injury. We discussed the various tests, such as MRI scanning, EEG, and neuropsychological testing. None were deemed necessary at the time. My personal bias was that some group counseling for victims of this event would be a very good idea, even though the patient acknowledged no personal distress.

In terms of symptomatic treatment, naproxen (Naprosyn), 375 mg PO bid, was prescribed as a prophylactic. I suggested that she avoid using acetaminophen, since its excessive employment can lead to analgesic rebound problems (Mathew, 1997). We also discussed the use of ginger as symptomatic treatment for nausea, dizziness, and headache (Mustafa and Srivastava, 1990). This treatment was well known in her mother's Oriental ethnic tradition and was acceptable to both of them on an as-needed basis. We also discussed and prescribed *Ginkgo biloba*, 40 mg bid, of a standardized preparation corresponding to EGb 761. Also suggested was simple sleep rationing, to 9 h a night, with cautious resumption of her aerobic activity.

One month later, she returned for evaluation of the posttraumatic syndrome. She had done quite well with satisfactory school performance. Headaches were less frequent, perhaps twice a week, or even a full week without any. They were also less severe. She still complained of a numb feeling in the left parietal area, but with no dizziness. It seemed as if she had to concentrate somewhat more on her homework but was managing well. The only thing she was taking regularly was the *Ginkgo biloba*, 40 mg bid. If she felt nauseated at night, her mother prepared some fresh ginger for her, and, although she did not like the taste, it was very effective for her symptoms and helped her sleep.

Repeat examination was normal.

The patient seemed to be progressing well. I felt that maintaining the status quo was reasonable. When she began having fewer headaches, a possible phased withdrawal of ginkgo was discussed.

The patient's mother called two weeks later to indicate an increase in headaches, accompanied by a flu virus. The girl had been off of her naproxen and was advised to resume.

Six months later, this thirteen-year-old girl returned. She had recently been in Paris with her mother, and they spent a lot of time on the plane. For about a week afterward she had problems with the left side of her neck and shoulder being sore. She rarely had head pain in the interim but did have spontaneous episodes of dizziness every couple of days that were self-limited and not very severe. She was not taking medicine for them. There had been no problems with her memory, and she got all As in the spring term. She came in second in a regional music competition despite having headaches. She had not taken ginkgo for the previous month. Eventually the naproxen bothered her stomach, and she had not been taking it or any regular medicine.

Exam was again normal.

We talked about the possibility of a shoulder X ray, but that was tabled. She was given some cervical exercises to practice. I instructed that she could take ibuprofen as needed for pain.

Editorial Comments

Did herbal treatment make a difference in this case? The patient and her mother felt that it did. The ultimate outcome likely would have been the same, but it is my feeling that the ginkgo and ginger provided some significant measure of symptomatic relief when the patient was most vulnerable. The available choices of herbal medicines were fortuitous in this case, since the patient's mother was familiar with the use of ginkgo and ginger in traditional Chinese medicine (TCM) and was eager to employ them.

Case Study 4

Head Injury Treated with Ginkgo

This female patient, twelve and a half years old, was brought in by her mom for neurological evaluation. She had been well until one week earlier, when she was involved in the same school bus accident described in the previous case. The vehicle slid on the ice and rolled over onto its side. The patient does not think she was knocked out but has little memory of the event. She ended up facedown against a broken window. She sustained a laceration and abrasion around the right eye and a fracture of the left wrist. She was seen in a local emergency room, x-rayed, casted, and released. The patient felt "shaken up" in the aftermath of this and suffered some daily headaches. These were located in the right temple or other areas, and she rated them as a 3 to 4 on a ten-point subjective pain scale with steady contour. The headache took on an occasional beating quality with exertion but caused no nausea. She denied visual change or photophobia. She seemed to get some benefit from Motrin (ibuprofen), 400 mg bid. The patient found her weekend homework took longer than usual, and she had returned to school only the previous day. She had not appeared particularly moody, in her mother's estimation. The patient had a prior history of infrequent headaches that did not require treatment.

The patient was born after a full-term pregnancy without illness, use of medications, or alcohol. The mother did smoke a little during the pregnancy. Labor was 14 h, and the birth weight was 8 lb 9 ounces (oz). There was some jaundice, treated with phototherapy for a couple of days. The patient was hospitalized at age three with orbital cellulitis. There was no history of other major head trauma, seizures, meningitis, etc. She was on no other medication and had no allergies. She was in the seventh grade, getting As and Bs, and was right-handed.

Family history was noteworthy: both the mother and an aunt suffered from headaches and fibromyalgia.

The patient's mom was a musician, and it was just the two of them at home. The patient was normally active in ballet and played cello. She was sleeping normally.

Physical examination recorded a weight of 110 lb and a height of 61.5 in. The patient was generally pleasant and cooperative. Head was normocephalic with bruising and abrasions around the right forehead and eye. Ear, nose, and throat examination was otherwise unremarkable. Neck was supple, carotids full without bruits. Heart sounds were normal without murmur.

Mental status: The patient was alert and fully oriented. Fund of knowledge, right-left orientation, praxis, and naming skills were normal. She read a sixth-grade-level passage well with good recall. Serial 3s were a little slow in a repetitive "7-4-1" sequence. She remembered two of three objects after 5 min, the third with a hint. She named sixteen animals in 30 sec, which was well above average. Speech and affect were normal.

Cranial nerves: I—Intact. II—Acuity was measured as 20/40 OD (right eye), 20/50 OS (left eye), with contacts. Fields and OKNs were normal. Fundi were benign. Pupils were equal and reactive, with full EOMs and no nystagmus. Remaining cranial nerves V and VII through XII were unremarkable.

Motor exam: The patient was casted on the left arm, but otherwise tone and strength seemed normal throughout. Sensation was intact to fine touch, sharp/dull, vibration, position, and graphesthesia, the latter only in the right hand. Finger-to-nose movement on the right and RAMs, as well as heel-to-shin movement, were normal. Gaits, including toe, heel, and tandem, were normal. Reflexes were 2+ to 3+, symmetric, where available, with down-going toes.

Assessment: This patient had a closed head injury with relatively mild posttraumatic headaches. This was predicted to be self-limited. I had suggested a switch to naproxen, but apparently she did not swallow pills and her current ibuprofen was chewable. We did not order any neurodiagnostic tests at the time. I was concerned about emotional fallout from this traumatic event as a possibility, but this youngster seemed to be well adjusted at the time and the mother agreed to closely monitor the situation, letting us know if any additional difficulties arose.

Two weeks later, her mother called. She continued to have interim headaches. While her cast was being removed, she had become faint and experienced a brief loss of consciousness, which was followed by increasing headache symptoms with vomiting. Ibuprofen or naproxen was suggested in conjunction with a strong ginger ale or ginger beer.

Two months later, the patient was seen for follow-up of posttraumatic syndrome. The patient continued to have headaches that occurred once or twice a day. Pain was right or left frontal, rating a 5 to 6 on a ten-point scale and lasting 60 to 90 min. Fortunately, there was little in the way of associated nausea, blurring, or other changes. She often took junior strength Advil (ibuprofen) or, rarely, Tylenol (acetaminophen) and seemed to require the medicine to rid herself of the headache symptoms. The mother noted some new issues. The patient remained on the honor roll, but her grades dropped from a 3.96 to a 3.53 grade point average (GPA). She was easily startled in the car. She was not riding the school bus; instead, her mother had been driving her to school. There were concerns about lack of safety equipment on the bus in light of the accident. The patient showed some decreased focus of attention as well as some shifting of moods and lability.

Follow-up examination revealed a weight of 113 lb and a BP of 100/60. The patient was alert, cooperative, and fully oriented. She followed directions well. She remembered two of three objects after 5 min, needing a hint for the third. She had full EOMs and fields. Pupils were equal and reactive, and fundi were benign. Finger-to-nose movement was normal. Reflexes were 1+ to 2+ and symmetric. Gaits, including tandem, were normal.

The patient was judged to be doing reasonably, but with some residual symptomatology. She had learned how to swallow pills in the interim. We discussed options and prophylaxis. Cyproheptadine did not seem attractive to her due to the possibility of weight gain so I suggested naproxen, 375 mg PO bid, with food. I suggested that she try this for a couple of months, and if she improved, the dosage could possibly be tapered off over a couple of weeks.

A month later, the patient had been taking naproxen, but only about once a day. Her grades had definitely dropped, for instance, a C in math and a D in social studies on the latest report. The patient felt that her focus was diminished, that she would drift off in class. She felt slightly overwhelmed at times. She was only having overt headaches about once or twice every other week, but there was some blurring in the right eye, with no changes on eye exam. There was no dizziness. Her mother noted some erratic mood changes and lack of organization and a need for repetition of requests.

Exam was normal, except for a blasé affect.

The patient was determined to have definite manifestations of posttraumatic syndrome, about three and a half months after the accident. Although she certainly had additional time to heal, I wished to try to treat her symptoms better. We discussed alternatives, including selective serotonin receptor inhibitors, chelated magnesium, and *Ginkgo biloba*. It was decided to go with the latter, a standardized preparation of EGb 761, 60 mg PO bid. Plans were to continue to see her monthly until we saw considerable improvement.

By the next visit, her recent report card showed a 3.3 GPA versus a 3.6. She had a C in math, with As and Bs in other classes. Apparently the patient was scheduled for follow-up on her neuropsychological testing, and no results were available. The patient had been on *Ginkgo biloba*, 60 mg bid, along with Aleve (naproxen), (just one) at night. Interestingly, although she had a headache the previous night without the Aleve, she had been fairly headache free in the interim. Her mother felt there had been a minimal improvement in her memory. The patient did not have a lot of somatic complaints.

She did give the date as Tuesday, April 18, instead of Wednesday, April 15. However, she knew the president, had normal praxis, and remembered three objects for 5 min. Remaining exam was normal.

The patient seemed to be doing well symptomatically, and I suggested continuing the status quo. If she remained reasonably headache free in the coming weeks, discontinuation of the naproxen was planned.

Neuropsychological test results subsequently revealed a Wechsler Intelligence Scale for Children (WISC-III) with verbal IQ at the sixty-seventh percentile, performance at the twenty-seventh, and full scale at the forty-seventh. A twenty-five-point drop in verbal and a twenty-four-point drop in full scale IQs were noted as compared to 1992 results (eight times the standard error of the measurement). This was definitely believed to be due to the intervening head trauma. Wide Range Assessment of Memory and Learning (WRAML) revealed the Visual Memory Index to be only at the second percentile, and Learning Index at the seventh percentile. These scores were far below expected performance in this youngster who previously had high academic achievement. Attention and concentration appeared fairly normal, in contrast. Some decrement was observed in tactile function in the left upper extremity, consistent with previous fracture. In addition, a greater than expected number of errors occurred in abstract reasoning, conceptualization, hypothesis generation, and testing. She was slow in the Trail Making Form B, and the Picture Arrangement subtest score was notably low. Perseverative errors on the Wisconsin Card Sorting Test brought her score down to the tenth percentile. Overall, these results were believed to support disruption of the right hemisphere and right anterior brain function.

The school was informed of temporarily reduced academic expectations in this patient. Further medical treatment was recommended.

Two months later, she was off naproxen and taking only ginkgo, 60 mg PO bid. She had headaches only when medication was missed. Dizziness symptoms were rare. Her grades were probably pretty good, but this was not known for sure. Her mood was improved. Occasionally, she would forget ground rules at home, but it did not sound like too radical a problem. She had baby-sitting duties planned, as well as music and dance camps for the summer.

Exam seemed normal.

The patient appeared stable. I saw no reason to change the ginkgo, since it seemed to have been helpful.

Subsequently, an MRI study was performed. This revealed punctate foci of abnormal signal along the gray-white matter junction, but also in the midbrain and pons. This was seen as consistent with traumatic shearing forces in the bus accident.

Two months later her mother called. The patient's grades had arrived late for some reason and showed a marked drop-off in performance, including a failure in math.

The patient returned for evaluation of posttraumatic syndrome that fall. She was in eighth grade, getting four As and two Bs. However, she still was having trouble with math and spending an inordinate amount of time on homework, often 2 or 3 h. She remained in orchestra (cello) and on student council but was not back at dance. She remained on *Ginkgo biloba,* 60 mg bid. She reported having headaches about weekly or a little less frequent. They often responded to ibuprofen or other over-the-counter agents but might last overnight. Generally there was benefit with the medication.

She did serial 3s with some hesitation, but accurately. She remembered three objects for 5 min. The rest of the exam was normal.

The patient seemed fairly stable. It was recommended to continue using analgesics on an as-needed basis. I preferred naproxen for its longer time of action and higher efficacy. Alternatively, if headaches increased to any degree, prophylaxis with Amino-Mag (chelated magnesium), 200 mg PO bid, with food, was suggested.

We planned to see her again about the anniversary date of her accident.

Editorial Comments

This case study demonstrates a couple of pitfalls in the treatment of traumatic head injury. Patients' assessment of their own status is often suspect, and the opinions of family and objective data from school or psychometric testing are frequently necessary. Although *Ginkgo biloba* clearly benefited the patient's cognitive function and sense of well-being and aided symptom reduction, it did not, nor can any medicine, eliminate morbid effects of such an injury.

Treatment of Varied Symptoms with 5-HTP

This fourteen-year-old male was first seen in 1996 for continuing evaluation of an unusual movement disorder. Excellent notes were available from prior caregivers, supplemented by information from the patient and his mother.

The patient first presented to a neurologist in 1995. He had suffered spells over the prior three to four years of involuntary movement lasting 10 sec at a time. This involved movements in the arms and legs of varying severity. He had a vague feeling before the spells, but no other specific aura. It would seem to occur most often when arising in the morning or anticipating the initiation of motor activity. Movements were controllable volitionally to some degree but spells of difficulty would supervene seven to eight times a day. They seemed to be associated with speech arrest, but no postictal confusion or other residua after a few seconds elapsed. He had noted two episodes of brief, left-sided numbness and occasional blurring of vision.

On previous physical examination, the only finding was an asymmetry of the brachioradial reflexes. The patient had an MRI that showed a left anterior temporal lobe arachnoid cyst, which was reportedly unchanged from a prior CT of May 4, 1991. It was thought that there might be mild compression of the temporal lobe. An EEG was read as negative. By December 28, 1995, the patient had several more spells precipitated by movement. A serum copper was a bit low, at 8.8, and ceruloplasmin was 21, just below lower limits. He was believed at the time to have a "kinesiogenic" seizure disorder versus paroxysmal dystonia. He was given the option of taking Tegretol (carbamazepine). On January 1, 1996, the patient underwent a four-hour video EEG study at Stanford. The patient experienced two ictal episodes during which he had increased muscle tone, but neither were full-blown typical spells, and he did identify them as the same kind of episodes he had been suffering. No EEG changes were documented.

By February 28, 1996, it was determined that his problem was a movement disorder and not seizures. By May 22, he acceded to taking medicine, 200 mg of Tegretol tid. He complained of some initial fatigue but seemed to have fewer episodes, and none that were visible to his mother. The carbamazepine level was 8.0 (in the middle of the therapeutic range). His dose was increased to 400 mg a.m., 200 mg p.m., and 200 mg at bedtime.

In the previous two months, he had finally acknowledged that the medicine was necessary for his condition and had adjusted to the fatigue, not complaining of any current side effects. He reported no full-blown spells, although occasionally he felt as if one might occur. Occasionally he vaguely noted "trouble getting started." The patient experienced very brief head pains, alleviated by acetaminophen or ibuprofen.

The patient was born to a multiparous mother after a full-term pregnancy, with no illnesses or use of medicines, alcohol, or tobacco. Labor lasted 5.5 h, and birth weight was just under 10 lb. There was some neonatal jaundice, which went untreated. In 1991, the patient had a bike wreck. He apparently was found unconscious and, upon awakening, was incoherent for awhile, but a CT scan was normal, aside from the aforementioned arachnoid cyst. He was observed overnight. He cracked his teeth in a subsequent bike accident, but he had no other history of head injuries, convulsions, meningitis, or encephalitis. He experienced periodic asthma and used Proventil or Intal inhalers. He had no allergies. His developmental milestones were normal. He was entering ninth grade and was a good student. He was right-handed.

Family history was noteworthy for maternal second cousins, one with seizures and one with multiple sclerosis.

The family had just moved from California. The patient denied use of alcohol or tobacco. He exercised normally and slept well.

Physical examination recorded a weight of 135 lb, height of 69 in, and occipitofrontal circumference of 59 cm. He was a pleasant, cooperative patient. Head was normocephalic without bruits. ENT exam was unremarkable. Neck was supple, carotids full without bruits. Cardiac and abdominal exam was normal. The patient's expiratory phase was slightly prolonged, but without wheezing. Skin was free of neurocutaneous syndromes.

Mental status: The patient was alert and fully oriented. Fund of knowledge, right-left orientation, praxis, and naming skills were normal. He read a sixth-grade-level passage well, with good recall. Serial 3s were well done. He remembered three objects for 5 min. Speech and affect were normal.

Cranial nerves: I—Intact. II—Acuity was measured as 20/20 OD and 20/25 OS. Fields and OKNs were normal. Fundi were benign. Pupils were equal and reactive with full EOMs and no nystagmus. Remaining cranial nerves V and VII through XII were unremarkable.

Motor exam: The patient had normal tone and strength with no drift. Sensation was intact to fine touch, sharp/dull, vibration, position, and graphesthesia. Romberg was negative. He performed finger-to-nose, heel-to-shin, and rapid alternating movements of the hands well. Fine finger movements showed a trace of mirroring. Toe gait was normal, with heel and tandem gait minimally awkward. Reflexes were 1+ and symmetric throughout with down-going toes.

Assessment: The examiner assessed the patient to have paroxysmal choreoathetosis. This is a rather rare syndrome that responds well to carbamazepine, although it is not a seizure disorder. The arachnoid cyst seemed to be a chance finding. It was agreed to look at an MRI after a year, and then perhaps two years after that, if no changes occurred. Tegretol dosing was maintained.

The patient returned six months later. He had done well, but during the football season, he felt as if he was close to having episodes periodically, so he raised his dose of Tegretol to 400 tid with no specific subsequent attacks. He recently had a drug level of 9.2 with no side effects. His asthma seemed well controlled. He was doing well in ninth grade.

Exam was stable. Without complaint of headaches, it was agreed to hold off on reimaging the brain in relation to the arachnoid cyst.

When seen six months later, the patient had some irregularity of dosing attributable to a move that the family made. At worst, he experienced times when he felt as if he might have an impending spell, but none occurred. However, he had a variety of other symptoms, including some lethargy and headaches, which he related to his braces, but which had increased since baseball season ended and he had become less active. These were generalized, seemingly of mild severity, without nausea or photophobia, but with an occasional beating quality. Pain occurred every day or two but went away with ibuprofen.

Examination was unchanged and unremarkable. It was determined that the patient still required the same dose of medicine. He was switched to a long-acting preparation of carbamazepine for bid dosing. He seemed to still have some adjustment issues after moving to Montana. I asked that he and his family think about that for a few weeks to consider whether he should have treatment for depression—counseling, medication, or both.

When seen six months later, the patient had experienced no spells of paroxysmal choreoathetosis for a year. He had recently seen his pediatrician with complaints of fatigue, but both he and his mother thought, in retrospect, that this was related to viral involvement. Basic labs were normal. It had come to light that his Tegretol use was only sporadic, actually half the time. More recently, he has taken 600 mg of Tegretol-XR just once a day. He was doing well in tenth grade, except for math. He noted some sleep latency and early morning awakening with rumination but denied other symptoms of depression. He had no current complaint of headache. Exam was again normal.

The patient seemed stable. It was an open question as to whether he needed to continue the medicine. He was asked to continue as prescribed or taper the dosage to see what might occur, bearing in mind the implications of additional spells. Some discussion occurred on sleep hygiene and depressive symptoms.

When seen six months later, the patient had tried to discontinue medicine. Although he did not have an overt attack, he felt as if he might. This consisted of a feeling of muscle spasms or having difficulty upon rising. When regular about taking Tegretol-XR, 200 mg bid, he seemed to do fine. His mother thought he was more cheerful. There were some nonspecific symptoms over the prior two years, including frequent headaches, with pain at the vertex, and perhaps some nausea, but no photophobia or visual change. He was prone to periodic bouts of abdominal cramping, nausea, and diarrhea. His sister and grandmother had history of IBS (idiopathic bowel syndrome, "spastic colon"). Exam was again unremarkable.

We talked about his headaches and other symptoms and mood, and how they might be related to a relative serotonin deficiency. We discussed possible treatments, such as an SSRI versus 5-hydroxy-tryptophan (5-HTP). After this discussion, he opted to try the latter, 50 mg at bedtime.

He returned in another six months. He had been quite ill in the meantime with strep throat and then pneumonia. He had remained on Tegretol-XR 200 mg bid, with a rare miss during this illness. There had been no interim spells of the choreoathetosis. He occasionally would dream of it, and that bothered him, but not unduly. Eleventh grade was going quite well. He had a good driver's record, with no accidents or tickets. He was active in drama and had a girlfriend. He was also working part-time at an ice cream parlor, up to 20 h a week.

The patient remained on 5-hydroxytryptophan, 50 mg a day. His mother felt he was sleeping well, with fewer stomach problems. The patient noticed no clear effect on anxiety levels, but his headaches were only occasional.

Exam was stable and unchanged. It was agreed we would continue his low dose of Tegretol-XR. He was encouraged to try to regard his condition as a minor problem rather than a major one.

We had a long discussion about 5-hydroxytryptophan, including the "Peak X" controversy. I suggested trying a higher dose of 100 mg at hs and seeing if there was any improvement in the symptomatology.

One month later, his mother called to say that he had seen a newsmagazine show on television on the dangers of 5-HTP, with his brand displayed on a table, giving the implication that it could be unsafe. I gave his mother ordering information on a 5-HTP brand that had been specifically tested as free of "Peak X."

The patient switched to a brand known to be "clean" and was doing quite well six months later. He had a girlfriend and was active in the local newspaper and acting.

Editor's Note

It is unfortunate that the media now dictate the practice of medicine, most commonly without substantiation. The consumer is bombarded with information about herbs and drugs, both pro and con, with little ability to sift through the information to make truly informed choices.

Case Study 6

Dementia Treated with Ginkgo

This eighty-year-old male was referred by his internist for cognitive evaluation. The patient saw his doctor in 1986 regarding a question of a stroke. The only thing he reported was an episode in which he had problems with word finding. He was on aspirin and dipyridamole at the time. It was noted that he walked on a wide base, with his legs splayed apart to maintain balance. His CT showed atrophy. His wife complained of possible Alzheimer's disease because he displayed memory problems. He had some rectal and urinary incontinence and loss of libido. He had dysarthria with fatigue. Subsequently, a carotid ultrasound was normal, as was an EEG. He was continued on aspirin.

The patient returned in a few months with continued short-term memory concerns and word-finding problems. The patient tended to deny a problem whenever his wife noted it. There was associated weight loss. An MRI showed multiple lacunes in the white matter, with atrophy and some thalamic involvement. The patient had an elevated MCV (mean corpuscular volume) and low serum vitamin B_{12}. It was thought he had a multi-infarct or alcohol-related dementia. An echocardiogram was negative, and a carotid ultrasound showed minimal disease. A chemistry panel and thyroid-stimulating hormone (TSH) test were negative. He did have elevated homocystine and methylmalonic acid. The patient had tried to limit his alcohol and went on Zyban (bupropion), with supplemental vitamin B_{12}. He reported having a seizure in October, by which he means, while on Zyban, he got shaky and may have passed out. There were no convulsions. He then quit the drug with its associated emesis.

One month previously, his wife reported that he had trouble finding his drinking glasses and was also having difficulty reconciling bank statements. He continued to lose weight. His B_{12} level then tested above normal. Again, the patient tended to minimize his memory problems but admitted that, at times, he could not remember where everyday items were located. He also admitted that he got confused about a business arrangement he had previously made. There was a ten-day lapse in his Hytrin medication. His wife admits that he may display a short temper but is not belligerent, and there were no major personality changes.

The patient had a previous appendectomy, sinus surgery, and hospitalization for alcohol treatment. He had BPH (benign prostatic hyperplasia). There was no diabetic, thyroid, seizure, trauma, or encephalitis history. Medications were Hytrin, aspirin, and vitamins. He was allergic to penicillin.

The patient had a business administration degree and was right-handed.

Family history was negative for neurological conditions. He had worked as a corporate troubleshooter for the Atomic Energy Commission. He had dropped his current intake of liquor from 8 oz a day down to 4 oz. His wife reported an intake of a fifth of liquor a day when he was younger. He slept well.

Physical examination gave his weight at 126 lb and his BP at 112/62. He was generally pleasant and cooperative, but a very thin eighty-year-old male. Head was normocephalic without bruits. ENT was noteworthy for arcus senilis. Neck was supple, carotids 1+ without bruits.

Mental status: The patient was alert and basically fully oriented. Fund of knowledge, right-left orientation, praxis, and naming skills were normal. He read a sixth-grade-level passage well, with diminished partial recall of the contents. Serial 3s were well done. He was able to draw a cube, and his writing was a little shaky. He remembered one of three objects for 5 min, the second with a hint, and failed to name the third with choice. Speech was normal. His affect was social, and he showed a nice sense of humor and ability to laugh at himself. There was occasional circumlocution. He was able to name only eight animals in 30 sec (average of ten to twelve), but there were no word intrusions.

Cranial nerves: I—Intact. II—Fields and OKNs were normal. Fundi were benign. The patient's pupils were quite miotic, right greater than left. The right side was irregular. EOMs were full with no nystagmus. Remaining cranial nerves were normal.

Motor exam: The patient had normal tone and strength within limits of his limited bulk. There was no drift. Sensation was intact to fine touch, sharp/dull, vibration, position, and graphesthesia. Romberg was negative. There was a fine tremor on finger-to-nose movement on the right, moderate on the left. Similarly, rapid alternating movements of the hands and fingers were impaired on the left to a mild degree. Heel-to-shin movement looked equal. Basic gait looked okay, as did toe gait. Heel gait was slightly awkward, and tandem gait was suspect. Reflexes were trace at the biceps and knees and absent elsewhere, with toes equivocal, probably upgoing, especially on the left.

Assessment: The patient was assessed as having mental status changes with mild left-body neurological changes. The latter was felt to be lacunar in nature. Overall, his dementia was more likely related to alcohol than Alzheimer's disease. This was on the basis of his retained sense of humor, intact praxis with obvious short-term memory difficulties, his self-realization, and the fact that Alzheimer's would usually not be present twelve years without marked deterioration. We discussed options. First, it was my feeling that the patient should quit alcohol. He did agree to a trial of *Ginkgo biloba* in the form of an EGb 761 product, 60 mg PO bid. We also discussed the options of donepezil and neuropsychological testing.

The patient returned two months later. He had quit drinking after his previous visit. He had been taking *Ginkgo biloba* as directed, with no side effects. He saw his internist in the meantime, with mutual agreement that he was a lot better.

He felt his memory was improved. He was now remembering things that he had forgotten. He read a variety of materials and retained their content. He was more aware when balancing his checkbook and saw improvements in accuracy. He was losing fewer things around the home and felt happier. He attributed his improvement to ginkgo. His wife was not so sure about what was responsible, but she certainly saw that he was smiling more and was more responsive socially with her.

On exam the patient was alert and cooperative, fully oriented, and able to name the president. We attempted to have him name animals for 30 sec, but he did not sustain his attention well. The best he could manage was seven very quickly before bailing out on the task. He did remember two of three objects after 5 min and the third with a hint. He had full eye movement, with small pupils. There was no arm drift, and only a mild tremor on finger-to-nose movement. Reflexes were 1+ in the arm, trace in the legs. Gait showed slight arm swing, and tandem gait was a little suspect.

The patient was assessed, subjectively and objectively, as mildly improved. He was commended for abstaining from alcohol, but with this kind of difference in this period of time, I strongly suspected a pharmacological basis. The patient did not wish to try other agents, such as donepezil. We agreed to pursue the status quo with *Ginkgo biloba.*

When seen six months later, he appeared to be quite stable on the ginkgo.

Editorial Comments

This case seems to be a good example of the benefits that may accrue when a person with an earlier or milder form of dementia takes *Ginkgo biloba.*

Case Study 7

Treatment with a Variety of Herbal Agents

This patient first sought medical care in 1984. A professional in his early thirties, he had begun to suffer increasingly frequent, even daily, migraines. However, his history suggested a number of important psychiatric issues.

He had suffered from a very significant anxiety disorder in his teens and had a cycle of winter-associated dysfunction that suggested at least the possibility of seasonal affective disorder. He had pursued no formal treatment beyond counseling. He also experinced intermittent, and occasionally severe, bouts of idiopathic bowel syndrome (IBS, or spastic colon), which had been recalcitrant to all standard medical treatment.

Through college and for some years subsequently, the patient had smoked cannabis on weekends and occasionally during the week. This use trailed off subsequent to his perceived responsibilities and legal constraints.

Family history was noteworthy for a strong thread of migraine and anxiety in the patient's mother and reported bipolar disorder in a paternal aunt.

The neurological exam was unremarkable, and a physical merely revealed mild obesity associated with an extended break from past levels of physical activity.

A variety of medicinal approaches for the headaches were attempted by the patient. Use of six to nine aspirin a day led to a worsening frequency of headaches (which we would now attribute to the "analgesic rebound syndrome" [Mathew, 1997]). Trazodone (Desyrel) was efficacious acutely but was attended by initial feelings of ataxia and spaciness. When taken chronically, it produced sedation and hangover.

He also tried atenolol (Tenormin), a beta-blocker preferred to propranolol (Inderal) due to a lower incidence of side effects (Stensrud and Sjaastad, 1980), but, nevertheless, he enjoyed only a mild, temporary decrement in the headache burden. At higher dosage levels, he complained of lassitude, and after a course of acupuncture, he tapered off the drug.

The patient was unable to tolerate prophylactic use of naproxen (Naprosyn) due to gastric upset. Subsequently, he tried protriptyline (Vivactil), and then nortriptyline (Pamelor), both tricyclic antidepressants. Both produced sedation and mild dry mouth. The patient also noted an ususual association with these medicines. He possessed a temper that sometimes would get the best of him, but under the influence of these agents, it became hair-trigger. (This tendency is a known pitfall of tricyclic use in patients with bipolarity, but he did not fulfill diagnostic criteria.) The nortriptyline was also tapered off after the patient enjoyed some improvement in headaches through prescription of a program of sleep rationing, to 7 h nightly, coupled with aggressive aerobic activity.

During this interval, the patient sought counseling periodically for marital and "job burnout" issues. His diagnosis was Adjustment Disorder, Not Otherwise Specified. Subsequently, some years later, marital discord became more acute. Though depressed by this turn of events, he did not fit diagnostic criteria of depression, and, as before, testing (MMPI, MCMI [Millon Clinical Multiaxial Inventory]) did not support a specific diagnosis. A psychiatrist, nevertheless, did recommend the use of sertraline (Zoloft). The patient reported prominent initial diarrhea, nausea, and dizziness but continued the medicine. Eventually, prolonged counseling led to gains in his relationship. Medication was continued. Higher doses lead to lassitude and other side effects. Whether cause and effect, when a dose was rarely missed, the patient reported associated anxiety. When on vacation a few years later, he missed the medicine for four days. He noticed the error when an "inexplicable sense of ennui and futility" arose. He reported improvement upon resumption of the prescription.

After four and a half years on sertraline, along with the use of phototherapy of seasonal affective disorder (SAD), he sought herbal alternatives. Initially, he began on three 300 mg tablets of a standardized hypericum product, with 0.3 percent total hypericins.

He stopped the sertraline two days later. For ten days, he barely slept and reported vivid dreaming when he did. Almost immediately, he felt less sedated. Eventually, he slept longer, but only some 5 to 6 h nightly as opposed to his normal 7. That notwithstanding, he reported feeling quite a bit better. However, he noticed a return of the hair-trigger temper. Eventually, after two months, he chose to discontinue the hypericum.

Additional trials of natural medicine ensued. *Ginkgo biloba* was taken in doses up to 240 mg per day of a standardized extract (EGb 761). He reported no change in his continued periodic headaches or mood beyond a subtle enhancement of alertness. A *Panax ginseng* preparation, 110 mg standardized to 7 percent ginsenosides, was taken bid for three months, with no subjective changes. Chelated magnesium was taken in repetitive trials. Initially it led to a marked reduction in headache frequency and intensity but was ultimately not tolerated from a gastrointestinal standpoint. Similar problems arose with vitamin/mineral supplements. A sublingual B-vitamin supplement was without apparent effect.

He took 5-hydroxytryptophan (5-HTP) in doses of 50 to 100 mg. Initially, it seemed to help sleep, gastric complaints, and headache frequency. Over time, however, benefits became inapparent, and sedation was notable. Once discontinued, the patient felt better than previously.

Further trials of feverfew *(Tanacetum partheniu)*, a standardized lyophilized extract containing 400 μg of parthenolide for two months were not helpful.

Subsequently, the patient underwent a gastrointestinal regimen, advised by a clinical nutritionist, comprised of a two-month course of goldenseal *(Hydrastis canadensis)* in conjuction with butyric acid, quercetin, and gamma-oryzanol. A marked reduction in gastrointestinal symptoms and food tolerance resulted, along with a mild improvement in "sense of well-being." Headaches continued intermittently but were controllable with 1,100 mg of ginger powder, as needed, or, rarely, anti-inflammatories or triptan preparations (sumatriptan nasal [Imitrex] or rizatriptan oral [Maxalt-MLT]).

The patient reported his usual baseline level of chronic unhappiness, what one colleague came to term "cultural dsyphoria." Once more, clinical criteria for no formal psychiatric diagnosis were met.

Eventually, improved symptom control was achieved with dietary changes, an exercise program, and a combination of fish oil and borage seed oil supplementation.

Editorial Comments

This case demonstrates a common scenario, that of the patient with definite clinical complaints, but whose formal diagnoses remain elusive and treatment suboptimal. Nothing works for everyone. We cannot prescribe happiness and fulfillment, always avoiding life's frustrations. On the plus side, many such clients manage to achieve at a high level.

One speculative item concerns previous use of cannabis. When the patient was partaking of this substance, he reported no significant ongoing problems with headaches or IBS. Both complaints became more acute and chronic upon abstinence. Inasmuch as both conditions are reported to benefit from "medical marijuana" (Grinspoon and Bakalar, 1997; Russo, 1998), it is interesting to speculate what reintroduction of cannabis might provide to the patient from a therapeutic standpoint. He may represent an example of "clinical endogenous cannabinoid deficiency." Legal considerations currently obviated the possibility of experimentation with cannabis.

Another point of interest revolves around the patient's reaction to hypericum. Although this has not previously been reported, his side effect of temper supports the idea of noradrenergic stimulation in relation to that agent. Other practitioners and patients should be wary of this possible relationship when hypericum is employed in patients with bipolar tendencies or a family history of such.

Case Study 8

Managing Mania
and Obsessive-Compulsive Disorder

Chanchal Cabrera

Ms. L. first consulted with me in early 1993. At that time, she was thirty-nine years old and single and had been employed for several years as a cashier in a large supermarket. Initially she complained about abdominal gas and bloating and confided that she was sure she had cancer. When I explored this with her, it became apparent that she lived in fear of cancer and was convinced it was going to get her. She had become obsessed with it while nursing her mother, who some years previously died of cancer. In fact, she admitted, she tended to obsess about her health in general and about other things too. She had a history of admissions for temporary stays in the psychiatric ward of the local hospital, for episodes of anxiety, hysteria, and mania. She attended a care center once a week where she received counseling and support. She had taken lithium, BuSpar (buspirone, an agent for anxiety), and Luvox (fluvoxamine, an SSRI antidepressant, marketed for OCD) in the past and presently used Rivotril (clonazepam) at night to help her sleep. She admitted that she did not really know what her natural sleep pattern was because she always took the drug anyway.

Ms. L. was very articulate and well presented. She lived with her brother in a house they had inherited, and she had good relations with her family, friends, and co-workers. She said she was very happy and contented and had a good quality of life. She had been a heavy coffee drinker in the past, but three months before the first consultation, she had decided to stop in case it was adversely affecting her stomach. Indeed, the gas and belching had diminished somewhat, but to her surprise, she also noticed such a decline in her manic symptoms that she decided to consult with a natural health care practitioner to see if other simple remedies could be effected.

She was about 5′ 6″ and weighed 113 lb, though she said she had been down to 97 lb a year previously when extremely anxious. Her general health seemed to be quite good. She mentioned occasional nasal congestion, especially if exposed to smoke, and had been born with almost no sense of smell. She had lumpy and occasionally tender breast tissue, especially premenstrually, and she complained of dry skin. She also described a fluttering sensation in the stomach that we identified as being anxiety related. She was having two to three bowel movements daily, which tended to be soft and occasionally urgent.

Her diet was not good, and her eating habits were very erratic. She would eat almost nothing one day, then overeat the next, and she made no effort to balance basic nutrients. She did eat vegetables as well as fish and meat, just none of it with any consistency. She had an insistent sweet tooth and ate lots of chocolate, candies, and baked goods. She drank about six cups of black tea daily, as well as several cups of herbal tea (store-bought tea bags), and she took 2 tablespoons daily of Flor-Essence, an Essiac-type product with a laxative and alterative action (that which restores healthy bodily function). She took no nutritional supplements.

On examination, she showed some signs of adrenergic over-stimulation, with a pulse of eighty-five beats per minute, slightly clammy skin, dry mouth, and thin, wiry hair. Her blood pressure was normal at 115/78 mm Hg. Her patellar and brachial reflexes were not hypertonic. The breast tissue was fibrous, and I diagnosed fibrocystic breast disease. Palpation of the thyroid did not reveal any goiter.

I recommended that she obtain blood work to assess thyroid and adrenal function and have an ultrasound to establish a baseline condition for the breasts. I suggested that she quit the black tea, to reduce both the xanthine (caffeine and related compounds) influence on the breasts and the caffeine influence on the nervous system. I also gave her handouts and discussed the basic components of a healthy diet and how to balance nutrient intake. I asked her to drastically reduce her sugar intake and to eat whole grains, not refined ones. I also suggested she stop taking the Flor-Essence, as it was probably too stimulating for the bowel at this time. She was reluctant to take any supplements, saying she had difficulty swallowing capsules and tablets, so I emphasized the importance of eating well, in addition to being relaxed when eating, to switch on the parasympathetic nervous system and promote good digestive function.

We discussed her use of Rivotril, and I suggested she continue to use it for a few weeks until she felt confident and comfortable with the herbs. I also obtained her permission to contact her psychiatrist and her therapist to discuss the future reduction or cessation of the drug.

Treatment

Tincture Blend

Stachys officinalis (wood betony)	20 ml
Matricaria recutita (German chamomile)	20 ml
Verbena hastata (blue vervain)	15 ml
Humulus lupulus (hops)	15 ml
Avena sativa (oats)	15 ml
Lavendula angustifolia (lavender)	15 ml
Total	100 ml

The dose was 5 ml twice daily in hot water before meals.

Tea Blend

Melissa officinalis (lemon balm)	30 g
Mentha × piperita (peppermint)	30 g
Scutellaria lateriflora (scullcap)	20 g
Tilia × europea (linden)	20 g
Total:	100 g

The dose was 1 teaspoon per cup of boiling water, two to three times daily.

Rationale

The intention in choosing these herbs was both to calm the mind and to relax the digestive system. I wanted to bring her digestive symptoms under control so that she could have peace of mind, while recognizing that this very lack of such was a contributory factor in the digestive upset. I believed that if we could break this cycle, it would be a helpful beginning, giving her renewed confidence to work with the herbs in the long term to achieve better mental balance and stability. Each of the herbs in the tincture, except the *Avena,* serves the dual purpose of quieting both mind and gastrointestinal system, while the *Avena* provides a long-term tonic, nourishing and supporting the nervous system. In the tea, *Mentha* is a powerful carminative (helping to expel gas), the *Scutellaria* and the *Tilia* are relaxing nervines, while the *Melissa* is both a digestive aid and a relaxing nervine.

Stachys officinalis is the English wood betony, not the American lousewort or betony, which is actually a *Pedicularis.* This plant has a long tradition of use as a bitter digestive tonic, appearing to adjust the vagal nerve supply and the autonomic regulation of the digestive system, as well as being a relaxing tonic nervine, but only very mildly sedative. It contains such compounds as stachydrine, trigonelline, and betaine, as well as a bitter substance, volatile oils, and choline. It is especially indicated in situations of anxiety and nervous tension, with accompanying digestive upsets. It is also helpful for chronic headaches, migraines, neuralgia, lack of energy, loss of memory, dizziness, and disordered thoughts.

German chamomile is a traditional remedy for anxiety, restlessness, and hysteria. Chamomile also contains a bitter element that acts as a gentle digestive stimulant and normalizer. Another reason to include chamomile is for its antiallergenic properties, which I hoped would benefit the sinus congestion and stuffiness.

Verbena was included both as a nervine and a stomachic. It is quite bitter and stimulates appetite; production of digestive enzymes, mucus, and hydrochloric acid; hepatic and biliary activity; and absorption of nutrients and elimination of wastes. In addition, it has long been considered a tonic nervine, being stimulating and relaxing at the same time. It is traditionally used for hysteria and anxiety. It has been shown to stimulate both sympathetic and parasympathetic tone, which herbalists believe points to the herb's intrinsically balancing or regulating effect upon the nervous system.

Hops are one of the best-known remedies for nervous digestive upsets, as well as being markedly sedative and relaxing. The female flowers are used in medicine. They contain a number of flavonoids as well as a phenolic oleoresin, tannins, a bitter principle, and volatile oils. Hops also contain isovalerianic acid, which yields a fishy smell on drying and aging. 2-methyl-3-buten-2-ol, a degradation product of the alpha and beta bitter acids in the oleoresin, has been shown to exhibit the strongest sedative effect, although other constituents may augment the effect. Only a small amount of this substance is present in the herb, but higher levels may be formed in vivo by metabolism of humulones and lupulones. Hops have also been shown to exert a strong antispasmodic effect on smooth muscles and, thus, a marked digestive regulating effect, presumably by mediating the nervous supply to the gut.

Oats are considered to be a powerful amphoteric (balancing and normalizing agent) to the nervous system, being both a stimulant tonic and a sedative, as required. In this case, we wanted to calm the mind and ease the anxiety without causing drowsiness—a situation well suited to the use of *Avena*. Avena is a nerve tonic, restorative, antidepressant, and tranquilizer, as well as being a rich source of minerals with a nutritive specificity for the brain. The presence of an indole alkaloid called gramine is not unlike the sedative and hypnotic harmine group found in passion flower. It is recommended especially for nervous depression and overanxiety. For maximum potency, I used a fresh plant extract of the unripe seed (in the milk stage) at a 1:1 strength.

Lavender has been shown to contain bitter principles that make it an excellent choleretic and cholagogue (agent that increases bile flow). It is also rich in volatile oils, which, when inhaled, stimulate the limbic system and the diencephalon and cause relaxation in anxious, tense, or hysterical states. Lavender is considered to be a nervous restorative and recommended for nervous agitation, restlessness, palpitations, and fainting. It is best combined with warming agents, such as nutmeg and coriander, as a carminative digestive tonic.

Lemon balm is one of the best-known carminative relaxing nervines, being safe for children but effective for even quite acute cases. It was mentioned by Dioscorides, Pliny, and Gerard, and

Shakespeare named it as a strewing herb in *The Merry Wives of Windsor.* It is recommended to strengthen the brain, for restlessness, anxiety, and neuroses. It is used also for dizziness, insomnia, nervous excitability, loss of energy, migraine, hyperthyroidism, stomach cramps, and a nervous sensation in the stomach. Lemon balm acts as a sedative, antispasmodic, and carminative, specifically a nerve remedy with a carminative element. The three main indications are nervous heart, nervous stomach, and difficulty going to sleep, and, for the digestion, it combines especially well with peppermint. *Melissa* is notably high in volatile oils, although these are very difficult to extract commercially, and, hence, true essential oil of *Melissa* is rare and costly. The commercially available product is often adulterated with lemongrass, lemon, or lemon verbena. For this reason, herbalists use the whole leaf as a tea rather than the extracted oil. Taken as a tea, the volatile oil will evaporate, so it is wise to inhale the steam from the cup. It is soothing, calming, and uplifting. Volatile oil components that have shown sedative activity include citral, limonene, citronellol, citronellal, and geraniol, with citronellal being the most potent. They are believed to work in the hippocampus of the limbic system and are effective in reducing symptoms of excitability, restlessness, headaches, and palpitations.

Peppermint is also rich in volatile oils, the most notable constituents being menthol and menthone. It was included in this formula for its strong carminative action, which is due to the volatile oils that are believed to cause vagal stimulation and, hence, improved peristaltic function as well as enhanced production of digestive secretions. Peppermint is traditionally called a stomachic and is recommended for dyspepsia, flatulence, abdominal cramping, and colic. It is known to relax the cardiac (or gastroesophageal) sphincter of the stomach and thus ease belching (although in some preparations, this may promote gastroesophageal reflux disease [GERD], or heartburn).

Scullcap may be usefully employed wherever there is overexcitability of the nervous system. It is recommended for nervous irritability and restlessness as well as nervous disorders characterized by irregular muscular activity, twitching, tremors, restlessness, and incoordination. The *British Herbal Compendium* lists it as a sedative, relaxant, and spasmolytic.

Linden contains a number of amino acids, as well as up to 1 percent volatile oils. That fraction is rich in citral, citronellal, citronellol, eugenol, limonene, nerol, and alpha-pinene. The volatile oil also contains a characterizing odorant called "linden ether." This herb acts as an antispasmodic, sedative, hypotensive, anxiolytic, and immune stimulant. It has a long history of use for colds and flu, especially those accompanied by feverish headaches, chills, and fretfulness or restlessness. It is also widely used as a sedative for hysteria, anxiety, phobias, and irrational fear. The antispasmodic and diaphoretic properties are attributed to the flavonoids and *p*-coumaric acid, and the diuretic, sedative properties to the volatile oil, which is also an antispasmodic.

Clinical Outcome

Ms. L. was highly motivated and followed the dietary recommendations very closely. Symptomatic improvement occurred rapidly. Within two weeks she reported a marked decrease in digestive symptoms and a feeling of greater calm and mental stability. She began doing relaxation exercises and tried to get more physical exercise as well. Over the first three months of treatment, her digestive symptoms were completely eliminated, and this contributed to a lessening of the anxiety. She continued to use Rivotril, initially every night, but after two months, she spontaneously reduced this to an as-needed basis that averaged once a week for the next several months. This was the least amount of pharmaceutical influence she had known for many years, and her psychiatrist and therapist were very pleased.

Six months after commencing treatment, her uncle died of cancer and she began obsessing about it again. This rapidly spiraled out of control, and she was admitted to the psychiatric ward for a two-week stay. While there, she was put on Luvox (fluvoxamine), 100 mg nightly, but her psychiatrist encouraged her to reduce this and to stop taking it within a few weeks of leaving the hospital.

Since that time, for the past four years, she has taken Rivotril only two or three times in total, during periods of acute stress, and has otherwise relied on herbal remedies.

In the meantime, her blood work had come back showing normal thyroid and adrenal function, but slightly elevated fasting blood sugar. I counseled her extensively about dietary management of this situation and also prescribed trivalent chromium (glucose tolerance factor [GTF]) at 200 µg daily, and a tincture of *Galega officinalis* (goat's rue) and *Oplopanax horridum* (devil's club), to be taken twice daily. She took these herbs consistently for three months, then reduced the dose to once a day for three more months. Subsequent blood work has been normal, including hemoglobin A1C (a blood component that reflects blood sugar levels over the prior three months; elevations are common in diabetic patients who are not well controlled). She continued to be careful with her diet. I also gave her evening primrose oil (3 g daily) and vitamin E (400 IU daily) for the breast lumps.

In the early stages of the treatment I prescribed a Bach Flower Remedy (a homeopathic preparation). This was based on her completion of a detailed questionnaire. Her prescription contained clematis for being dreamy, inattentive, lost in thought, and impractical; honeysuckle for being nostalgic and unable to shut off memories; mimulus for fear of known cause; olive for feeling burned out, exhausted, and fatigued after a long ordeal, and white chestnut for persistent unwanted thoughts and being unable to shut off the chatter of the mind. She took this daily for a couple of months, then sporadically for several more months. I also gave her Rescue Remedy (a Bach homeopathic), for use as needed, that she reported was quite helpful.

Ms. L. continued on the full dose of tincture and tea for three months after the last psychiatric episode (nine months in total). We then dropped the dose of tincture to twice a day for three months, then down to once a day. She took this for several months and still used it sporadically thereafter, if she felt stress and tensions accumulating. Since July 1996, she has not used any herbs regularly, except the occasional cup of her tea blend, and has been more or less stable. She still tends to magnify things out of proportion and finds her weekly therapy session to be very important to prevent her from obsessing about things. She clearly notices the connection between her state of mind and her digestive system and no longer worries unduly when she has a minor digestive upset (usually triggered by poor eating habits). She took classes in assertiveness as well as art therapy, and this has helped her emotionally. I gave her instructions on breathing therapy as a means of stress control.

I still see Ms. L. every two months for a breast exam because she does not trust herself to do it. We always have a long chat about her life, emotions, and so on, but she receives no medications, except the chromium, evening primrose oil, and vitamin E. She remains in extremely good general health and very good spirits.

In conclusion, the biggest challenge in this case was the chronicity of her problems. Ms. L. had developed a habit of anxiety that was wired into her system. It was necessary to prescribe herbs over a long period of time, and even at the end of treatment, she still needed their support on occasion. This, however, seems preferable to the daily tranquilizers she had been taking for many years.

This case illustrates the vital importance of appropriate counseling and psychotherapy in managing mental illness. The herbs alone would not have been adequate, but they provided a nourishing tonic and strengthening adjunct to the therapy.

In this case I was fortunate to be able to consult closely with her psychiatrist and her therapist and to have their absolute support in attempting to keep the patient off prescription pharmaceuticals. It is likely that Ms. L. will always have a nervous disposition and tend to be a worrier. It is hoped that with the judicious use of herbs she can remain drug free and fully functioning.

Editorial Comments

This case is commendable in that a skilled herbalist does a thorough history and examination, taking into account the "whole person," collaborates with other caregivers, prescribes a specific regimen of herbal remedies, and adjusts therapy subsequently according to the patient's needs.

One point of interest is worthy of mention. A patient's difficulty with smell, or anosmia, may have diagnostic relevance. Such an affliction is frequently associated with depression and may be a deteriorating function as schizophrenia develops.

Case Study 9

Cases of Treatment with Ginkgo and Kava

Rebecca A. Wittenberg

This may sound apocryphal, but it actually happened. While I was working in Jackson, Wyoming, with herbalist Clarissa Smith, she decided that she would try to find out, to her own satisfaction, if *Ginkgo biloba* extract really had an appreciable effect on memory loss among the aged. She gave a 1 oz bottle of extract to every member of the local nursing home, with instructions to take three times a day and respond in a month with any effects they or their nurses noticed. She got an identical response from all. Without fail, each person had forgotten to take it.

This is actually a personal experience. I know nobody should prescribe for himself or herself, and it is absolutely true for me. I am the world's worst patient. I whine, I cry, I want somebody to make it all better and let me throw soup. The worst is, I cannot think straight about my own problem. I have long thought that two types of people are drawn to work in medicine: hypochondriacs and people who ignore their own health. I fall firmly into the latter category.

Several years ago, I hurt my back. I woke up one morning and could not stand up or roll over without assistance. It was a very scary feeling. I had had no trauma and had no idea if this was muscular or structural; I simply could not move. So I went to my doctor, who handed me muscle relaxants, took X rays, encouragingly said that if the problem was arthritis, it would not show up on an X ray for five years, and sent me on my way. I could not concentrate to read, but I could watch movies, if someone laid out pillows for me to lie on.

After six months, a pattern had been established. For about five days every four to six weeks, I could not move. During the rest of the month, I hurt. By this time I was getting desperate. So I went to more doctors. I went to general practitioners, orthopedic surgeons, chiropractors, and acupuncturists. I was poked and prodded, X-rayed, and handed medicines, told to apply heat, cold, alternating, but in the end, it all boiled down to the same response: "We don't know what's wrong; we can't find anything; it looks perfectly simple; there doesn't really seem to be a problem here. We think you're fine; you're just in a hell of a lot of pain."

The thing about long-term pain is it changes your personality. I am a fairly cheerful, happy-go-lucky sort of person, but during this time, I was consistently tired, discouraged, could not care about my friends' problems. I felt as if my self had been taken away from me.

I dimly remembered (I did, after all, have lots of time to think, though I was not doing so too efficiently) Kevin Spellman (an Ayurvedic practitioner) saying that kava *(Piper methysticum)* was useful for people in chronic pain with the sort of personality loss I was experiencing.

So I tried it. One day while well enough to go to work and sick of slathering wintergreen essential oil on my back (which helped mildly with the pain), I made a strong infusion of dried kava root (1 oz dried herb to 6 oz water). It perhaps worked a little too well. I spent my afternoon giggling so hard, everyone around me thought I was on marijuana. So I went home.

I now thought kava might help, but clearly I needed to work on doses, so I tried a formula I had made long ago for a potter who had back pain while working clay. (I can only say in defense of my having not tried this before, I do not do well when I am sick.) This is a tincture consisting of four parts kava fresh root extract, two parts *Pedicularis* fresh leaf and flower extract, one part scullcap *(Scutellaria lateriflora)* fresh plant extract, one-half part black cohosh *(Cimicifuga racemosa)* dried root extract. It was really wonderful. It did not help with range of motion or pain per se, but it really did give me that sense of self back. Although it hurt, I could carry on, with an occasional laugh and some caring for others.

A young lady was working with me at the time. I will call her Ruth. She was generally a very efficient and even-tempered person, but while working with her one morning, I noticed she seemed agitated. Although she was in no sense a client of mine, I asked what was wrong and was told she and her partner (I will call him Greg) were flying home for the holidays. This did not sound like cause for alarm, so I asked her whether she got along with her family. I was totally on the wrong track. It turns out that they were both frightened of flying, but as these trips were two thousand miles, no other alternative was available. I told her all the logical pap—that flying is perfectly safe—but they both were so concerned because the trauma was mental as well as physical. They described symptoms such as headaches and vomiting before, during, and after flights. This was compounded by the fact that Ruth had actually been in a minor plane accident as a child. So we talked about various relaxants, from chamomile tea to physical relaxation exercises.

Later that day, for an unrelated reason, we were talking about kava and how its place among neurological drugs is rather ambiguous. Although it is touted for sleep, I have personally found it more helpful in relaxation, mental clarity, and smoothing deeper pains one cannot change. So we tried it.

Now when they fly, starting three days beforehand, each of them takes kava tincture (fresh root extract 1:2) three times a day, and up to every three hours on the day of the flight. Although I cannot claim either of them feels easy about flying, the vomiting has stopped and other physical symptoms have lessened.

I think the kava is an effective therapy, but I do think that, in this case, some of that therapy is giving them something to do to help themselves rather than sitting there helpless.

Afterword

In this book, we have examined more than two dozen herbal alternatives in psychiatry. It is the author's fervent hope that this effort will contribute to the promulgation of knowledge of these psychotropic herbs.

Of the agents discussed, hypericum, ginkgo, and kava appear destined for phytotherapeutic superstardom. Whereas the former two have received broad public acceptance already, kava would certainly seem to be on the ascendancy, although it has not yet achieved similar market penetration. Its potential is truly great.

Additional herbs of considerable promise include valerian, German chamomile, linden, cannabis, and the essential oils. Similarly, it is hoped that research will soon allow us to understand the nutritional error of our ways and lead to a more rational diet, emphasizing helpful plant products that may ameliorate or prevent a degree of our current burden of depression and related ills. More botanical miracles portend; they merely need bold and adventurous scientists to seek them out in the fields and forests of our planet.

This book has attempted to present a balanced picture of herbal benefits and risks. The latter are greater in the underregulated U.S. market but must be examined in context. This text will serve as testimony to the extraordinary safety of quality standardized herbal psychotropic products. Their promulgation and usage may contribute greatly to the collective mental health of our society.

With continued research, it is hoped that herbal medicine may be reintegrated into its rightful place as a valued part of our modern pharmacopeia.

Ethan Russo

Glossary

AA: Arachidonic acid, an essential fatty acid (see Chapter 4).

acetylcholine: Neurotransmitter involved in movement and memory.

adaptogen: An agent that enhances everyday adjustment (see Chapter 8).

ADHD: Attention-deficit hyperactivity disorder (see Chapter 3).

adjunct: An added ingredient to enhance efficacy.

agonist: A stimulator of receptor or other function.

alkaloid: Bitter chemicals from plants with physiological activity (e.g., morphine).

ANOVA: Analysis of variance between groups.

antagonist: An inhibitor of receptor or other function.

anticholinergic: Activity in opposition to acetylcholine.

anxiolytic: An agent that "cuts" or treats anxiety.

BDI: Beck Depression Inventory (see Chapter 3).

Bender-Gestalt: A test of visual-spatial function (see Chapter 3).

benzodiazepine: Anxiolytic sedatives related to diazepam (Valium).

bid: Twice a day.

bioavailability: How much of an ingested substance is absorbed.

botanical: A plant medicine (see Chapter 1).

cerebral insufficiency: European term encompassing dementia (see Chapter 6).

CGI: Clinical Global Impressions scale (see Chapter 3).

CGIC: Clinical Global Impressions of Change (see Chapter 3).

chemotype: Plant variety with a certain chemical composition.

chemovar: A chemical variety of a plant.

cholinergic: Activity serving to stimulate acetylcholine.

chromatography: One of a variety of techniques to separate out chemical components (gas, liquid, thin-layer) (see Chapter 1).

CITES: Commission on International Trade in Endangered Species.

CNV: Contingent negative variation, an EEG measure of expectation.

Commission E: German agency regulating herbal safety and efficacy.

comorbid: Medical condition occurring concomitantly with another.

Conner's scales: Test employed to assess ADHD (see Chapter 3).

CT: Computed tomography, or "CAT scan," a computerized X ray technique.

cultivar: A cultivated variety of plant.

DHA: Docosahexanoic acid, an essential fatty acid (see Chapter 4).

dioecious: Type of plant with distinct sexual forms (e.g., ginkgo, cannabis).

dopamine: Neurotransmitter involved in movement and mood.

down-regulation: A decrease over time in neurotransmitter activity.

DRS: Dementia Rating Scale (see Chapter 3).

DSHEA: Dietary Supplement Health and Education Act (see Chapter 2).

DSI: A depressive mood scale.

DSM: *Diagnostic and Statistical Manual of Mental Disorders,* currently in its fourth edition (DSM-IV), employed in diagnosis of psychiatric and psychological conditions (see Chapter 3).

EAPC: European-American Phytomedicine Coalition (see Chapter 2).

EEG: Electroencephalography (brain wave test), employed in assessment of cerebral function.

EFA: Essential fatty acid, dietary requirement not synthesized in the human body (see Chapter 4).

EGb: Extract of *Ginkgo biloba* (see Chapter 6).

endorphin: "Endogenous morphine," neurotransmitter of opiate system modulating pain and, perhaps, depression.

enkephalin: Peptide neurotransmitter of opiate system.

ENT: Ear, nose, and throat.

enteric-coated: Treatment that allows passage through the stomach prior to digestion.

entheogen: Modern synonym for hallucinogen, a drug or plant producing "the divine within."

EOM: External ocular movements (or muscles).

EPA: Eicosapentanoic acid, an essential fatty acid (see Chapter 4).

ESCOP: European Scientific Cooperative on Phytotherapy (see Chapters 1 and 2).

FDA: Food and Drug Administration (United States).

flavonoid: Plant chemical components, often yellow, frequently displaying antioxidant activity.

free radicals: Chemical forms producing oxidation of lipids or membranes.

g: Gram.

G 115: Standardized extract of ginseng (see Chapter 8).

GABA: Gamma-aminobutyric acid, an inhibitory neurotransmitter.

GC-MS: Gas chromatography/mass spectrometry (see Chapter 1).

GLA: Gamma-linolenic acid, an essential fatty acid (see Chapter 4).

glycoside: Chemical combining a sugar and nonsugar.

GRAS: Generally Recognized As Safe.

ha: Hectare, approximately 2.5 acres.

half-life: Time needed for 50 percent of a chemical to be metabolized.

hallucinogenic: A drug or plant that induces hallucinations.

Halstead-Reitan: A battery of tests employed in neuropsychological assessment.

HAMA: Hamilton Rating Scale for Anxiety (see Chapter 3).

HAMD: Hamilton Rating Scale for Depression (see Chapter 3).

hypericism: Toxicity in grazing animals due to ingestion of *Hypericum perforatum* (see Chapter 4).

hypnotic: Agent to promote sleep.

ICD: International Classification of Diseases.

im: Intramuscular.

infusion: Herbal brew, as for tea.

ip: Intraperitoneal injection of a drug.

iv: Intravenous.

kg: Kilogram.

l: Liter.

LA: Linoleic acid, an essential fatty acid (see Chapter 4).

learned helplessness: An animal experimental technique designed to test states of anxiety.

LI 160: A standardized extract of *Hypericum perforatum* based on hypericin content.

lipophilic: "Fat loving" property of a chemical.

LNA: Linolenic acid, an essential fatty acid (see Chapter 4).

locomotor: Pertaining to movement.

MAO: Monoamine oxidase, an enzyme cleaving norepinephrine and dopamine.

MAOI: Monoamine oxidase inhibitor.

MCMI: Millon Clinical Multiaxial Inventory.

mean: In statistics, an average, the sum of scores divided by the number of scores (see Chapter 3).

median: The midpoint of a distribution; half of scores are above and half below this point.

Meta-analysis: An evaluation of a cohort of related studies (see Chapter 3).

mg: Milligram, 1/1000 of a gram.

ml: Milliliter, 1/1000 of a liter, equivalent to cc, or cubic centimeter.

MMPI: Minnesota Multiphasic Personality Inventory.

motility: Relative movement.

nervine: Agent taken for "nerves" or anxiety.

NF: *National Formulary.*

ng: Nanogram, one billionth of a gram.

NMDA: A type of neural receptor, N-methyl-D-aspartate.

nocebo: Opposite of placebo, a factor that produces side effects, although it should be inactive.

N-of-1: Type of drug study in which a subject serves as his or her own control.

nonpolar: Chemical property, preferring water.

nootropic: Agent enhancing thought or cognition (see Chapter 6).

norepinephrine: Noradrenaline, a stimulatory neurotransmitter involved in alertness and mood.

OCD: Obsessive-compulsive disorder.

ODS: Office of Dietary Supplements (see Chapter 2).

OKN: Optokinetic nystagmus, a railway following movement of the eyes that is a sensitive measure of visual pathway function.

OTC: Over the counter, drugs or supplements sold without prescription.

p: A probability value, stated as a decimal (see Chapter 3).

panacea: "Cure-all."

pharmacopoeia: A collection of drugs.

phytochemistry: Plant chemistry.

phytomedicine: Plant medicine (see Chapter 1).

placebo: False or inactive medicine, used as a control.

po: *Per oris,* by mouth.

polar: Chemical property, preferring fat or lipid.

polysomnogram: Test employing EEG and other measures to assess sleep (see Chapter 5).

ppm: Parts per million.

precursor: Previous step or compound in a metabolic pathway.

psychedelic: "Mind manifesting," a synonym for hallucinogen or entheogen.

psychometric: Test of mental function.

psychotropic: An agent that "turns the mind" (see Chapter 1).

PUFA: Polyunsaturated fatty acid (see Chapter 4).

qd: Once a day.

qid: Four times a day.

receptor: Cellular target of a neurotransmitter or drug molecule.

REM: Rapid eye movement or dream sleep (see Chapter 5).

SAD: Seasonal affective disorder, a type of depression aggravated by winter.

serotonergic: Affecting serotonin.

serotonin: 5-hydroxytryptamine, a regulatory neurotransmitter.

SFC: Structure-function claim (see Chapter 2).

Spielberger: A trait anxiety scale (see Chapter 3).

SSRI: Selective serotonin reuptake inhibitor, a kind of antidepressant (e.g., Prozac).

standard deviation: The square root of the average squared deviation from the mean.

standardized: Uniform composition and activity.

synaptosomes: Packets of neurotransmitters released to stimulate the downstream neuron process.

synergy: The quality of ingredients to enhance effects beyond a mere additive benefit.

tachyphylaxis: The loss of clinical effect of a drug with continued use.

tannin: Chemical plant component, often unstable.

TCA: Tricyclic antidepressant (e.g., amitriptyline).

terpene: Chemical component, especially of essential oils (see Chapter 9).

theriaca: Mixture of many herbal (and nonherbal) ingredients.

tid: Three times a day.

tincture: Plant extract in alcohol.

tonic: Agent designed to improve strength and well-being (e.g., ginseng).

T-score: A normalized score with a mean of 50 and a standard deviation of 10.

TSH: Thyroid-stimulating hormone, a pituitary hormone stimulating the thyroid.

up-regulation: Activity enhancing a metabolic pathway.

USP: *United States Pharmacopeia.*

verum: "True" or actual drug, as opposed to placebo.

WS 1490: Standardized extract of *Piper methysticum.*

WS 5572: Standardized extract of *Hypericum perforatum* based on hyperforin content (see Chapter 4).

Bibliography

Ackerman, D. 1990. *A natural history of the senses,* First edition. New York: Random House.

Adams, P.B., S. Lawson, A. Sanigorski, and A.J. Sinclair. 1996. Arachidonic acid to eicosapentaenoic acid ratio in blood correlates positively with clinical symptoms of depression. *Lipids* 31(Suppl.):S157-S161.

Ahmad, A. and L.N. Misra. 1997. Isolation of herniarin and other constituents from *Matricaria chamomilla* flowers. *International Journal of Pharmacognosy* 35:121-125.

Ainslie, W. 1826. *Materia indica; or, some account of those articles which are employed by the Hindoos and other Eastern nations, in their medicine, arts, and agriculture.* London: Longman, Rees, Orme, and Brown.

Allain, H., P. Raoul, A. Lieury, F. LeCoz, J.M. Gandon, and P. d'Arbigny. 1993. Effect of two doses of *Ginkgo biloba* extract (EGb 761) on the dual-coding test in elderly subjects. *Clinical Therapy* 15(3):549-558.

Almeida, J.C. and E.W. Grimsley. 1996. Coma from the health food store: Interaction between kava and alprazolam. *Annals of Internal Medicine* 125(11):940-941.

American Psychiatric Association. 1994. *The diagnostic and statistical manual of mental disorders,* Fourth edition. Washington, DC: American Psychiatric Association.

Anderson, E.F. 1993. *Plants and people of the Golden Triangle: Ethnobotany of the hill tribes of northern Thailand.* Portland, OR: Dioscorides Press.

Anderson, R.C., J.S. Fralish, J.E. Armstrong, and P.K. Benjamin. 1993. Ecology and biology of *Panax quinquefolius* L. (Araliaceae) in Illinois. *American Midland Naturalist* 129:357-372.

Anonymous. 1898. Ginseng in Korea. *Journal of the American Medical Association* 31:1491-1492.

Anonymous. 1995. Herbal roulette. *Consumer Reports* (November):698-705.

Anonymous. 1996a. *Centella asiatica* (Gotu kola). *American Journal of Natural Medicine* 3(6):22-25.

Anonymous. 1996b. Eleutherococcus. *Lawrence Review of Natural Products* (May):1-4.

Anonymous. 1996c. Survey indicates increasing herb use. *HerbalGram* 37:56.

Anonymous. 1997. "fx": Chemically adulterated product does not contain kava. *HerbalGram* 39:9.

Anonymous. 1999. AHPA reissues kava label warning. *HerbalGram* 45:15.

Aoyagi, N., R. Kimura, and T. Murata. 1974. Studies on *Passiflora incarnata* dry extract. I. Isolation of maltol and pharmacological action of maltol and ethyl maltol. *Chemical and Pharmaceutical Bulletin (Tokyo)* 22(5):1008-1013.

Appa Rao, M.V.R., K. Srinivasan, and R.T.L. Koteswara. 1977. The effect of Centella asiatica on the general mental ability of mentally retarded children. *Indian Journal of Psychiatry* 19:54-59.

Arenz, A., M. Klein, K. Fiehe, J. Gross, C. Drewke, T. Hernscheidt, and E. Leistner. 1996. Occurrence of neurotoxic 4'-*O*-methylpyridoxine in *Ginkgo biloba* leaves, *ginkgo* medications and Japanese *ginkgo* food. *Planta Medica* 62:548-551.

Arrigo, A. 1986. Behandlung der chronischen zerebrovaskulären Insuffizienz mit Ginkgo-biloba-Extrakt. *Therapiewoche* 36:5202-5218.

Arvigo, R., and M.J. Balick. 1993. *Rainforest remedies: One hundred healing herbs of Belize,* First edition. Twin Lakes, WI: Lotus Press.

Astin, J.A. 1998. Why patients use alternative medicine: Results of a national study. *Journal of the American Medical Association* 279(19):1548-1553.

Atanassova-Shopova, S. and K. Roussinov. 1970a. Experimental studies on certain effects of the essential oil of *Salvia sclarea* L. on the central nervous system. *Bulletin of the Institute of Physiology of the Bulgarian Academy of Sciences* 13:89-95.

Atanassova-Shopova, S. and K.S. Roussinov. 1970b. On certain central neurotropic effects of lavender essential oil. *Bulletin of the Institute of Physiology of the Bulgarian Academy of Sciences* 13:69-76.

Aulde, J. 1890. Studies in therapeutics—*Cannabis indica. Therapeutic Gazette* 14:523-526.

Awang, D.V.C. 1991. Herbal medicine: St. John's wort. *Canadian Pharmaceutical Journal* 124(January):33-35.

Awang, D.V.C. 1998. The anti-stress potential of North American ginseng (*Panax quinquefolius* L.). *Journal of Herbs, Spices and Medicinal Plants* 6(2):87-91.

Ayensu, Edward S. 1978. *Medicinal plants of West Africa.* Algonac, MI: Reference Publications.

Bahrke, M.S. and W.P. Morgan. 1994. Evaluation of the ergogenic properties of ginseng. *Sports Medicine* 18(4):229-248.

Balderer, G. and A.A. Borbély. 1985. Effect of valerian on human sleep. *Psychopharmacology* 87(4):406-409.

Beck, A.T. 1967. *Depression: Clinical, experimental and theoretical aspects.* New York: Harper & Row.

Beck, A.T. 1970. *Depression: Causes and treatment.* Philadelphia: University of Pennsylvania Press.

Beck, M.A. and H. Haberlain. 1999. Flavonol glycosides from Eschscholzia californica. *Phytochemistry* 50(2):329-332.

Becker, B.N., J. Greene, J. Evanson, G. Chidsey, and W.J. Stone. 1996. Ginseng-induced diuretic resistance. *Journal of the American Medical Association* 276(8):606-607.

Bell, E.A. and E.A. Fellows. 1966. Occurrence of 5-hydroxy-L-tryptophan as a free plant amino acid. *Nature* 210:529.

Bennett, D.A., L. Phun, J.F. Polk, S.A. Voglino, V. Zlotnik, and R.B. Raffa. 1998. Neuropharmacology of St. John's wort (*Hypericum*). *Annals of Psychiatry* 32:1201-1208.

Bernasconi, R. and J. Gebistorf. 1968. Ein Beitrag zur Kenntnis des ätherischen Lindenblütenöles und zur Chemotaxonomie der Gattung Tilia (A contribution to the knowledge of the essential oils of linden blossoms and to the chemotaxonomy of the genus *Tilia*). *Pharmaceutica Acta Helvetiae* 43 (10):677-688.

Biber, A., H. Fischer, A. Romer, and S.S. Chatterjee. 1998. Oral bioavailability of hyperforin from hypericum extracts in rats and human volunteers. *Pharmacopsychiatry* 31(Suppl. 1):36-43.

Binet, L., P. Binet, M. Miocque, M. Roux, and A. Bernier. 1972. Recherches sur les propriétés pharmcodynamiques (action sédative et action spasmolytique) de quelques alcools terpéniques aliphatiques. *Annales Pharmaceutiques Françaises* 30(9):611-616.

Birdsall, T.C. 1998. 5-hydroxytryptophan: A clinically-effective serotonin precursor. *Alternative Medicine Review* 3(4):271-280.

Bisset, N.G. and M. Wichtl. 1994. *Herbal drugs and phytopharmaceuticals: A handbook for practice on a scientific basis*. Stuttgart, Boca Raton, FL: Medpharm Scientific Publishers, CRC Press.

Bladt, S. and H. Wagner. 1994. Inhibition of MAO by fractions and constituents of hypericum extract. *Journal of Geriatric Psychiatry and Neurology* 7(Suppl. 1): S57-S59.

Blumenthal, M. 1997. Kava: The peaceful herb of the South Pacific. *Natural Pharmacy* (April):12, 15.

Blumenthal, M., W.R. Busse, A. Goldberg, J. Gruenwald, T. Hall, C.W. Riggins, and R.S. Rister. 1998. *The complete German Commission E monographs: Therapeutic guide to herbal medicines*. Trans. S. Klein. Austin, TX: American Botanical Council.

Bokstaller, S. and P.C. Schmidt. 1997. A comparative study on the content of passionflower flavonoids and sesquiterpenes from valerian root extracts in pharmaceutical preparations by HPLC. *Pharmazie* 52:552-557.

Bombardelli, E. and P. Morazzoni. 1995. *Hypericum perforatum. Fitoterapia* 66(1):43-68.

Bone, K. 1993-1994. Kava—A safe herbal treatment for anxiety. *British Journal of Phytotherapy* 3(4):147-153.

Borkman, M., L.H. Storlien, D.A. Pan, A.B. Jenkins, D.J. Chisholm, and L.V. Campbell. 1993. The relation between insulin sensitivity and the fatty-acid composition of skeletal-muscle phospholipids. *New England Journal of Medicine* 328(4):238-244.

Bos, R., H. Hendriks, J.C. Scheffer, and H.J Woerdenbag. 1998. Cytotoxic potential of valerian constituents and valerian tinctures. *Phytomedicine* 5(3):219-225.

Bos, R., H.J. Woerdenbag, F.M.S. van Putten, H. Hendriks, and J.C. Scheffer. 1998. Seasonal variation of the essential oil, valerenic acid and derivatives, and valepotriates in *Valeriana officinalis* roots and rhizomes, and the selection of plants suitable for phytomedicines. *Planta Medica* 64:143-147.

Boswell, J. 1960. *Boswell's life of Johnson,* New edition. London, New York: Oxford University Press.

Bove, G.M. 1998. Acute neuropathy after exposure to sun in a patient treated with St John's wort. *Lancet* 352(9134):1121-1122.

Brako, L. and J.L. Zarucchi. 1993. *Catalogue of the flowering plants and gymnosperms of Peru, Monographs in systematic botany from the Missouri Botanical Garden,* Volume 45. St. Louis, MO: Missouri Botanical Garden.

Braquet, P.G. 1997. Platelet-activating factor and its antagonists: Scientific background and clinical applications of ginkgolides. In *Ginkgo biloba: A global treasure: From biology to medicine,* Eds. T. Hori, R.W. Ridge, W. Tulecke, P. Del Tredici, J. Tremouillaux-Guiller, and H. Tobe. Tokyo: Springer-Verlag, pp. 359-369.

Brasseur, T. and L. Angenot. 1984. Contribution à l'étude pharmacognostique de la passiflore (The pharmacognosy of the passion flower). *Journal de Pharmacie de Belgique* 39(1):15-22.

Bravo, L., J. Cabo, A. Fraile, J. Jimenez, and A. Villar. 1974. Estudio farmacodinamico del lupulo (*Humulus lupulus* L.). Accion tranquilizante (Pharmacodynamic study of the lupulus' [*Humulus lupulus* L.] tranquilizing action). *Bolletino Chimico Farmaceutico* 113(5):310-315.

Brevoort, P. 1996. The U.S. botanical market—An overview. *HerbalGram* 36:49-57.

Brink, T.L., J.A. Yesavage, L. Owen, P.H. Heersema, M. Adey, and T.L. Rose. 1982. Screening tests for geriatric depression. *Clinical Gerontology* 1:37-43.

Bronaugh, R.L., R.C. Wester, D. Bucks, H.I. Maibach, and R. Sarason. 1990. In vivo percutaneous absorption of fragrance ingredients in rhesus monkeys and humans. *Food and Chemical Toxicology* 28(5):369-373.

Brooker, D.J., M. Snape, E. Johnson, D. Ward, and M. Payne. 1997. Single case evaluation of the effects of aromatherapy and massage on disturbed behaviour in severe dementia. *British Journal of Clinical Psychology* 36(Pt. 2):287-296.

Brynne, N., C. Svanstrom, A. Aberg-Wistedt, B. Hallen, and L. Bertilsson. 1999. Fluoxetine inhibits the metabolism of tolterodine-pharmacokinetic implications and proposed clinical relevance. *British Journal of Clinical Pharmacology* 4(4):553-563.

Buchbauer, G., L. Jirovetz, and W. Jäger. 1992. Passiflora and lime-blossoms: Motility effects after inhalation of the essential oils and of some of the main constituents in animal experiment. *Archive der Pharmazie (Weinheim Germany)* 325(4):247-248.

Buchbauer, G., L. Jirovetz, W. Jäger, H. Dietrich, and C. Plank. 1991. Aromatherapy: Evidence for sedative effects of the essential oil of lavender after inhalation. *Zeitschrift für Naturforschung [C]* 46(11/12):1067-1072.

Buchbauer, G., L. Jirovetz, W. Jäger, C. Plank, and H. Dietrich. 1993. Fragrance compounds and essential oils with sedative effects upon inhalation. *Journal of Pharmaceutical Sciences* 82(6):660-664.

Bullington, S.D. 1897. Passion flower *(Passiflora incarnata)* in epilepsy and other neuroses. *Nashville Journal of Medicine and Surgery* 107-109.

Burton, R. 1907. *The anatomy of melancholy.* London: Chatto and Windus.

Butters, N., D.P. Salmon, C.M. Culmin, P. Carins, A.I. Troester, D. Jacobs, M. Moss, and L.S. Cermak. 1988. Differentiation of amnestic and demented patients with the Wechsler Memory Scale-Revised (WMS-R). *The Clinical Neuropsychologist* 2:133-148.

Byerley, W.F., L.L. Judd, F.W. Reimherr, and B.I. Grosser. 1987. 5-hydroxytryptophan: A review of its antidepressant efficacy and adverse effects. *Journal of Clinical Psychopharmacology* 7(3):127-137.

Cabral, G.A., D.M. Toney, K. Fischer-Stenger, M.P. Harrison, and F. Marciano-Cabral. 1995. Anandamide inhibits macrophage-mediated killing of tumor necrosis factor-sensitive cells. *Life Sciences* 56(23/24):2065-2072.

Callaway, J.C., R.A. Weeks, L.P. Raymon, H.C. Walls, and W.L. Hearn. 1997. A positive THC urinalysis from hemp (cannabis) seed oil. *Journal of Analytical Toxicology* 21(4):319-320.

Capasso, A., V. de Feo, F. de Simone, and L. Sorrentino. 1996. Pharmacological effects of aqueous extracts from *Valeriana adscendens*. *Phytotherapy Research* 10:309-312.

Capasso, L. 1998. 5300 years ago, the Ice Man used natural laxatives and antibiotics. *Lancet* 352(9143):1864.

Caso Marasco, A., R. Vargas Ruiz, A. Salas Villagomez, and C. Begona Infante. 1996. Double-blind study of a multivitamin complex supplemented with ginseng extract. *Drugs Under Experimental and Clinical Research* 22(6):323-329.

Caughey, G.E., E. Mantzioris, R.A. Gibson, L.G. Cleland, and M.J. James. 1996. The effect on human tumor necrosis factor alpha and interleukin 1 beta production of diets enriched in n-3 fatty acids from vegetable oil or fish oil. *American Journal of Clinical Nutrition* 63(1):116-122.

Cavadas, C., I. Araujo, M.D. Cotrim, T. Amaral, A.P. Cunha, T. Macedo, and C.F. Ribeiro. 1995. In vitro study on the interaction of *Valeriana officinalis* L. extracts and their amino acids on GABA$_A$ receptor in rat brain. *Arzneimittelforschung* 45(7):753-755.

Cawthorn, A. 1995. A review of the literature surrounding the research into aromatherapy. *Complementary Therapies in Nursing and Midwifery* 1(4):118-120.

Chalone, G.P. and R.A. Bornstein. 1988a. Memory characteristics of patients with unilateral temporal and nontemporal lesions. *The Clinical Neuropsychologist* 2:275.

Chalone G.P. and R.A. Bornstein. 1988b. WMS-R patterns among patients with unilateral brain lesions: *The Clinical Neuropsychologist* 2:121-132.

Chan, T.Y.K. 1998. An assessment of the delayed effects associated with valerian overdose. *International Journal of Clinical Pharmacology and Therapeutics* 36(10):569.

Chatterjee, S.S., S.K. Bhattacharya, M. Wonnemann, A. Singer, and W.E. Müller. 1998. Hyperforin as a possible antidepressant component of hypericum extracts. *Life Sciences* 63(6):499-510.

Chatterjee, S.S., M. Noldner, E. Koch, and C. Erdelmeier. 1998. Antidepressant activity of *Hypericum perforatum* and hyperforin: The neglected possibility. *Pharmacopsychiatry* 31(Suppl. 1):7-15.

Chopra, I.C. and R.W. Chopra. 1957. The use of cannabis drugs in India. *Bulletin on Narcotics* 9:4-29.

Clendinning, J. 1843. Observation on the medicinal properties of *Cannabis sativa* of India. *Medico-Chirurgical Transactions* 26:188-210.

Cohen, A.J. and B. Bartlik. 1998. *Ginkgo biloba* for antidepressant-induced sexual dysfunction. *Journal of Sexual and Marital Therapy* 24(2):139-143.

Collura, J.O. 1997. Ginseng: Prince of tonics. *Vegetarian Times* (March):94-97.

Conners, C.K. 1990. *Conners rating scales manual.* North Tonawanda, NY: Multi-Health Systems.

Conquer, J.A. and B.J. Holub. 1996. Supplementation with an algae source of docosahexaenoic acid increases (n-3) fatty acid status and alters selected risk factors for heart disease in vegetarian subjects. *Journal of Nutrition* 126(12): 3032-3039.

Conrad, C. 1997. *Hemp for health: The medicinal and nutritional uses of* Cannabis sativa. Rochester, VT: Healing Arts Press.

Consroe, P. 1998. Brain cannabinoid systems as targets for the therapy of neurological disorders. *Neurobiology of Disease* 5(6)(Pt. B):534-551.

Cook, J. 1955. *The Journals of Captain James Cook on his voyages of discovery, Works issued by the Hakluyt Society,* Extra series, no. 34-37. Ed. J.C. Beaglehole. Cambridge: Published for the Hakluyt Society at the Cambridge University Press.

Cott, J. 1995. Medicinal plants and dietary supplements: Sources for innovative treatment or adjuncts? *Psychopharmacology Bulletin* 31(1):131-137.

Cott, J.M. 1997. *In vitro* receptor binding and enzyme inhibition by *Hypericum perforatum* extract. *Pharmacopsychiatry* 30(Suppl. 2):108-112.

Cott, J.M. and A. Fugh-Berman. 1998. Is St. John's wort (*Hypericum perforatum*) an effective antidepressant? *Journal of Nervous and Mental Disorders* 186(8):500-501.

Cross-National Collaborative Group. 1992. The changing rate of major depression: Cross-national comparisons. *Journal of the American Medical Association* 268 (21):3098-3105.

Culpeper, N. 1994. *Culpeper's complete herbal: Consisting of a comprehensive description of nearly all herbs with their medicinal properties and directions for compounding the medicines extracted from them.* London, New York: W. Foulsham, distributed by Sterling Publishing Company.

D'Angelo, L., R. Grimaldi, M. Caravaggi, M. Marcoli, E. Perucca, S. Lecchini, G.M. Frigo, and A. Crema. 1986. A double-blind, placebo-controlled clinical study on the effect of a standardized ginseng extract on psychomotor performance in healthy volunteers. *Journal of Ethnopharmacology* 16(1):15-22.

da Orta, G. 1913. *Colloquies on the simples and drugs of India.* London: Henry Sotheran.

Dastur, J.F. 1962. *Medicinal plants of India and Pakistan: A concise work describing plants used for drugs and remedies according to Ayurvedic, Unani and Tibbi systems and mentioned in British and American pharmacopoeias,* Second edition. Bombay, India: D.B. Taraporevala Sons.

Davies, L.P., C.A. Drew, P. Duffield, G.A. Johnston, and D.D. Jamieson. 1992. Kava pyrones and resin: Studies on GABA$_A$, GABA$_B$ and benzodiazepine binding sites in rodent brain. *Pharmacology and Toxicology* 71(2):120-126.

De Smet, P.A. and W.A. Nolen. 1996. St John's wort as an antidepressant. *British Medical Journal* 313(7052):241-242.

Delaveau, P., J. Guillemain, G. Narcisse, and A. Rousseau. 1989. Sur les propriétés neuro-dépressives de l'huile essentielle de Lavande (Neuro-depressive properties of essential oil of lavender). *Comptes Rendues de la Societé de Biologie* 183(4):342-348.

Dellis, C., J.H. Kramer, E. Caplan, and B.A. Ober. 1987. *California verbal learning test adult version manual.* San Antonio, TX: The Psychological Corporation.

Denke, A., H. Schempp, E. Mann, W. Schneider, and E.F. Elstner. 1999. Biochemical activities of extracts from *Hypericum perforatum* L. 4th communication: Influence of different cultivation methods. *Arzneimittelforschung* 49(2): 120-125.

Denke, A., W. Schneider, and E.F. Elstner. 1999. Biochemical activities of extracts from *Hypericum perforatum* L. 2nd communication: Inhibition of metenkephaline- and tyrosine-dimerization. *Arzneimittelforschung* 49(2):109-114.

Devane, W.A., L. Hanus, A. Breuer, R.G. Pertwee, L.A. Stevenson, G. Griffin, D. Gibson, A. Mandelbaum, A. Etinger, and R. Mechoulam. 1992. Isolation and structure of a brain constituent that binds to the cannabinoid receptor. *Science* 258(5090):1946-1949.

Diwan, P.V. and I. Karwande. 1991. Anti-anxiety profile of manduk parni *(Centella asiatica)* in animals. *Fitoterapia* 62(3):253-257.

Dixon, W.E. 1899. The pharmacology of *Cannabis indica. British Medical Journal* 2:1354-1357.

Dolan, J.P. 1971. A note on the use of *Cannabis sativa* in the 17th century (Engelbert Kaempfer). *Journal of the South Carolina Medical Association* 67(10):424-427.

Domínguez, X.A. and M. Hinojosa. 1976. Mexican medicinal plants. XXVIII. Isolation of 5-hydroxy-7,3',4'- trimethoxy-flavone from *Turnera diffusa. Planta Medica* 30(1):68-71.

Duke, J.A. 1985. *CRC handbook of medicinal herbs.* Boca Raton, FL: CRC Press.

Duke, J.A. 1997. *The green pharmacy: New discoveries in herbal remedies for common diseases and conditions from the world's foremost authority on healing herbs.* Emmaus, PA: Rodale Press.

Dwuma-Badu, D., W.H. Watson, E.M. Gopalakrishna, T.U. Okarter, J.E. Knapp, P.L. Schiff, and D.J. Slatkin. 1976. Constituents of West African medicinal plants. XVI. Griffonin and griffonilide, novel constituents of *Griffonia simplicifolia. Lloydia* 39(6):385-390.

Eagles, J.M. 1990. Treatment of depression with pumpkin seeds. *British Journal of Psychiatry* 157:937-938.

Eaton, S.B. 1990. What did our late paleolithic (preagricultural) ancestors eat? *Nutrition Reviews* 48(5):227-230.

Eaton, S.B., S.B. Eaton III, and M.J. Konner. 1997. Paleolithic nutrition revisited: A twelve-year retrospective on its nature and implications. *European Journal of Clinical Nutrition* 51(4):207-216.

Eaton, S.B., S.B. Eaton III, A.J. Sinclair, L. Cordain, and N.J. Mann. 1998. Dietary intake of long-chain polyunsaturated fatty acids during the paleolithic. *World Review of Nutrition and Dietetics* 83:12-23.

Eaton, S.B. and M. Konner. 1985. Paleolithic nutrition. A consideration of its nature and current implications. *New England Journal of Medicine* 312(5):283-289.

Eaton, S.B., M. Shostak, and M. Konner. 1988. *The Paleolithic prescription: A program of diet and exercise and a design for living,* First edition. New York: Harper & Row.

Edwards, R., M. Peet, J. Shay, and D. Horrobin. 1998. Omega-3 polyunsaturated fatty acid levels in the diet and in red blood cell membranes of depressed patients. *Journal of Affective Disorders* 48(2/3):149-155.

Ehrlichman, H. and J.N. Halpern. 1988. Affect and memory: Effects of pleasant and unpleasant odors on retrieval of happy and unhappy memories. *Journal of Personality and Social Psychology* 55(5):769-779.

Eisenberg, D.M., R.C. Kessler, C. Foster, F.E. Norlock, D.R. Calkins, and T.L. Delbanco. 1993. Unconventional medicine in the United States. Prevalence, costs, and patterns of use. *New England Journal of Medicine* 328(4):246-252.

Ellison, J.M. and P. DeLuca. 1998. Fluoxetine-induced genital anesthesia relieved by *Ginkgo biloba* extract. *Journal of Clinical Psychiatry* 59(4):199-200.

Emerit, I., R. Arutyunyan, N. Oganesian, A. Levy, L. Cernjavsky, T. Sarkisian, A. Pogosian, and K. Asrian. 1995. Radiation-induced clastogenic factors: Anticlastogenic effect of *Ginkgo biloba* extract. *Free Radical Biology and Medicine* 18(6):985-991.

Emerit, I., N. Oganesian, T. Sarkisian, R. Arutyunyan, A. Pogosian, K. Asrian, A. Levy, and L. Cernjavski. 1995. Clastogenic factors in the plasma of Chernobyl accident recovery workers: Anticlastogenic effect of *Ginkgo biloba* extract. *Radiation Research* 144(2):198-205.

Erasmus, U. 1993. *Fats that heal, fats that kill: The complete guide to fats, oils, cholesterol, and human health,* Revised, updated, and expanded edition. Burnaby, BC, Canada: Alive Books.

Ernst, E., J.I. Rand, and C. Stevinson. 1998a. Adverse effects profile of the herbal antidepressant St. John's wort (*Hypericum perforatum* L.). *European Journal of Clinical Pharmacology* 54:589-594.

Ernst, E., J.I. Rand, and C. Stevinson. 1998b. Complementary therapies for depression: An overview. *Archives of General Psychiatry* 55(11):1026-1032.

European Scientific Cooperative on Phytotherapy. 1996-1997. *Monographs on the medicinal uses of plant drugs.* Exeter, UK: European Scientific Cooperative on Phytotherapy.

European Scientific Cooperative on Phytotherapy. 1997. *Monographs on the medicinal uses of plant drugs.* Exeter, UK: European Scientific Cooperative on Phytotherapy.

Farnsworth, N.R., O. Akerele, A.S. Bingel, D.D. Soejarto, and Z. Guo. 1985. Medicinal plants in therapy. *Bulletin of the World Health Organization* 63(6):965-981.

Federal Register. 1998. FDA rules and regulations, dated April 29, 1998, concerning supplements, pp. 23623-23628. Available online: <wais.access.gpo.gov>.

Fellows, L.E. and E.A. Bell. 1970. 5-hydroxy-L-tryptophan, 5-hydroxytryptamine and L-tryptophan-5-hydroxylase in *Griffonia simplicifolia. Phytochemistry* 9:2389-2396.

Felter, H.W. and J.U. Lloyd. 1900. *King's American Dispensatory.* Cincinnati, OH: Ohio Valley Co.

Flanagan, N. 1995. The clinical use of aromatherapy in Alzheimer's patients. *Alternative and Complementary Therapies* (November/December):377-380.

Folstein, M.F., S.E. Folstein, and P.R. McHugh. 1975. Mini-mental state. A practical method for grading the cognitive state of patients for the clinician. *Journal of Psychiatric Research* 12:189-198.

Food and Drug Administration. 1980. *Unsafe herbs.* Washington, DC: U.S. Food and Drug Administration.

Foster, S. 1996a. *American ginseng:* Panax quinquefolius. Austin, TX: American Botanical Council.

Foster, S. 1996b. *Asian ginseng:* Panax ginseng. Austin, TX: American Botanical Council.

Foster, S. 1996c. *Chamomile:* Matricaria recutita and Chamaemelum nobile. Austin, TX: American Botanical Council.

Foster, S. 1996d. Scullcap: An herbal enigma. *The Business of Herbs* (May/June): 14-16.

Foster, S. 1996e. *Siberian ginseng:* Eleutherococcus senticosus. Austin, TX: American Botanical Council.

Foster, S. 1996f. *Valerian:* Valeriana officinalis. Austin, TX: American Botanical Council.

Foster, S. and V.E. Tyler. 1999. *Tyler's honest herbal: A sensible guide to the use of herbs and related remedies,* Fourth edition. Binghamton, NY: The Haworth Herbal Press.

Freud, S. 1930. *Civilization and its discontents.* London: Hogarth Press.

Fundaro, A. and M.C. Cassone. 1980. Azione degli olii essenziali di camomilla, canella, assenzio, macis e origano su un comportamento operativo nel ratto (Action of essential oils of chamomile, cinnamon, absinthium, mace and origanum on operant conditioning behavior of the rat). *Bollettino—Societa Italiana Biologia Sperimentale (Napoli)* 56(22):2375-2380.

Galli, C. and F. Marangoni. 1997. Recent advances in the biology of n-6 fatty acids. *Nutrition* 13(11/12):978-985.

Garges, H.P., I. Varia, and P.M. Doraiswamy. 1998. Cardiac complications and delirium associated with valerian root withdrawal. *Journal of the American Medical Association* 280(18):1566-1567.

Gattefossé, R.-M. 1993. *Gattefossé's aromatherapy.* Trans. R.W. Tisserand. Essex: C.W. Daniel.

Gerard, J. 1931. *Leaves from Gerard's herball.* Ed. M. Woodward. Boston: Houghton Mifflin.

Gerard, J. 1975. *The herbal: or, general history of plants.* New York: Dover Publications.

Gerhard, U., N. Linnenbrink, C. Georghiadou, and V. Hobi. 1996. Vigilanzmindernde Effekte zweier pflanzlicher Schlafmittel (Vigilance-decreasing effects of 2 plant-derived sedatives). *Schweizerische Rundschau für Medizin Praxis* 85(15):473-481.

Gerhardt, G., K. Rogalla, and J. Jaeger. 1990. Medikamentöse Therapie von Hirnleistungsstören. Randomisierte Vergleichstudie mit Dihydroergotoxin und *Ginkgo-biloba* Extrakt (Drug therapy of disorders of cerebral performance. Randomized comparative study of dihydroergotoxine and *Ginkgo biloba* extract). *Fortschritte der Medizin* 108(19):384-388.

Gibbons, E. 1966. *Stalking the healthful herbs.* New York: David McKay.

Gillis, C.N. 1997. *Panax ginseng* pharmacology: A nitric oxide link? *Biochemical Pharmacology* 54(1):1-8.

Golsch, S., E. Vocks, J. Rakoski, K. Brockow, and J. Ring. 1997. Reversible increase in photosensitivity to UV-B caused by St. John's wort extract. *Hautarzt* 48(4):249-252.

Gordon, J.B. 1998. SSRIs and St. John's wort: Possible toxicity? *American Family Physician* 57(5):950, 953.

Grässel, E. 1992. Einfluss von Ginkgo-biloba Extrakt auf die gestige Leistungsfähigkeit (Effect of ginkgo-biloba extract on mental performance. Double-blind study using computerized measurement conditions in patients with cerebral insufficiency). *Fortschritte der Medizin* 110(5):73-76.

Grauds, C. 1999. *Everything you need to know about kava and anxiety, the natural pharmacist.* Rocklin, CA: Prima Health.

Greenberg, J.H., A. Mellors, and J.C. McGowan. 1978. Molar volume relationships and the specific inhibition of a synaptosomal enzyme by psychoactive cannabinoids. *Journal of Medicinal Chemistry* 21(12):1208-1212.

Grieve, M. 1971. *A modern herbal: The medicinal, culinary, cosmetic and economic properties, cultivation and folk-lore of herbs, grasses, fungi, shrubs, and trees with all their modern scientific uses.* New York: Dover Publications.

Grieve, M. 1974. *A modern herbal: The medicinal, culinary, cosmetic, and economic properties, cultivation, and folklore of herbs, grasses, fungi, shrubs, and trees with all their modern scientific uses.* New York: Hafner Press.

Griffiths, M. 1994. *Index of garden plants.* Portland, OR: Timber Press.

Grinspoon, L. and J.B. Bakalar. 1997. *Marihuana, the forbidden medicine,* Revised and expanded edition. New Haven, CT: Yale University Press.

Grinspoon, L., and J.B. Bakalar. 1998. The use of cannabis as a mood stabilizer in bipolar disorder: Anecdotal evidence and the need for clinical research. *Journal of Psychoactive Drugs* 30(2):171-177.

Gruenwald, J. 1997. Standardized St. John's wort extract clinical monograph. *Quarterly Review of Natural Medicine* (Winter):289-299.

Guillemain, J., A. Rousseau, and P. Delaveau. 1989. Effets Neurodépresseurs de l'huile essentielle de *Lavandula angustifolia* Mill (Neurodepressive effects of the essential oil of *Lavandula angustifolia* Mill.). *Annales Pharmaceutiques Francaises* 47(6):337-343.

Guy, W. Ed. 1976. *Clinical global assessment scale (CGI). ECDEU assessment manual for psychopharmacology.* Rockville, MD: U.S. Department of Health, Education and Welfare, National Institute of Mental Health, pp. 218-222.

Halama, P. 1990. Was leistet der Spezialextrakt (EGb 761)?: Ergebnisse einer placebokontrollierten, randomisierten doppelblinden Pilotstudie. *Therapiewoche* 40:3760-3765.

Hamazaki, T., S. Sawazaki, M. Itomura, E. Asaoka, Y. Nagao, N. Nishimura, K. Yazawa, T. Kuwamori, and M. Kobayashi. 1996. The effect of docosahexaenoic acid on aggression in young adults. A placebo-controlled double-blind study. *Journal of Clinical Investigation* 97(4):1129-1133.

Hamilton, M. 1959. The assessment of anxiety states by rating. *British Journal of Medical Psychology* 32:50-55.

Hamilton, M. 1960. A rating scale for depression. *Journal of Neurology, Neurosurgery and Psychiatry* 23:56-62.

Hänsel, R. 1968. Characterization and physiological activity of some *Kawa* constituents. *Pacific Science* 22:293-313.

Hänsel, R. 1997-1998. Kava-kava (*Piper methysticum* G. Forster) in contemporary medical research. Portrait of a medicinal plant. *European Journal of Herbal Medicine* 3(3):17-23.

Hänsel, R., R. Wohlfart, and H. Coper. 1980. Versuche, sedativ-hypnotische Wirkstogge im Hopfen nachzuwesein, II (Sedative-hypnotic compounds in the exhalation of hops, II). *Zeitschrift fuer Naturforschung [C]* 35(11/12):1096-1097.

Hänsen, H.S. 1994. New biological and clinical roles for the n-6 and n-3 fatty acids. *Nutrition Reviews* 52(5):162-167.

Hänsgen, K.D., J. Vesper, and M. Ploch. 1994. Multicenter double-blind study examining the antidepressant effectiveness of the hypericum extract LI 160. *Journal of Geriatric Psychiatry and Neurology* 7(Suppl. 1):S15-S18.

Hardy, M. 1991. Sweet scented dreams: Vaporised lavender oil as a nocturnal sedative for elderly patients with sleeping difficulties. *International Journal of Aromatherapy* 3(2):12-13.

Harnsberger, S. 1898. Partial blindness following the administration of potassium bromide and passion flower. *Virginia Medical Semi-Monthly* (October 7):392.

Harrer, G., W.D. Hübner, and H. Podzuweit. 1994. Effectiveness and tolerance of the hypericum extract LI 160 compared to maprotiline: A multicenter double-blind study. *Journal of Geriatric Psychiatry and Neurology* 7(Suppl. 1): S24-S28.

Harrer, G. and V. Schulz. 1994. Clinical investigation of the antidepressant effectiveness of hypericum. *Journal of Geriatric Psychiatry and Neurology* 7(Suppl. 1): S6-S8.

Hathaway, S.R. and J.C. McKinley. 1943. *Booklet for the Minnesota multiphasic personality inventory (MMPI).* New York: The Psychological Corporation.

Hathaway, S.R., J.C. McKinley, J.N. Butcher, W.G. Dalstrom, J.R. Graham, A. Tellegen, and B. Kramer. 1989. *Minnesota multiphasic personality inventory, Second edition (MMPI-2): Manual for administration and scoring.* Minneapolis: University of Minnesota Press.

Heaton, R.K., I. Grant, C.G. Matthews. 1991. *Comprehensive norms for an expanded Halstead-Reitan battery: Demographic corrections, research findings, and clinical applications.* Odessa, FL: Psychological Assessment Resources.

Heiligenstein, E. and G. Guenther. 1998. Over-the-counter psychotropics: A review of melatonin, St. John's wort, valerian, and kava-kava. *Journal of American College Health* 46(6):271-276.

Hemming, M. and P.M. Yellowlees. 1993. Effective treatment of Tourette's syndrome with marijuana. *Journal of Psychopharmacology* 7(4):389-391.

Hendriks, H., R. Bos, D.P. Allersma, T.M. Malingre, and A.S. Koster. 1981. Pharmacological screening of valerenal and some other components of essential oil of *Valeriana officinalis. Planta Medica* 42(1):62-68.

Herkenham, M.A. 1993. Localization of cannabinoid receptors in brain: Relationship to motor and reward systems. In *Biological Basis of Substance Abuse*, Eds. S.G. Korman and J.D. Barchas. London: Oxford University, pp. 187-200.

Herkenham, M., A.B. Lynn, M.D. Little, M.R. Johnson, L.S. Melvin, B.R. de Costa, and K.C. Rice. 1990. Cannabinoid receptor localization in brain. *Proceedings National Academy of Sciences, USA* 87(5):1932-1936.

Herodotus. 1954. *Herodotus: The histories.* Trans. A. De Sélincourt. Harmondsworth, Middlesex, Baltimore: Penguin Books.

Hess, F.G., Jr., R.A. Parent, K.R. Stevens, G.E. Cox, and P.J. Becci. 1983. Effects of subchronic feeding of ginseng extract G115 in beagle dogs. *Food and Chemical Toxicology* 21(1):95-97.

Hibbeln, J.R. 1998. Fish consumption and major depression. *Lancet* 351(9110): 1213.

Hibbeln, J.R. and N. Salem Jr. 1995. Dietary polyunsaturated fatty acids and depression: When cholesterol does not satisfy. *American Journal of Clinical Nutrition* 62(1):1-9.

Hibbeln, J.R., J.C. Umhau, D.T. George, and N. Salem Jr. 1997. Do plasma polyunsaturates predict hostility and depression? *World Review of Nutrition and Dietetics* 82:175-186.

Hibbeln, J.R., J.C. Umhau, M. Linnoila, D.T. George, P.W. Ragan, S.E. Shoaf, M.R. Vaughan, R. Rawlings, and N. Salem Jr. 1998. A replication study of violent and nonviolent subjects: Cerebrospinal fluid metabolites of serotonin and dopamine are predicted by plasma essential fatty acids. *Biological Psychiatry* 44(4):243-249.

Hildegard. 1998. *Hildegard von Bingen's physica: The complete English translation of her classic work on health and healing.* Trans. Priscilla Throop. Rochester, VT: Healing Arts Press.

Hiller, K.-O. and G. Zetler. 1996. Neuropharmacological studies on ethanol extracts of *Valeriana officinalis* L.: Behavioural and anticonvulsant properties. *Phytotherapy Research* 10:145-151.

Hippius, H. 1998. St. John's wort (*Hypericum perforatum*)—An herbal antidepressant. *Current Medical Research and Opinion* 14(3):171-184.

Hirase, S. 1895. Études sur la fecondation et l'embryogenie du Ginkgo biloba. *Journal of the College of Sciences of the University of Tokyo* 8:307-322.

Hobbs, C. 1988-1989. St. John's wort: *Hypericum perforatum* L. *HerbalGram* 18/19:24-33.

Hofferberth, B. 1994. The efficacy of EGb 761 in patients with senile dementia of the Alzheimer type: A double-blind placebo-controlled study on different levels of investigation. *Human Psychopharmacology* 9:215-222.

Holzl, J. and P. Godau. 1989. Receptor binding studies with *Valeriana officinalis* on the benzodiazepine receptor. *Planta Medica* 55:642.

Houghton, P.J. 1988. The biological activity of valerian and related plants. *Journal of Ethnopharmacology* 22(2):121-142.

Houghton, P. 1994. Valerian. *Pharmaceutical Journal* 253:95-96.

Hu, S.-Y. 1976. The genus *Panax* (ginseng) in Chinese medicine. *Economic Botany* 30:11-28.

Hu, S.-Y. 1977. A contribution to our knowledge of ginseng. *American Journal of Chinese Medicine* 5(1):1-23.

Hübner, W.D., S. Lande, and H. Podzuweit. 1994. Hypericum treatment of mild depressions with somatic symptoms. *Journal of Geriatric Psychiatry and Neurology* 7(Suppl. 1):S12-S14.

Huh, H. and E.J. Staba. 1990. The botany and chemistry *of Ginkgo biloba* L. *Journal of Herbs, Spices and Medicinal Plants* 1(1/2):91-124.

Hutt, M. 1969. *Hutt adaptation of the Bender-Gestalt test,* Second edition. New York: Gruen and Stratton.

Indian Hemp Drugs Commission. 1893-1894. *Indian Hemp Drugs Commission Report,* India: Simla, seven volumes.

Irvine, F.R. 1961. *Woody plants of Ghana: With special reference to their uses,* Revised edition. London: Oxford University Press.

Israël, L., E. Dell'accio, G. Martin, and R. Hugonot. 1987. Extrait de Ginkgo biloba et exercises d'entraînement de la mémoire. Evaluation comparative chez des personnes agées ambulatoires. *Psychologie Medicale* 19(8):1431-1439.

Itil, T. M., E. Eralp, I. Ahmed, A. Kunitz, and K.Z. Itil. 1998. The pharmacological effects of *Ginkgo biloba*, a plant extract, on the brain of dementia patients in comparison with tacrine. *Psychopharmacology Bulletin* 34(3):391-397.

Itil, T.M., E. Eralp, E. Tsambis, K. Itil, and U. Stein. 1996. Central nervous system effects of *Ginkgo biloba*, a plant extract. *American Journal of Therapeutics* 3:63-73.

Itil, T. and D. Martorano. 1995. Natural substances in psychiatry (*Ginkgo biloba* in dementia). *Psychopharmacology Bulletin* 31(1):147-158.

Iwu, M.M. 1986. *African ethnomedicine: Based on a seminar delivered at Institute for Medical Research, Yaba, Lagos, February 10, 1982.* Nsukka, Nigeria: Ups.

Jäger, W., G. Buchbauer, L. Jirovetz, H. Dietrich, and C. Plank. 1992. Evidence of the sedative effect of neroli oil, citronellal and phenylethyl acetate on mice. *Journal of Essential Oil Research* 4:387-394.

Jamieson, D.D., P.H. Duffield, D. Cheng, and A.M. Duffield. 1989. Comparison of the central nervous system activity of the aqueous and lipid extract of kava

(*Piper methysticum*). *Archives Internationales de Pharmacodynamie et de Thérapie* 301:66-80.

Janetzky, K. and A.P. Morreale. 1997. Probable interaction between warfarin and ginseng. *American Journal of Health-System Pharmacy* 54:692-693.

Jappe, U., I. Franke, D. Reinhold, and H.P. Gollnick. 1998. Sebotropic drug reaction resulting from kava-kava extract therapy: A new entity? *Journal of the American Academy of Dermatology* 38(1):104-106.

Jartoux, P. 1714. The description of a Tartarian plant, call'd gin-seng; with an account of its virtues. In a letter from Father Jartoux, to the Procurator General of the millions of India and China. Taken from the Tenth Volume of Letters of the Missionary Jesuits, Printed at Paris in Octavo, 1713. *Philosophical Transaction for the Royal Society of London* 28:237-247.

Jensen-Jarolim, E., N. Reider, R. Fritsch, and H. Breiteneder. 1998. Fatal outcome of anaphylaxis to camomile-containing enema during labor: A case study. *Journal of Allergy and Clinical Immunology* 102(6 Pt. 1):1041-1042.

Jirovetz, L., G. Buchbauer, W. Jäger, V. Raverdino, and A. Nikiforov. 1990. Determination of lavender oil fragrance compounds in blood samples. *Fresenius Journal of Analytic Chemistry* 338:922-923.

Jobst, K.A., M. McIntyre, D. St. George, and M. Whitelegg. 2000. Safety of St. John's wort (*Hypericum perforatum*). *Lancet* 355(9203):575.

Johnston, B. 1997. One-third of a nation's adults use herbal remedies: Market estimated at $3.24 billion. *HerbalGram* 40:49.

Joy, J.E., S.J. Watson, and J.A. Benson Jr. 1999. *Marijuana and medicine: Assessing the science base.* Washington, DC: Institute of Medicine.

Kaempfer, E. 1712. *Amoenitatum Exoticarum,* Fasciculus V. Lemgo, Westphalia: Lemgoviae.

Kaempfer, E. Trans. R. W. Carrubba. 1996. *Exotic pleasures, The Library of Renaissance Humanism.* Carbondale, IL: Southern Illinois University Press.

Kahn, R.S., H.G. Westenberg, W.M. Verhoeven, C.C. Gispen-de Wied, and W.D. Kamerbeek. 1987. Effect of a serotonin precursor and uptake inhibitor in anxiety disorders: A double-blind comparison of 5-hydroxytryptophan, clomipramine and placebo. *International Clinical Psychopharmacology* 2(1):33-45.

Kanowski, S., W.M. Herrmann, K. Stephan, W. Wierich, and R. Horr. 1996. Proof of efficacy of the Ginkgo biloba special extract EGb 761 in outpatients suffering from mild to moderate primary degenerative dementia of the Alzheimer type or multi-infarct dementia. *Pharmacopsychiatry* 29(2):47-56.

Karamat, E., J. Ilmberger, G. Buchbauer, K. Rösslhuber, and C. Rupp. 1992. Excitatory and sedative effects of essential oils on human reaction time performance. *Chemical Senses* 17:847.

Kartnig, T. 1988. Clinical applications of *Centella asiatica* (L.) Urb. *Herbs, Spices and Medicinal Plants* 3:145-173.

Kessler, R.C., K.A. McGonagle, S. Zhao, C.B. Nelson, M. Hughes, S. Eshleman, H.U. Wittchen, and K.S. Kendler. 1994. Lifetime and 12-month prevalence of DSM-III-R psychiatric disorders in the United States. Results from the national comorbidity survey. *Archives of General Psychiatry* 51(1):8-19.

Keville, Kathi. 1996. *Herbs for Health and Healing*. Emmaus, PA: Rodale Press.

Kimmens, Andrew C. 1977. *Tales of hashish*. New York: William Morrow.

King, J.R. 1994. Scientific status of aromatherapy. *Perspectives in Biology and Medicine* 37(3):409-415.

Kinzler, E., J. Krömer, and E. Lehmann. 1991. Wirksamkeit eines Kava-Spezial-Extractes bei Patienten mit Angst-, Spannungs-, und Erregungszuständen nicht-psychotischer Genese. Doppelblind-Studie gegen Plazebo über 4 Wochen (Effect of a special kava extract in patients with anxiety, tension, and excitation states of non-psychotic genesis. Double-blind study with placebos over four weeks). *Arzneimittelforschung* 41:584-588.

Kirk-Smith, M.D., C. Van Toller, and G.H. Dodd. 1983. Unconscious odour conditioning in human subjects. *Biological Psychology* 17(2/3):221-231.

Kleber, E., T. Obry, S. Hippeli, W. Schneider, and E.F. Elstner. 1999. Biochemical activities of extracts from *Hypericum perforatum* L. 1st communication: Inhibition of dopamine-beta-hydroxylase. *Arzneimittelforschung* 49(2):106-109.

Kleber, E., W. Schneider, H.L. Schäfer, and E.F. Elstner. 1995. Modulation of key reactions of the catecholamine metabolism by extracts from *Eschscholtzia californica* and *Corydalis cava*. *Arzneimittelforschung* 45(2):127-131.

Kleijnen, J. and P. Knipschild. 1992a. *Ginkgo biloba*. *Lancet* 340(8828):1136-1139.

Kleijnen, J. and P. Knipschild. 1992b. *Ginkgo biloba* for cerebral insufficiency. *British Journal of Clinical Pharmacology* 34(4):352-358.

Kleijnen, J., P. Knipschild, and G. ter Riet. 1991. Clinical trials of homoeopathy. *British Medical Journal* 302(6772):316-323.

Klerman, G.L. and M.M. Weissman. 1989. Increasing rates of depression. *Journal of the American Medical Association* 261(15):2229-2235.

Kloss, J. 1975. *Back to Eden: American herbs for pleasure and health: Natural nutrition with recipes and instruction for living the Edenic life,* Fifth edition. Santa Barbara, CA: Lifeline Books.

Knasko, S.C. 1992. Ambient odor's effect on creativity, mood, and perceived health. *Chemical Senses* 17(1):27-35.

Knasko, S.C. 1993. Performance, mood, and health during exposure to intermittent odors. *Archives of Environmental Health* 48(5):305-308.

Komori, T., R. Fujiwara, M. Tanida, J. Nomura, and M.M. Yokoyama. 1995. Effects of citrus fragrance on immune function and depressive states. *Neuroimmunomodulation* 2(3):174-180.

Kovar, K.A., B. Gropper, D. Friess, and H.P.T. Ammon. 1987. Blood levels of 1,8-cineole and locomotor activity of mice after inhalation and oral administration of rosemary oil. *Planta Medica* 53(4):315-318.

Kramer, P.D. 1993. *Listening to Prozac*. New York: Viking.

Laakmann, G., C. Schüle, T. Baghai, and M. Kieser. 1998. St. John's wort in mild to moderate depression: The relevance of hyperforin for the clinical efficacy. *Pharmacopsychiatry* 31(Suppl. 1):54-59.

Lawless, J. 1994. *Aromatherapy and the mind: An exploration into the psychological and emotional effects of essential oils*. London: Thorsons.

Lawless, J. 1995. *The illustrated encyclopedia of essential oils: The complete guide to the use of oils in aromatherapy and herbalism.* Shaftesbury, Dorset, England; Rockport, MA: Element.

Le Bars, P.L., M.M. Katz, N. Berman, T.M. Itil, A.M. Freedman, and A.F. Schatzberg. 1997. A placebo-controlled, double-blind, randomized trial of an extract of *Ginkgo biloba* for dementia. North American EGb study group. *Journal of the American Medical Association* 278(16):1327-1332.

Leathwood, P.D. and F. Chauffard. 1985. Aqueous extract of valerian reduces latency to fall asleep in man. *Planta Medica* 50(2):144-148.

Leathwood, P.D., F. Chauffard, E. Heck, and R. Munoz-Box. 1982. Aqueous extract of valerian root (*Valeriana officinalis* L.) improves sleep quality in man. *Pharmacology Biochemistry and Behavior* 17(1):65-71.

Lebot, V. 1991. Kava (*Piper methysticum* Forst f.): The Polynesian dispersal of an Oceanian plant. In *Islands, plants and Polynesians: An introduction to Polynesian ethnobotany,* Eds. P.A. Cox and S.A. Bannack. Portland, OR: Dioscorides Press, pp. 169-201.

Lebot, V. and P. Cabalion. 1986. *Les Kavas de Vanuatu: Cultivars de* Piper methysticum *Forst.* Paris: Editions de l'ORSTOM.

Lebot, V. and J. Lévesque. 1989. *The origin and distribution of Kava (*Piper methysticum Forst. F., Piperaceae)*: A phytochemical approach.* Lawai, Kauai, Hawaii: National Tropical Botanical Garden.

Lebot, V., M.D. Merlin, and L. Lindstrom. 1997. *Kava: The Pacific elixir: The definitive guide to its ethnobotany, history, and chemistry.* Rochester, VT: Healing Arts Press.

Leclerc, H. 1920. La passiflore. *Bulletin des Sciences Pharmacologiques* 27: 548-553.

Leclerc, L. 1881. *Notices et extraits des manuscrits de la Bibliothèque Nationale,* Volume 2. Paris: Imprimerie Nationale.

Lehmann, E., E. Kinzler, and J. Friedemann. 1996. Efficacy of a special kava extract (*Piper methysticum*) in patients with states of anxiety, tension and excitedness of non-mental origin—A double-blind placebo-controlled study of four weeks treatment. *Phytomedicine* 3:113-119.

Lemert, E.M. 1967. Secular use of kava in Tonga. *Quarterly Journal of Studies on Alcohol* 28(2):328-341.

Lewin, L. 1998. *Phantastica.* Rochester, VT: Park Street Press.

Lewis, B., V.L. Ménage, C.H. Pellat, and J. Schacht. 1971. *The encyclopedia of Islam.* Leiden, Netherlands: E.J. Brill.

Lewis, H.E. 1900. *Cannabis Indica*: A study of its physiologic action, toxic effects and therapeutic indications. *Merck's archives of materia medica and its uses* 2:247-251.

Li, H.-L. 1956. A horticultural and botanical history of ginkgo. *Morris Arboretum Bulletin* 7:3-12.

Li, H.-L. 1974. An archaeological and historical account of cannabis in China. *Economic Botany* 28:437-448.

Li, T.S.C. and D. Harries. 1996. Medicinal values of ginseng. *Herb, Spice, and Medicinal Plant Digest* 14(3):1-5.

Lindahl, O. and L. Lindwall. 1989. Double blind study of a valerian preparation. *Pharmacology, Biochemistry and Behavior* 32(4):1065-1066.

Linde, K., N. Clausius, G. Ramirez, D. Melchart, F. Eitel, L.V. Hedges, and W.B. Jonas. 1997. Are the clinical effects of homeopathy placebo effects? A meta-analysis of placebo-controlled trials. *Lancet* 350(9081):834-843.

Linde, K., G. Ramirez, C.D. Mulrow, A. Pauls, W. Weidenhammer, and D. Melchart. 1996. St. John's wort for depression—An overview and meta-analysis of randomised clinical trials. *British Medical Journal* 313(7052):253-258.

Lindsay, W.R., D. Pitcaithly, N. Geelen, L. Buntin, S. Broxholme, and M. Ashby. 1997. A comparison of the effects of four therapy procedures on concentration and responsiveness in people with profound learning disabilities. *Journal of Intellectual Disability Research* 41(Pt. 3):201-207.

Liu, C.-X. and P.-G. Xiao. 1992. Recent advances on ginseng research in China. *Journal of Ethnopharmacology* 36(1):27-38.

Long, D., N.H. Ballentine, and J.G. Marks Jr. 1997. Treatment of poison ivy/oak allergic contact dermatitis with an extract of jewelweed. *Americal Journal of Contact Dermatitis* 8(3):150-153.

Lorig, T.S. and M. Roberts. 1990. Odor and cognitive alteration of the contingent negative variation. *Chemical Senses* 15(5):537-545.

Lowry, T.P. 1984. Damiana. *Journal of Psychoactive Drugs* 16(3):267-268.

Lozano Camara, I. and Instituto de Cooperación con el Mundo Arabe. 1990. *Tres tratados Árabes sobre el cannabis indica: Textos para la historia del hachis en las sociedades Islamicas S. XIII-XVI.* Madrid: Agencia Española de Cooperacion Internacional Instituto de Cooperación con el Mundo Árabe.

Ludvigson, H.W. and T.R. Rottman. 1989. Effects of ambient odors of lavender and cloves on cognition, memory, affect and mood. *Chemical Senses* 14(4):525-536. Quoted material reprinted with permission of Oxford University Press.

Luthringer, R., P. d'Arbigny, and J.P. Macher. 1995. *Ginkgo biloba* extract (EGb 761), EEG and event-related potentials mapping profile. In *Advances in* Ginkgo biloba *extract research: Effect of* Ginkgo biloba *extract (EGb 761) on aging and age-related disorders*, Eds. Y. Christen, Y. Courtois, and M.-T. Droy-Lefaix. Paris: Elsevier.

Lyketsos, C.G., E. Garrett, K.Y. Liang, and J.C. Anthony. 1999. Cannabis use and cognitive decline in persons under 65 years of age. *American Journal of Epidemiology* 149(9):794-800.

Ma, Y.-C., J. Zhu, L. Benkrima, M. Luo, L. Sun, S. Sain, K. Kont, and Y.Y. Plaut-Carcasson. 1996. A comparative evaluation of ginsenosides in commercial ginseng products and tissue culture samples using HPLC. *Journal of Herbs, Spices and Medicinal Plants* 3(4):41-50.

Macht, D.I. and G.C. Ting. 1921. Experimental inquiry into the sedative properties of some aromatic drugs and fumes. *Journal of Pharmacology and Experimental Therapeutics* 18(5):361-372.

Maes, M., R. Smith, A. Christophe, P. Cosyns, R. Desnyder, and H. Meltzer. 1996. Fatty acid composition in major depression: Decreased omega 3 fractions in cholesteryl esters and increased C20: 4 omega 6/C20:5 omega 3 ratio in cholesteryl esters and phospholipids. *Journal of Affective Disorders* 38(1):35-46.

Mahadik, S.P., N.S. Shendarkar, R.E. Scheffer, S. Mukherjee, and E.E. Correnti. 1996. Utilization of precursor essential fatty acids in culture by skin fibroblasts from schizophrenic patients and normal controls. *Prostaglandins Leukotrienes and Essential Fatty Acids* 55(1/2):65-70.

Maluf, E., H.M.T. Barros, M.L. Frochtengarten, R. Benti, and J.R. Leite. 1991. Assessment of the hypnotic/sedative effects and toxicity of *Passiflora edulis* aqueous extract in rodents and humans. *Phytotherapy Research* 5:262-266.

Mantzioris, E., M.J. James, R.A. Gibson, and L.G. Cleland. 1994. Dietary substitution with an alpha-linolenic acid-rich vegetable oil increases eicosapentaenoic acid concentrations in tissues. *American Journal of Clinical Nutrition* 59(6): 1304-1309.

Mantzioris, E., M.J. James, R.A. Gibson, and L.G. Cleland. 1995. Differences exist in the relationships between dietary linoleic and alpha-linolenic acids and their respective long-chain metabolites. *American Journal of Clinical Nutrition* 61(2):320-324.

Martin, G.N. 1996. Olfactory remediation: Current evidence and possible applications. *Social Science Medicine* 43(1):63-70.

Martin, M.A. 1975. Ethnobotanical aspects of cannabis in Southeast Asia. In *Cannabis and culture*, Ed. V. Rubin. The Hague, Paris: Mouton Publishers.

Martinez, B., S. Kasper, S. Ruhrmann, and H.J. Moller. 1994. Hypericum in the treatment of seasonal affective disorders. *Journal of Geriatric Psychiatry and Neurology* 7(Suppl. 1):S29-S33.

Mathew, N.T. 1997. Transformed migraine, analgesic rebound, and other chronic daily headaches. *Neurologic Clinics* 15(1):167-186.

Matthews, M.K., Jr. 1998. Association of *Ginkgo biloba* with intracerebral hemorrhage. *Neurology* 50(6):1933.

Mattis, S. 1988. *Dementia rating scale: Professional manual.* Odessa, FL: Psychological Assessment Resources.

Mattison, J.B. 1891. *Cannabis indica* as an anodyne and hypnotic. *St. Louis Medical and Surgical Journal* 61:265-271.

Maury, M. 1989. *Marguerite Maury's guide to aromatherapy.* Trans. D. Ryman. Essex: Saffron Waldon.

Mayor's Committee on Marihuana. 1944. *The marihuana problem in the city of New York: Sociological, medical, psychological and pharmacological studies.* Lancaster, PA: Jacques Cattell Press.

McMeens, R.R. 1860. Report of the Ohio State medical committee on *Cannabis indica.* White Sulphur Springs, OH: Ohio State Medical Society.

McPartland, John M. and P.L. Pruitt. 1999. Side effects of pharmaceuticals not elicited by comparable herbal medicines: The case of tetrahydrocannabinol and marijuana. *Alternative Therapies in Health and Medicine* 5(4):57-62.

Mechoulam, R. and S. Ben-Shabat. 1999. From gan-zi-gun-nu to anandamide and 2-arachidonylglycerol: The ongoing story of cannabis. *Natural Product Reports* 16(2):131-143.

Mechoulam, R. and S.H. Burstein. 1973. *Marijuana; chemistry, pharmacology, metabolism and clinical effects*. New York: Academic Press.

Medical Economics Company. 1998. *PDR for herbal medicines*. 1st ed. Montvale, NJ: Medical Economics Company.

Medical Letter. 1997. St. John's wort. *Medical Letter* 39(1014):107-108.

Medical Letter. 1998. *Ginkgo biloba* for dementia. *Medical Letter on Drugs and Therapeutics* 40(1029):63-64.

Medical Letter. 1999a. Drugs for depression and anxiety. *Medical Letter* 41(1050): 33-38.

Medical Letter. 1999b. Homeopathic products. *Medical Letter* 41(1047):20-21.

Mehta, S., D.N. Stone, and H.F. Whitehead. 1998. Use of essential oil to promote induction of anaesthesia in children. *Anaesthesia* 53(7):720-721.

Mennini, T. and P. Bernasconi. 1993. In vitro study on the interaction of extracts and pure compounds from *Valeriana officinalis* roots with GABA, benzodiazepine and barbiturate receptors. *Fitoterapia* 64:291-300.

Menon, M.K. and A. Kar. 1971. Analgesic and psychopharmacological effects of the gum resin of *Boswellia serrata*. *Planta Medica* 19(4):333-341.

Meschler, J.P. and A.C. Howlett. 1999. Thujone exhibits low affinity for cannabinoid receptors but fails to evoke cannabimimetic responses. *Pharmacology, Biochemistry and Behavior* 62(3):473-480.

Meyerhof, M. 1940. *Sarh Asma al-Uqqar (l'Explication de Noms des Drogues): Un Glossaire de Matière Médicale Composé par Maimonide*. Cairo: Imprimerie de l'Institut Français d'Archéologie Orientale.

Mikuriya, T.H. 1970. Cannabis substitution. An adjunctive therapeutic tool in the treatment of alcoholism. *Medical Times* 98(4):187-191.

Millis, S.R., S.H. Putnam, K.M. Adams, and J.H. Ricker. 1995. The California verbal learning test in the detection of incomplete effort in neuropsychological evaluation. *Psychological Assessment* 7:463-471.

Mitchell, S. 1993. Dementia: Aromatherapy's effectiveness in disorders associated with dementia. *International Journal of Aromatherapy* 5(2):20-23.

Miyake, Y., M. Nakagawa, and Y. Asakura. 1991. Effects of odors on humans. I. Effects on sleep latency. *Chemical Senses* 16(2):183.

Moerman, D.E. 1998. *Native American ethnobotany*. Portland, OR: Timber Press.

Moore, M. 1979. *Medicinal plants of the mountain West: A guide to the identification, preparation, and uses of traditional medicinal plants found in the mountains, foothills, and upland areas of the American West*. Santa Fe, NM: Museum of New Mexico Press.

Morazzoni, P. and E Bombardelli. 1995. *Valeriana officinalis:* Traditional use and recent evaluation of activity. *Fitoterapia* 66(2):99-112.

Moreau, J.-J. Joseph. 1845. *Du hachisch et de l'aliénation mentale: Études psychologiques*. Paris: Fortin Masson.

Moreau, J.-J. 1857. Lypemanie avec stupeur; tendance a la demence. Traitement par l'extract (principe resineux) de *Cannabis indica*. Guerison. *Gazette des Hopitaux Civils et Militaires* 30:391.

Moreau, J.-J. 1973. *Hashish and mental illness*. New York: Raven Press.

Morgenthaler, J. and L. Lenard. 1998. *5-HTP (5-hydroxytryptophan): The natural alternative to Prozac*. Petaluma, CA: Smart Publications.

Morphy, M.A., G.A. Fava, and N. Sonino. 1993. Beta-endorphin responsiveness in depression. *Archives of General Psychiatry* 50(5):406.

Moss, D.E., P.Z. Manderscheid, S.P. Montgomery, A.B. Norman, and P.R. Sanberg. 1989. Nicotine and cannabinoids as adjuncts to neuroleptics in the treatment of Tourette syndrome and other motor disorders. *Life Sciences* 44(21):1521-1525.

Mulkens, A. and I. Kapetanidis. 1987. Flavonoïdes des feuilles de *Melissa officinalis* L. (Lamiaceae) (Flavonoids of the leaves of *Melissa officinalis* L. [Lamiaceae]). *Pharmaceutica Acta Helvetiae* 62(1):19-22.

Müller, W.E., M. Rolli, C. Schäfer, and U. Hafner. 1997. Effects of hypericum extract (LI 160) in biochemical models of antidepressant activity. *Pharmacopsychiatry* 30(Suppl. 2):102-107.

Müller, W.E. and R. Rossol. 1994. Effects of hypericum extract on the expression of serotonin receptors. *Journal of Geriatric Psychiatry and Neurology* 7(Suppl. 1): S63-S64.

Müller-Vahl, K.R., H. Kolbe, and R. Dengler. 1997. Gilles de la Tourette-Syndrom Einfluss von Nikotin, Alkohol und Marihuana auf die klinische Symptomatik (Gilles de la Tourette syndrome. Effect of nicotine, alcohol and marihuana on clinical symptoms). *Der Nervenarzt* 68(12):985-989.

Müller-Vahl, K.R., H. Kolbe, U. Schneider, and H.M. Emrich. 1998. Cannabinoids: Possible role in patho-physiology and therapy of Gilles de la Tourette syndrome. *Acta Psychiatrica Scandinavica* 98(6):502-506.

Müller-Vahl, K.R., U. Schneider, H. Kolbe, and H.M. Emrich. 1999. Treatment of Tourette's syndrome with delta-9-tetrahydrocannabinol. *American Journal of Psychiatry* 156(3):495.

Münte, T.F., H.J. Heinze, M. Matzke, and J. Steitz. 1993. Effects of oxazepam and an extract of kava roots (*Piper methysticum*) on event-related potentials in a word recognition task. *Neuropsychobiology* 27(1):46-53.

Murkovic, M., A. Hillebrand, J. Winkler, E. Leitner, and W. Pfannhauser. 1996. Variability of fatty acid content in pumpkin seeds (*Cucurbita pepo* L.). *Zeitschrift für Lebensmitteluntersuchung und-forschung* 203(3):216-219.

Murray, M. 1995. *Ginkgo biloba* extract vs. phosphatidylserine in the treatment of depression and Alzheimer's disease. *American Journal of Natural Medicine* 2(10):8-9.

Mustafa, T. and K.C. Srivastava. 1990. Ginger (*Zingiber officinale*) in migraine headache. *Journal of Ethnopharmacology* 29(3):267-273.

Nadkarni, K.M. and A.K. Nadkarni. 1954. *Indian materia medica with Ayurvedic, Unani-Tibbi, Siddha, allopathic, homeopathic, naturopathic and home remedies, appendices and indexes,* Third, revised edition. Bombay: Popular Book Depot.

Nagai, H., M. Nakagawa, W. Fujii, T. Inui, and Y. Asakura. 1991. Effects of odors on humans. II. Reducing effects of mental stress and fatigue. *Chemical Senses* 16(2):183.

Nahrstedt, A. and V. Butterweck. 1997. Biologically active and other chemical constituents of the herb of *Hypericum perforatum* L. *Pharmacopsychiatry* 30(Suppl. 2):129-134.

Neary, J.T. and Y. Bu. 1999. Hypericum LI 160 inhibits uptake of serotonin and norepinephrine in astrocytes. *Brain Research* 816:358-363.

Nebel, A., B.J. Schneider, R.K. Baker, and D.J. Kroll. 1999. Potential metabolic interaction between St. John's wort and theophylline. *Annals of Pharmacotherapy* 33(4):502.

Nikaido, T., T. Ohmoto, U. Sankawa, O. Tanaka, R. Kasai, J. Shoji, S. Sanada, S. Hiai, H. Yokoyama, H. Oura, et al. 1984. Inhibitors of cyclic AMP phosphodiesterase in *Panax ginseng* C. A. Meyer and *Panax japonicus* C. A. Meyer. *Chemical and Pharmaceutical Bulletin (Tokyo)* 32(4):1477-1483.

Norton, S.A. and P. Ruze. 1994. Kava dermopathy. *Journal of the American Academy of Dermatology* 31(1):89-97.

Oken, B.S., D.M. Storzbach, and J.A. Kaye. 1998. The efficacy of *Ginkgo biloba* on cognitive function in Alzheimer disease. *Archives of Neurology* 55(11): 1409-1415.

Orth, H.C., C. Rentel, and P.C. Schmidt. 1999. Isolation, purity analysis and stability of hyperforin as a standard material from *Hypericum perforatum* L. *Journal of Pharmacy and Pharmacology* 51(2):193-200.

Ortiz de Urbina, A.V., M.L. Martin, M.J. Montero, A. Moran, and L. San Roman. 1989. Sedating and antipyretic activity of the essential oil of *Calamintha sylvatica* subsp. *ascendens*. *Journal of Ethnopharmacology* 25(2):165-171.

O'Shaughnessy, W.B. 1838-1840. On the preparations of the Indian hemp, or gunjah (*Cannabis indica*): Their effects on the animal system in health, and their utility in the treatment of tetanus and other convulsive diseases. *Transactions of the Medical and Physical Society of Bengal*:71-102, 421-461.

Ott, J. 1994. *Ayahuasca analogues: Pangæan entheogens,* First edition. Kennewick, WA: Natural Products Company.

Ott, J. 1996. *Pharmacotheon: Entheogenic drugs, their plant sources and history,* Second edition. Kennewick, WA: Natural Products Company.

Oyama, Y., P.A. Fuchs, N. Katayama, and K. Noda. 1994. Myricetin and quercetin, the flavonoid constituents of *Ginkgo biloba* extract, greatly reduce oxidative metabolism in both resting and Ca(2+)-loaded brain neurons. *Brain Research* 635(1/2):125-129.

Pang, Z., F. Pan, and S. He. 1996. *Ginkgo biloba* L.: History, current status, and future prospects. *Journal of Alternative and Complementary Medicine* 2(3):359-363.

Paolo, A.M., A.I. Troester, and J.J. Ryan. 1997. California verbal learning test normative data for the elderly. *Journal of Clinical and Experimental Neuropsychology* 19:220-234.

Parkinson, S. 1773. *A journal of a voyage to the South Seas in His Majesty's ship the Endeavour (1768)*. London: S. Parkinson.

Patocka, J. 1998. Huperzine A—An interesting anticholinesterase compound from the Chinese herbal medicine. *Acta Medica* 41(4):155-157.

Patrick, J.1988. Concordance of the MCMI and the MMPI in the diagnosis of three DSM-III Axis I disorders. *Journal of Clinical Psychology* 44:186-190.

Payk, T.R. 1994. Treatment of depression. *Journal of Geriatric Psychiatry and Neurology* 7(Suppl. 1):S3-S5.

Peet, M., B. Murphy, J. Shay, and D. Horrobin. 1998. Depletion of omega-3 fatty acid levels in red blood cell membranes of depressive patients. *Biological Psychiatry* 43(5):315-319.

Pereira, J. and J. Carson. 1852. *The elements of materia medica and therapeutics*, Third American edition. Philadelphia: Blanchard and Lea.

Perovic, S. and W.E. Müller. 1995. Pharmacological profile of hypericum extract. Effect on serotonin uptake by postsynaptic receptors. *Arzneimittelforschung* 45(11):1145-1148.

Petkov, V. 1978. Effect of ginseng on the brain biogenic monoamines and 3′, 5′-AMP system. Experiments on rats. *Arzneimittelforschung* 28(3):388-393.

Pierre, S., I. Jamme, M.T. Droy-Lefaix, A. Nouvelot, and J.M. Maixent. 1999. *Ginkgo biloba* extract (EGb 761) protects Na,K-ATPase activity during cerebral ischemia in mice. *Neuroreport* 10(1):47-51.

Piscitelli, S.C., A.H. Burstein, D. Chaitt, R.M. Alfaro, and J. Falloon. 2000. Indinavir concentrations and St. John's wort. *Lancet* 355(9203):547-548.

Pöldinger, W., B. Calanchini, and W. Schwarz. 1991. A functional-dimensional approach to depression: Serotonin deficiency as a target syndrome in a comparison of 5-hydroxytryptophan and fluvoxamine. *Psychopathology* 24(2):53-81.

Polli, G. 1870. Further observations on haschish in medicine. *St. Andrew's Medical Graduates Association Transactions* 3:98-101.

Powers, K.A. and V.R. Beasley. 1985. Toxicological aspects of linalool: A review. *Veterinary and Human Toxicology* 27(6):484-486.

Practice Management Information Corporation. 1999. ICD-9-CM, Millennium Edition, *International Classification of Diseases*, Ninth revision, *Clinical Modification*, Fifth edition. Los Angeles, CA: Practice Management Information Corporation.

Price, S. 1998. Using essential oils in professional practice. *Complementary Therapies in Nursing and Midwifery* 4(5):144-147.

Rahman, K., L. Krenn, B. Kopp, M. Schubert-Zsilavecz, K.K. Mayer, and W. Kubelka. 1997. Isoscoparin-2″-O-glucoside from *Passiflora incarnata*. *Phytochemistry* 45(5):1093-1094.

Ramassamy, C., Y. Christen, F. Clostre, and J. Costentin. 1992. The *Ginkgo biloba* extract, EGb 761, increases synaptosomal uptake of 5-hydroxytryptamine: In-vitro and ex-vivo studies. *Journal of Pharmacy and Pharmacology* 44(11): 943-945.

Ramaswamy, A.S., S.M. Periyasamy, and N. Basu. 1970. Pharmacological studies on *Centella asiatica* Linn (Brahma Manduki) (N.O. Umbeliferae). *Journal of Research in Indian Medicine* 4(2):160-175.

Regelson, W., J.R. Butler, J. Schulz, T. Kirk, L. Peek, M.L. Green, and M.O. Zalis. 1976. Delta 9-tetrahydrocannabinol as an effective antidepressant and appetite-stimulating agent in advanced cancer patients. In *Pharmacology of marihuana*, Volume 2, Eds. M.C. Braude and S. Szara. New York: Raven Press, pp. 763-776.

Reimeier, C., I. Schneider, W. Schneider, H.L. Schäfer, and E.F. Elstner. 1995. Effects of ethanolic extracts from *Eschscholtzia californica* and *Corydalis cava* on dimerization and oxidation of enkephalins. *Arzneimittelforschung* 45(2): 132-136.

Reynolds, J.R. 1868. On some of the therapeutical uses of Indian hemp. *Archives of Medicine* 2:154-160.

Reynolds, J.R. 1890. Therapeutical uses and toxic effects of *Cannabis indica*. *Lancet* 1:637-638.

Reynolds, L.B. 1998a. Effects of drying on chemical and physical characteristics of American ginseng (*Panax quinquefolius* L.). *Journal of Herbs, Spices and Medicinal Plants* 6(2):9-21.

Reynolds, L.B. 1998b. Effects of harvest date on some chemical and physical characteristics of American ginseng (*Panax quinquefolius* L.). *Journal of Herbs, Spices and Medicinal Plants* 6(2):63-69.

Robbers, J.E., M.K. Speedie, and V.E. Tyler. 1996. *Pharmacognosy and Pharmacobiotechnology*. Baltimore, MD: Williams and Wilkins.

Robbers, J.E., and V.E. Tyler. 1999. *Tyler's Herbs of choice: The therapeutic use of phytomedicinals*. New York: The Haworth Herbal Press.

Rolland, A., J. Fleurentin, M.C. Lanhers, C. Younos, R. Misslin, F. Mortier, and J.M. Pelt. 1991. Behavioural effects of the American traditional plant *Eschscholzia californica*: Sedative and anxiolytic properties. *Planta Medica* 57(3): 212-216.

Rose, J.E. and F.M. Behm. 1994. Inhalation of vapor from black pepper extract reduces smoking withdrawal symptoms. *Drug and Alcohol Dependence* 34(3): 225-229.

Rosenblatt, M. and J. Mindel. 1997. Spontaneous hyphema associated with ingestion of *Ginkgo biloba* extract. *New England Journal of Medicine* 336(15):1108.

Rossi, T., M. Melegari, A. Bianchi, A. Albasini, and G. Vampa. 1988. Sedative, anti-inflammatory and anti-diuretic effects induced in rats by essential oils of varieties of *Anthemis nobilis*: A comparative study. *Pharmacological Research Communications* 20(Suppl. 5):71-74.

Rouhier, A. 1975. *Le peyotl: La plante qui fait les yeux émerveillés*. Paris: Guy Trédaniel.

Rowin, J. and S.L. Lewis. 1996. Spontaneous bilateral subdural hematomas associated with chronic *Ginkgo biloba* ingestion. *Neurology* 46(6):1775-1776.

Rumpf, G.E. and E.M. Beekman. 1981. *The poison tree: Selected writings of Rumphius on the natural history of the Indies, Library of the Indies*. Amherst: University of Massachusetts Press.

Ruschitzka, F., P.J. Meier, M. Turina, T.F. Luscher, and G. Noll. 2000. Acute heart transplant rejection due to Saint John's wort. *Lancet* 355(9203):548-549.

Russo, E. 1998. Cannabis for migraine treatment: The once and future prescription? An historical and scientific review. *Pain* 76(1/2):3-8.

Russo, E.B. 2001. Hemp for headache. *Journal of Cannabis Therapeutics* 1(2).

Ruze, P. 1990. Kava-induced dermopathy: A niacin deficiency? *Lancet* 335(8703): 1442-1445.

Salem, N. Jr. and C.D. Niebylski. 1995. The nervous system has an absolute molecular species requirement for proper function. *Molecular Membrane Biology* 12(1):131-134.

Salgueiro, J.B., P. Ardenghi, M. Dias, M.B. Ferreira, I. Izquierdo, and J.H. Medina. 1997. Anxiolytic natural and synthetic flavonoid ligands of the central benzodiazepine receptor have no effect on memory tasks in rats. *Pharmacology, Biochemistry and Behavior* 58(4):887-891.

Sanders, T.A. and S. Reddy. 1994. Vegetarian diets and children. *American Journal of Clinical Nutrition* 59(5)(Suppl.):S1176-S1181.

Sandyk, R. and G. Awerbuch. 1988. Marijuana and Tourette's syndrome. *Journal of Clinical Psychopharmacology* 8(6):444-445.

Sano, A., H. Sei, H. Seno, Y. Morita, and H. Moritoki. 1998. Influence of cedar essence on spontaneous activity and sleep of rats and human daytime nap. *Psychiatry and Clinical Neuroscience* 52(2):133-135.

Santos, M.S., F. Ferreira, A.P. Cunha, A.P. Carvalho, and T. Macedo. 1994. An aqueous extract of valerian influences the transport of GABA in synaptosomes. *Planta Medica* 60(3):278-279.

Sasaki, K., S. Hatta, M. Haga, and H. Ohshika. 1999. Effects of bilobalide on gamma-aminobutyric acid levels and glutamic acid decarboxylase in mouse brain. *European Journal of Pharmacology* 367(2/3):165-173.

Schäfer, H.L., H. Schäfer, W. Schneider, and E.F. Elstner. 1995. Sedative action of extract combinations of *Eschscholtzia californica* and *Corydalis cava*. *Arzneimittelforschung* 45(2):124-126.

Schellenberg, R., S. Sauer, and W. Dimpfel. 1998. Pharmacodynamic effects of two different hypericum extracts in healthy volunteers measured by quantitative EEG. *Pharmacopsychiatry* 31(Suppl. 1):44-53.

Schelosky, L., C. Raffauf, K. Jendroska, and W. Poewe. 1995. Kava and dopamine antagonism. *Journal of Neurology, Neurosurgery and Psychiatry* 58(5):639-640.

Schempp, H., A. Denke, E. Mann, W. Schneider, and E.F. Elstner. 1999. Biochemical activities of extracts from *Hypericum perforatum* L. 3rd communication: Modulation of peroxidase activity as a simple method for standardization. *Arzneimittelforschung* 49(2):115-119.

Schirrmacher, K., D. Büsselberg, J.M. Langosch, J. Walden, U. Winter, and D. Bingmann. 1999. Effects of (+/-)-kavain on voltage-activated inward currents of dorsal root ganglion cells from neonatal rats. *European Neuropsychopharmacology* 9(1/2):171-176.

Schmidt, M. 1997. Some cautions on interpreting qualitative indices for word-list learning tests. *The Clinical Neuropsychologist* 11:81-86.

Schnaubelt, K. 1998. *Advanced aromatherapy: The science of essential oil therapy,* First U.S. edition. Rochester, VT: Healing Arts Press.

Schneider L.S. and J.T. Olin. 1996. Clinical global impressions in Alzheimer's clinical trials. *International Journal of Psychogeriatrics* 8(2):277-288.

Schouten, W. 1771. The voyage of James Le Mair and William Schouten, 1616. In *A historical collection of the several voyages and discoveries in the South Pacific Ocean: Dutch voyages,* Volume 2. Ed. A. Dalrymple. Amsterdam: N. Israel, pp. 1-64.

Schubert, D.S. and R.H. Foliart. 1993. Increased depression in multiple sclerosis patients. A meta-analysis. *Psychosomatics* 34(2):124-130.

Schultes, R.E. 1988. *Where the gods reign: Plants and peoples of the Colombian Amazon.* Oracle, AZ: Synergetic Press.

Schultes, R.E. and A. Hofmann. 1980. *The botany and chemistry of hallucinogens,* Revised, second edition. Springfield, IL: Thomas.

Schultes, R.E. and A. Hofmann. 1992. *Plants of the gods: Their sacred, healing, and hallucinogenic powers.* Rochester, VT: Healing Arts Press.

Schultes, R.E. and R.F. Raffauf. 1990. *The healing forest: Medicinal and toxic plants of the northwest Amazonia.* Portland, OR: Dioscorides Press.

Schultes, R.E., R.F. Raffauf. 1992. *Vine of the soul: Medicine men, their plants and rituals in the Colombian Amazon.* Oracle, AZ: Synergetic Press.

Schultes, R.E. and E.W. Smith. 1976. *Hallucinogenic plants.* New York: Golden Press.

Schulz, H. and M. Jobert. 1994. Effects of hypericum extract on the sleep EEG in older volunteers. *Journal of Geriatric Psychiatry and Neurology* 7(Suppl. 1): S39-S43.

Schulz, H., C. Stolz, and J. Müller. 1994. The effect of valerian extract on sleep polygraphy in poor sleepers: A pilot study. *Pharmacopsychiatry* 27(4):147-151.

Schulz, V., R. Hänsel, and V.E. Tyler. 1998. *Rational phytotherapy: A physicians' guide to herbal medicine,* Third edition. Berlin, New York: Springer.

Seitz, U., A. Schüle, and J. Gleitz. 1997. [3H]-monoamine uptake inhibition properties of kava pyrones. *Planta Medica* 63(6):548-549.

Seto, T.A. and W. Keup. 1969. Effects of alkylmethoxybenzene and alkylmethylenedioxybenzene essential oils on pentobarbital and ethanol sleeping time. *Archives Internationales de Pharmacodynamie et de Thérapie* 180(1):232-240.

Seward, A. 1938. The story of the maidenhair tree. *Science Progress* 32:420-440.

Sharma, R., A.N. Jaiswal, S. Kumar, C. Chaturvedi, and P.V. Tewari. 1985. Role of bhrahmi *(Centella asiatica)* in educable mentally retarded children. *Journal of Research and Education in Indian Medicine* 4(January-June):55-57.

Sharpley, A.L., C.L. McGavin, R. Whale, and P.J. Cowen. 1998. Antidepressant-like effect of *Hypericum perforatum* (St. John's wort) on the sleep polysomnogram. *Psychopharmacology (Berlin)* 139(3):286-287.

Sherry, C.J. and R.E. Burnett. 1978. Enhancement of ethanol-induced sleep by whole oil of nutmeg. *Experientia* 34(4):492-493.

Shipochliev, T. 1981. Extracts from a group of medicinal plants enhancing uterine tonus. *Veterinarno-Meditsinski Naukit* 18:94-98.

Shulgin, A. and A. Shulgin. 1991. *PIHKAL: A chemical love story.* Berkeley, CA: Transform Press.

Shulgin, A.T. 1973. The narcotic pepper—The chemistry and pharmacology of *Piper methysticum* and related species. *Bulletin on Narcotics* 25:59-74.

Siegel, R.K. 1976. Herbal intoxication. Psychoactive effects from herbal cigarettes, tea, and capsules. *Journal of the American Medical Association* 236(5):473-476.

Siegel, R.K. 1979. Ginseng abuse syndrome. Problems with the panacea. *Journal of the American Medical Association* 241(15):1614-1615.

Singh, N.C., C. Ellis, A. Best, K. Eakin, C. Parsons, and I. Sharp. 1997. *Kavatrol (TM) reduces daily stress and anxiety in adults.* Paper read at Third Annual Alternative Therapies Symposium.

Singh, Y.N. 1983. Effects of kava on neuromuscular transmission and muscle contractility. *Journal of Ethnopharmacology* 7(3):267-276.

Singh, Y.N. 1992. Kava: An overview. *Journal of Ethnopharmacology* 37(1):13-45.

Singh, Y.N. and M. Blumenthal. 1997. Kava: An overview. *HerbalGram* 39:33-56.

Skogh, M. 1998. Extracts of *Ginkgo biloba* and bleeding or haemorrhage. *Lancet* 352(9134):1145-1146.

Skolnick, A.A. 1997. Old Chinese herbal medicine used for fever yields possible new Alzheimer disease therapy. *Journal of the American Medical Association* 277(10):776.

Smith, D.B., T. Allison, W.R. Goff, and J.J. Principato. 1971. Human odorant evoked responses: Effects of trigeminal or olfactory deficit. *Electroencephalography and Clinical Neurophysiology* 30:313-317.

Smith, G.W., T.M. Chalmers, and G. Nuki. 1993. Vasculitis associated with herbal preparation containing *Passiflora* extract. *British Journal of Rheumatology* 32(1):87-88.

Smith, R.S. 1991. The macrophage theory of depression. *Medical Hypotheses* 35(4):298-306.

Soejarto, D.D. and N.R. Farnsworth. 1989. Tropical rain forests: Potential source of new drugs? *Perspectives in Biology and Medicine* 32(2):244-256.

Sommer, H. and G. Harrer. 1994. Placebo-controlled double-blind study examining the effectiveness of an hypericum preparation in 105 mildly depressed patients. *Journal of Geriatric Psychiatry and Neurology* 7(Suppl. 1):S9-S11.

Sopranzi, N., G. De Feo, G. Mazzanti, and L. Tolu. 1990. Parametri biologici ed elettroencefalografici nel ratto correlati a *Passiflora incarnata* L. (Biological and electroencephalographic parameters in rats in relation to *Passiflora incarnata* L.). *Clinica Therapeutica* 132(5):329-333.

Sørensen, H. and J. Sonne. 1996. A double-masked study of the effects of ginseng on cognitive functions. *Current Therapeutic Research* 57(12):959-968.

Soulimani, R., J. Fleurentin, F. Mortier, R. Misslin, G. Derrieu, and J.M. Pelt. 1991. Neurotropic action of the hydroalcoholic extract of *Melissa officinalis* in the mouse. *Planta Medica* 57(2):105-109.

Soulimani, R., C. Younos, S. Jarmouni, D. Bousta, R. Misslin, and F. Mortier. 1997. Behavioural effects of *Passiflora incarnata* L. and its indole alkaloid and flavonoid derivatives and maltol in the mouse. *Journal of Ethnopharmacology* 57(1):11-20.

Speroni, E. and A. Minghetti. 1988. Neuropharmacological activity of extracts from *Passiflora incarnata*. *Planta Medica* 54(6):488-491.

Spielberger, C.D. 1983. *State-trait anxiety inventory*. Palo Alto, CA: Mind Garden.

Spreen, A. and E. Straus. 1998. *A compendium of neuropsychological tests: Administration, norms, and commentary*, Second edition. New York: Oxford University Press.

Squires, R. 1995. Ginkgo biloba. *ATOMS Journal (Australian Traditional-Medicine Society Journal)* (Autumn):9-14.

Staffeldt, B., R. Kerb, J. Brockmoller, M. Ploch, and I. Roots. 1994. Pharmacokinetics of hypericin and pseudohypericin after oral intake of the *Hypericum perforatum* extract LI 160 in healthy volunteers. *Journal of Geriatric Psychiatry and Neurology* 7(Suppl. 1):S47-S53.

Stapleton, W.J. 1904. The action of *Passiflora incarnata*. *Detroit Medical Journal* 4:17-18.

Steele, J. 1984. Brain research and essential oils. *Aromatherapy Quarterly* (Spring).

Stensrud, P. and O. Sjaastad. 1980. Comparative trial of Tenormin (atenolol) and Inderal (propranolol) in migraine. *Headache* 20(4):204-207.

Stevens, L.J., S.S. Zentall, M.L. Abate, T. Kuczek, and J.R. Burgess. 1996. Omega-3 fatty acids in boys with behavior, learning, and health problems. *Physiology and Behavior* 59(4/5):915-920.

Stevens, L.J., S.S. Zentall, J.L. Deck, M.L. Abate, B.A. Watkins, S.R. Lipp, and J.R. Burgess. 1995. Essential fatty acid metabolism in boys with attention-deficit hyperactivity disorder. *American Journal of Clinical Nutrition* 62(4):761-768.

Strange, W. 1883. *Cannabis indica:* As a medicine and as a poison. *British Medical Journal* 2(July 7):14.

Suckling, C.W. 1891. On the therapeutic value of Indian hemp. *British Medical Journal* 2:12.

Sushruta. 1991. *The Sushruta Samhita. An English translation of the* Sushruta Samhita *based on original Sanskrit text*. Trans. K.K. Bhishagratna. Varanasi, India: Chowkhamba Sanskrit Series Office.

Suzuki, O., Y. Katsumata, M. Oya, S. Bladt, and H. Wagner. 1984. Inhibition of monoamine oxidase by hypericin. *Planta Medica* 50(3):272-274.

Svanidze, N., A. Sanchez, V. Lanovenki, B. Soler, P. Rodriguez, A. Suarez, and G. Mendez. 1974. Resultados de la intraducción y estudio farmacognosico de la *Passiflora incarnata* L. en las condiciónes de Cuba. *Revista Cubana de Farmacia* 8:309-314.

Tang, X.C. 1996. Huperzine A (Shuangyiping): A promising drug for Alzheimer's disease [in Chinese]. *Chung Kuo Yao Li Hsueh Pao (Acta Pharmacologica Sinica)* 17(6):481-484.

Theophrastus. 1948. *Enquiry into plants and minor works on odours and weather signs*. Trans. A. Hort. Cambridge, MA: Harvard University Press.

Thiede, H.M., and A. Walper. 1994. Inhibition of MAO and COMT by hypericum extracts and hypericin. *Journal of Geriatric Psychiatry and Neurology* 7(Suppl. 1):S54-S56.

Thiele, B., I. Brink, and M. Ploch. 1994. Modulation of cytokine expression by hypericum extract. *Journal of Geriatric Psychiatry and Neurology* 7(Suppl. 1): S60-S62.

Thompson, R.C. 1924. *The Assyrian herbal.* London: Luzac and Company.

Thompson, R.C. 1949. *A dictionary of Assyrian botany by R. Campbell Thompson.* London: British Academy.

Tilford, G.L. 1997. *Edible and medicinal plants of the West.* Missoula, MT: Mountain Press Publishing.

Tisserand, R. 1977. *The art of aromatherapy: The healing and beautifying properties of the essential oils of flowers and herbs.* Rochester, VT: Destiny Books.

Tisserand, R. 1985. *The art of aromatherapy: The healing and beautifying properties of the essential oils of flowers and herbs,* Revised edition. Rochester, VT: Healing Arts Press.

Tisserand, R. 1988. *Aromatherapy: To heal and tend the body.* Santa Fe, NM: Lotus Press.

Tisserand, R. 1995. Aromatherapy as mind-body medicine. *International Journal of Aromatherapy* 6(3):14-19.

Tisserand, R. and T. Balacs. 1995. *Essential oil safety: A guide for health care professionals.* Edinburgh: Churchill Livingstone.

Titcomb, M. 1948. Kava in Hawaii. *Journal of the Polynesian Society* 57:105-171.

Tobin, P. 1995. Aromatherapy and its application in the management of people with dementia. *Lamp* 52(5):34.

Torii, S., H. Fukuda, R. Miyanchi, Y. Hamauzu, and M. Kawasaki. 1991. Contingent negative variation (CNV) and the psychologic effects of odor. In *Perfumery: The psychology and biology of fragrance,* Eds. S. Van Toller and G. Dodd. London: Chapman and Hall, pp. 107-120.

Trevelyan, J. 1993. Aromatherapy. *Nursing Times* 89(25):38-40.

Trevelyan, J. and B. Booth. 1994. Complementary medicine. Aromatherapy. *Nursing Times* 90(38):(Suppl.)1-16.

Troester, A.I., N. Butters, D.P. Salmon, C.M. Cullum, D. Jacobs, J. Brandt, and R.F. White. 1993. The diagnostic utility of saving scores: Differentiating Alzheimer's and Huntington's disease with the logical memory and visual reproduction tests. *Journal of Clinical and Experimental Neuropsychology* 15:773-788.

Tsang, D., H.W. Yeung, W.W. Tso, and H. Peck. 1985. Ginseng saponins: Influence on neurotransmitter uptake in rat brain synaptosomes. *Planta Medica* 51(3): 221-224.

Tufik, S., K. Fuhita, M.D.L. Seabra, and L.L. Lobo. 1994. Effects of prolonged administration of valepotriates in rats on the mothers and their offspring. *Journal of Ethnopharmacology* 41(1/2):39-44.

Turner, W., G.T.L. Chapman, M.N. Tweddle, and F. McCombie. 1995. *A new herball.* Cambridge, England; New York: Cambridge University Press.

Tyler, V.E. 1993. Phytomedicines in Western Europe: Potential impact on herbal medicine in the United States. In *Human medicinal agents from plants,* Eds.A.D. Kinghorn and M. F. Balandrin. Washington, DC: American Chemical Society, pp. 25-37.

Tyrell, H.J. 1867. On the treatment of delirium tremens by Indian hemp. *Medical Press and Circular* 17(March 13):243-244.

Uldry, P.A. and F. Regli. 1987. Indications du L-5-hydroxytryptophane en neurologie (Indications for L-5-hydroxytryptophan in neurology). *Revue Médicale de la Suisse Romande* 107(9):703-707.

Upton, R. 1997. St. John's wort monograph. *HerbalGram* 40:1-32.

U.S. Congress. 1994. Dietary Supplement Health and Education Act of 1994 (DSHEA). Public Law 103-417. 108 Stat. 4325. October 25.

Vale, S. 1998. Subarachnoid haemorrhage associated with *Ginkgo biloba. Lancet* 352:36.

Valnet, J. and R. Tisserand. 1990. *The practice of aromatherapy: A classic compendium of plant medicines and their healing properties.* Rochester, VT: Healing Arts Press.

Valpiani, C. 1995. *Valeriana officinalis. ATOMS Journal* (Australian Traditional-Medicine Society Journal) 1(2):57-62.

van Praag, H.M. and R.S. Kahn. 1988. L-5-hydroxytryptophan in depression and anxiety. *Schweizerische Rundschau für Medizin Praxis* 77(34A):40-46.

Vanderplank, J. 1996. *Passion flowers,* Second edition. Cambridge, MA: MIT Press.

Vesper, J. and K.D. Hänsgen. 1994. Efficacy of *Ginkgo biloba* in 90 outpatients with cerebral insufficiency caused by old age. *Phytomedicine* 1:9-16.

Vickers, A. 1997. Yes, but how do we know it's true? Knowledge claims in massage and aromatherapy. *Complementary Therapies in Nursing and Midwifery* 3(3): 63-65.

Vickers, A., S. Van Toller, and C. Stevensen. 1996. *Massage and aromatherapy: A guide for health professionals,* First edition. London: Chapman and Hall.

Vincieri, F.F., S. Celli, N. Mulinacci, and E. Speroni. 1988. An approach to the study of the biological activity of *Eschscholtzia californica* Cham. *Pharmacological Research Communications* 20(Suppl. 5):41-44.

Viola, H., C. Wasowski, M. Levi de Stein, C. Wolfman, R. Silveira, F. Dajas, J.H. Medina, and A.C. Paladini. 1995. Apigenin, a component of *Matricaria recutita* flowers, is a central benzodiazepine receptors-ligand with anxiolytic effects. *Planta Medica* 61(3):213-216.

Viola, H., C. Wolfman, M. Levi de Stein, C. Wasowski, C. Pena, J.H. Medina, and A.C. Paladini. 1994. Isolation of pharmacologically active benzodiazepine receptor ligands from *Tilia tomentosa* (Tiliaceae). *Journal of Ethnopharmacology* 44(1):47-53.

Volicer, L., M. Stelly, J. Morris, J. McLaughlin, and B.J. Volicer. 1997. Effects of dronabinol on anorexia and disturbed behavior in patients with Alzheimer's disease. *International Journal of Geriatric Psychiatry* 12(9):913-919.

Volz, H.P. 1996. The anxiolytic efficacy of the kava special extract WS 1490 using long-term therapy—A randomized double-blind study. *Quarterly Review of Natural Medicine* (Fall):186.

Volz, H.P. 1997. Controlled clinical trials of hypericum extracts in depressed patients—An overview. *Pharmacopsychiatry* 30(Suppl. 2):72-76.

Volz, H.P. and M. Kieser. 1997. Kava-kava extract WS 1490 versus placebo in anxiety disorders—A randomized placebo-controlled 25-week outpatient trial. *Pharmacopsychiatry* 30(1):1-5.

von Ardenne, M. and W. Klemm. 1987. Measurements of the increase in the difference between the arterial and venous Hb-O$_2$ saturation obtained with daily administration of 200 mg standardized ginseng extract G115 for four weeks. Long-term increase of the O$_2$ transport into the organs and tissues of the organism through biologically active substances. *Panminerva Medica* 29(2):143-150.

Vorbach, E.-U., K.H. Arnoldt, and W.D. Hubner. 1997. Efficacy and tolerability of St. John's wort extract LI 160 versus imipramine in patients with severe depressive episodes according to ICD-10. *Pharmacopsychiatry* 30(Suppl. 2):81-85.

Vorbach, E.-U., R. Görtelmayer, and J. Bruning. 1996. Therapie von insomnien: Wirksamkeit und vertraglichkeit eines Baldrian-Praparates. *Psychopharmakotherapie* 3:109-115.

Vorbach, E.-U., W.D. Hübner, and K.H. Arnoldt. 1994. Effectiveness and tolerance of the hypericum extract LI 160 in comparison with imipramine: Randomized double-blind study with 135 outpatients. *Journal of Geriatric Psychiatry and Neurology* 7(Suppl. 1):S19-S23.

Wagner, J., M.L. Wagner, and W.A Hening. 1998. Beyond benzodiazepines: Alternative pharmacologic agents for the treatment of insomnia. *Annals of Pharmacotherapy* 32:680-691.

Wagner, W. and U. Nootbaar-Wagner. 1997. Prophylactic treatment of migraine with gamma-linolenic and alpha-linolenic acids. *Cephalalgia* 17(2):127-130.

Warm, J.S., W.M. Dember, and R. Parasuraman. 1990. Effects of fragrances on vigilance performance and stress. *Perfumer & Flavorist* 15(January/February):15-18.

Warnecke, G. 1991. Psychosomatische Dysfunktionen im Weiblishen Klimakterium. Klinische Wirksamkeit und Verträglichkeit von Kava-Extrakt WS 1490. (Psychosomatic dysfunctions in the female climacteric. Clinical effectiveness and tolerance of Kava Extract WS 1490). *Forschritte de Medizin* 109(4): 119-122.

Warner, R., D. Taylor, J. Wright, A. Sloat, G. Springett, S. Arnold, and H. Weinberg. 1994. Substance use among the mentally ill: Prevalence, reasons for use, and effects on illness. *American Journal of Orthopsychiatry* 64(1):30-39.

Warot, D., L. Lacomblez, P. Danjou, E. Weiller, C. Payan, and A.J. Puech. 1991. Comparaison des effets d'extraits de *Ginkgo biloba* sur les performances psychomotrices et la mémoire chez le sujet sain (Comparative effects of *Ginkgo biloba* extracts on psychomotor performances and memory in healthy subjects). *Thérapie* 46(1):33-36.

Warrenburg, S. and G. Schwartz. 1990. A psychophysiological study of three odorants. *Chemical Senses* 13:744.

Webb, G. 1997. Kava improperly implicated in semi-comatose patient using conventional drugs. *Herb Clip,* September 11, 1997, 2 pp. Austin, TX: American
Botanical Council.

Welsh, C. 1997. Touch with oils: A pertinent part of holistic hospice care. *American
Journal of Hospice and Palliative Care* 14(1):42-44.

Wesnes, K., D. Simmons, M. Rook, and P Simpson. 1987. A double-blind placebo-
controlled trial of Tanakan in the treatment of idiopathic cognitive impairment in
the elderly. *Human Psychopharmacology* 2:159-169.

West, M.E. 1991. Cannabis and night vision. *Nature* 351:703-704.

Wheatley, D. 1997. LI 160, an extract of St. John's wort, versus amitriptyline in
mildly to moderately depressed outpatients—A controlled 6-week clinical trial.
Pharmacopsychiatry 30(Suppl. 2):77-80.

Wiklund, I., J. Karlberg, and B. Lund. 1994. A double-blind comparison of the
effect on quality of life of a combination of vital substances including standardized ginseng G115 and placebo. *Current Therapeutic Research* 55(1):32-42.

Willey, L.B., S.P. Mady, D.J. Cobaugh, and P.M. Wax. 1995. Valerian overdose: A
case report. *Veterinary and Human Toxicology* 37(4):364-365.

Williamson, B.L., K. Klarskov, A.J. Tomlinson, G.J. Gleich, and S. Naylor. 1998.
Problems with over-the-counter 5-hydroxy-L-tryptophan. *Nature Medicine* 4(9):
983.

Winslow, L.C. and D.J. Kroll. 1998. Herbs as medicines. *Archives of Internal
Medicine* 158(20):2192-2199.

Winter, J.C. and D. Timineri. 1999. The discriminative stimulus properties of EGb
761, an extract of *Ginkgo biloba. Pharmacology, Biochemistry and Behavior*
62(3):543-547.

Wirtshafter, D. 1997. Nutritional value of hemp seed and hemp seed oil. In *Cannabis in medical practice: A legal, historical and pharmacological overview of the
therapeutic use of marijuana,* Ed. M.L. Mathre. Jefferson, NC: McFarland and
Company, pp. 181-191.

Woelk, H., G. Burkard, and J. Grünwald. 1994. Benefits and risks of the hypericum
extract LI 160: Drug monitoring study with 3250 patients. *Journal of Geriatric
Psychiatry and Neurology* 7(Suppl. 1):S34-S38.

Woelk, H., O. Kapoula, S. Lehrl, K. Schröter, and P. Weinholz. 1993. Behandlung
von Angst-Patienten: Doppelblindstudie: Kava-Spezialextrakt WS 1490 versus
Benzodiazepine. *Zeitschrift für Allgemeinmedizin* 69:271-277.

Wolfman, C., H. Viola, A. Paladini, F. Dajas, and J.H. Medina. 1994. Possible
anxiolytic effects of chrysin, a central benzodiazepine receptor ligand isolated
from *Passiflora coerulea. Pharmacology, Biochemistry and Behavior* 47(1):1-4.

Wong, A.H., M. Smith, and H.S. Boon. 1998. Herbal remedies in psychiatric
practice. *Archives of General Psychiatry* 55(11):1033-1044.

Zhang, G.B., M.Y. Wang, J.Q. Zheng, and X.C. Tang. 1994. Facilitation of cholinergic transmission by huperzine A in toad paravertebral ganglia in vitro [in

Chinese]. *Chung Kuo Yao Li Hsueh Pao (Acta Pharmacologica Sinica)* 15(2):158-161.

Zhang, R.W., X.C. Tang, Y.Y. Han, G.W. Sang, Y.D. Zhang, Y.X. Ma, C.L. Zhang, and R.M. Yang. 1991. Drug evaluation of huperzine A in the treatment of senile memory disorders [in Chinese]. *Chung Kuo Yao Li Hsueh Pao (Acta Pharmacologica Sinica)* 12(3):250-252.

Zhu, L., J. Wu, J. Gao, X.N. Zhao, and Z.X. Shang. 1997. Antagonistic effects of extract from leaves of *Ginkgo biloba* on glutamate neurotoxicity. *Chung Kuo Yao Li Hsueh Pao (Acta Pharmacologica Sinica)* 18(4):344-347.

Zhu, X.D. and E. Giacobini. 1995. Second generation cholinesterase inhibitors: Effect of (L)-huperzine-A on cortical biogenic amines. *Journal of Neuroscience Research* 41(6):828-835.

Zhu, X.-Z. 1991. Development of natural products as drugs acting on central nervous system. *Memórias do Instituto Oswaldo Cruz* 86(Suppl. 2):173-175.

Zimmer, L.E. and J.P. Morgan. 1997. *Marijuana myths, marijuana facts: A review of the scientific evidence.* New York: Lindesmith Center.

Zuardi, A.W., R.A. Cosme, F.G. Graeff, and F.S. Guimaraes. 1993. Effects of ipsapirone and cannabidiol on human experimental anxiety. *Journal of Psychopharmacology* 7(1):82-88.

Zuardi, A.W., E. Finkelfarb, O.F. Bueno, R.E. Musty, and I.G. Karniol. 1981. Characteristics of the stimulus produced by the mixture of cannabidiol with delta 9-tetrahydrocannabinol. *Archives Internationales de Pharmacodynamie et de Thérapie* 249(1):137-146.

Zuardi, A.W. and F.S. Guimaraes. 1997. Cannabidiol as an anxiolytic and antipsychotic. In *Cannabis in medical practice: A legal, historical and pharmacological overview of the therapeutic use of marijuana,* Ed. M. L. Mathre. Jefferson, NC: McFarland and Company, pp. 133-139.

Zuardi, A.W., F.S. Guimaraes, and A.C. Moreira. 1993. Effect of cannabidiol on plasma prolactin, growth hormone and cortisol in human volunteers. *Brazilian Journal of Medical and Biological Research* 26(2):213-217.

Zuardi, A.W. and I.G. Karniol. 1983. Effects on variable-interval performance in rats of delta 9-tetrahydrocannabinol and cannabidiol, separately and in combination. *Brazilian Journal of Medical and Biological Research* 16(2):141-146.

Zuardi, A.W., S.L. Morais, F.S. Guimaraes, and R. Mechoulam. 1995. Antipsychotic effect of cannabidiol. *Journal of Clinical Psychiatry* 56(10):485-486.

Zuardi, A.W., J.A. Rodrigues, and J.M. Cunha. 1991. Effects of cannabidiol in animal models predictive of antipsychotic activity. *Psychopharmacology* 104(2):260-264.

Zuardi, A.W., I. Shirakawa, E. Finkelfarb, and I.G. Karniol. 1982. Action of cannabidiol on the anxiety and other effects produced by delta 9-THC in normal subjects. *Psychopharmacology* 76(3):245-250.

Index

THE HAWORTH HERBAL PRESS
Varro E. Tyler, PhD
Executive Editor

TYLER'S TIPS: THE SHOPPER'S GUIDE FOR HERBAL REMEDIES by George H. Constantine (2000). "George Constantine has given us a common sense, easily read, well-organized shopper's guide to the most frequently utilized and best-documented herbal remedies." *Paul L. Schiff Jr., PhD, Professor of Pharmaceutical Sciences, School of Pharmacy, University of Pittsburgh, Pennsylvania*

HANDBOOK OF PSYCHOTROPIC HERBS: A SCIENTIFIC ANALYSIS OF HERBAL REMEDIES FOR PSYCHIATRIC CONDITIONS by Ethan B. Russo (2000). "Sound advice on the rational use of safe and effective herbs to help alleviate a wide range of neurological disorders. An authoritative guide in an area where solid, reliable information is often difficult to obtain." *Mark Blumenthal, Founder and Executive Director, American Botanical Council; Editor,* HerbalGram; *Senior Editor,* The Complete German Commission E Monographs

UNDERSTANDING ALTERNATIVE MEDICINE: NEW HEALTH PATHS IN AMERICA by Lawrence Tyler. "An eye-opening account of the emerging health paths in the United States and other parts of the Western world. . . . Contains thoughtful discussions on the perception of nonspecific factors in healing." *Mark Bender, Assistant Professor of Chinese, Department of East Asian Languages and Literatures, The Ohio State University, Columbus*

SEASONING SAVVY: HOW TO COOK WITH HERBS, SPICES, AND OTHER FLAVORINGS by Alice Arndt. "Well-written and wonderfully comprehensive exploration of the world of herbs, spices and aromatics—at once authorative and easy to use." *Nancy Harmon Jenkins, Author of* The Mediterranean Diet Cookbook

TYLER'S HONEST HERBAL: A SENSIBLE GUIDE TO THE USE OF HERBS AND RELATED REMEDIES, Fourth Edition by Steven Foster and Varro E. Tyler. "An up-to-date revision of the most reliable source for the layperson on herbal medicines. Excellent as a starting point for scientists who desire more information on herbal medicines." *Norman R. Farnsworth, PhD, Research Professor of Pharmacognosy, College of Pharmacy, University of Illinois at Chicago*

TYLER'S HERBS OF CHOICE: THE THERAPEUTIC USE OF PHYTOMEDICINALS, Second Edition by James E. Robbers and Varro E. Tyler. "The first edition of this book was a landmark publication. . . . This new edition will no doubt become one of the most often-used references by health practitioners of all types." *Mark Blumenthal, Founder and Executive Director, American Botanical Council; Editor,* HerbalGram

Order Your Own Copy of
This Important Book for Your Personal Library!

HANDBOOK OF PSYCHOTROPIC HERBS
A Scientific Analysis of Herbal Remedies for Psychiatric Conditions

_____ in hardbound at $69.95 (ISBN: 0-7890-0718-5)

_____ in softbound at $29.95 (ISBN: 0-7890-1088-7)

COST OF BOOKS_____

OUTSIDE USA/CANADA/
MEXICO: ADD 20%_____

POSTAGE & HANDLING_____
*(US: $4.00 for first book & $1.50
for each additional book*
*Outside US: $5.00 for first book
& $2.00 for each additional book)*

SUBTOTAL_____

IN CANADA: ADD 7% GST_____

STATE TAX_____
*(NY, OH & MN residents, please
add appropriate local sales tax)*

FINAL TOTAL_____
*(If paying in Canadian funds,
convert using the current
exchange rate. UNESCO
coupons welcome.)*

☐ **BILL ME LATER:** ($5 service charge will be added)
(Bill-me option is good on US/Canada/Mexico orders only;
not good to jobbers, wholesalers, or subscription agencies.)

☐ Check here if billing address is different from
shipping address and attach purchase order and
billing address information.

Signature_____

☐ **PAYMENT ENCLOSED: $**_____

☐ **PLEASE CHARGE TO MY CREDIT CARD.**

☐ Visa   ☐ MasterCard   ☐ AmEx   ☐ Discover
☐ Diner's Club   ☐ Eurocard   ☐ JCB

Account #_____

Exp. Date_____

Signature_____

Prices in US dollars and subject to change without notice.

NAME_____
INSTITUTION_____
ADDRESS_____
CITY_____
STATE/ZIP_____
COUNTRY_____   COUNTY (NY residents only)_____
TEL_____   FAX_____
E-MAIL_____

May we use your e-mail address for confirmations and other types of information? ☐ Yes   ☐ No
We appreciate receiving your e-mail address and fax number. Haworth would like to e-mail or fax special
discount offers to you, as a preferred customer. **We will never share, rent, or exchange your e-mail
address or fax number.** We regard such actions as an invasion of your privacy.

Order From Your Local Bookstore or Directly From
The Haworth Press, Inc.
10 Alice Street, Binghamton, New York 13904-1580 • USA
TELEPHONE: 1-800-HAWORTH (1-800-429-6784) / Outside US/Canada: (607) 722-5857
FAX: 1-800-895-0582 / Outside US/Canada: (607) 772-6362
E-mail: getinfo@haworthpressinc.com
PLEASE PHOTOCOPY THIS FORM FOR YOUR PERSONAL USE.
www.HaworthPress.com

BOF00